DR. HUW PARRY
DEPARTMENT OF CLINICAL
HAEMATOLOGY AND ONCOLOGY
YSBYTY GWYNEDD
BANGOR,
GWYNEDD. LL57 2PW

FLOW CYTOMETRY
CLINICAL APPLICATIONS

FLOW CYTOMETRY

CLINICAL APPLICATIONS

EDITED BY

MARION G. MACEY

BSc, MSc, PhD, FIMLS
Honorary Lecturer, Department of Haematology,
The Royal London Hospital

OXFORD

BLACKWELL SCIENTIFIC PUBLICATIONS

LONDON EDINBURGH BOSTON

MELBOURNE PARIS BERLIN VIENNA

© 1994 by
Blackwell Scientific Publications
Editorial Offices:
Osney Mead, Oxford OX2 0EL
25 John Street, London WC1N 2BL
23 Ainslie Place, Edinburgh EH3 6AJ
238 Main Street, Cambridge
  Massachusetts 02142, USA
54 University Street, Carlton
  Victoria 3053, Australia

Other Editorial Offices:
Librairie Arnette SA
1, rue de Lille
75007 Paris
France

Blackwell Wissenschafts-Verlag GmbH
Düsseldorfer Str. 38
D-10707 Berlin
Germany

Blackwell MZV
Feldgasse 13
A-1238 Wien
Austria

First published 1994

Set by Setrite Typesetters, Hong Kong
Printed and bound in Great Britain
at the University Press, Cambridge

DISTRIBUTORS

Marston Book Services Ltd
PO Box 87
Oxford OX2 0DT
(*Orders*: Tel: 0865 791155
        Fax: 0865 791927
        Telex: 837515)

USA
Blackwell Scientific Publications, Inc.
238 Main Street
Cambridge, Massachusetts 02142
(*Orders*: Tel: 800 759−6102
        617 876−7000)

Canada
Times Mirror
Professional Publishing, Ltd
130 Flaska Drive
Markham, Ontario L6G 1B8
(*Orders*: Tel: 800 268−4178
        416 470−6739)

Australia
Blackwell Scientific Publications
Pty Ltd
54 University Street
Carlton, Victoria 3053
(*Orders*: Tel: 03 347−5552)

A catalogue record for this title
is available from the British Library
and the Library of Congress

ISBN 0-632-03673-7

Contents

List of Contributors

R. S. CAMPLEJOHN PhD, *Senior Lecturer, Richard Dimbleby Department of Cancer Research, UMDS, St Thomas' Hospital, Lambeth Palace Road, London SE1 7EH*

L. S. CRAM PhD, *Deputy Division Leader, Life Sciences Division, Los Alamos National Laboratory, Los Alamos, New Mexico 87545, USA*

A. H. GOODALL PhD, *Senior Lecturer, Department of Chemical Pathology, The Royal Free Hospital School of Medicine, Pond Street, Hampstead, London NW3 2QG*

T. HOY PhD, MRCPath, *Principal Research Officer, Department of Haematology, University of Wales College of Medicine, Heath Park, Cardiff CF4 4XN*

J. LAWRY PhD, FIMLS, *Department of Experimental and Clinical Immunology, University Medical School, Sheffield S10 2RX*

M. W. LOWDELL PhD, *Department of Immunology, The Royal London Hospital, Whitechapel, London E1 1BB*

M. G. MACEY PhD, FIMLS, *Clinical Scientist (Honorary Lecturer), Department of Haematology, The Royal London Hospital, Whitechapel, London E1 1BB*

L. W. M. M. TERSTAPPEN MD, PhD, *Becton Dickinson Fellow, Becton Dickinson Immunocytometry Systems, 2350 Qume Drive, San Jose, California 95131–1807, USA*

P. A. VEYS MRCP, MRCPath, *Consultant Haematologist, Department of Haematology, The Hospital for Sick Children, Great Ormond Street, London, WC1N 3JH*

Preface

Numerous books on flow cytometry have been published in the past few years. Most have concentrated on introducing the reader to the subject, or have detailed cell sorting or data analysis or indeed how to build your own flow cytometer. During the past 10 years flow cytometry has developed from a purely research tool to a major adjunct to clinical practice. This book is aimed at those working in a clinical setting and those interested in the molecular analysis of cells. The question of quality control is also addressed — a topic which all flow cytometrists should be aware of, not just those in a clinical environment.

Flow cytometry is recognized as the principal tool for immunophenotypic analysis of cell types, but its use to measure cell function — in particular cell-mediated cytotoxicity and calcium flux studies — is now rapidly becoming appreciated. The analysis of cell cycle events and DNA aberrations are now easy to assess by flow cytometry. Karyotypic analysis for the diagnosis of leukaemias and lymphomas is also feasible. Add to this its advent in the realms of molecular biology and one is presented with an essential tool for biomedical analysis.

Recently, much interest has focused on the measurement of molecules associated with adhesion on neutrophils, particularly in inflammatory conditions, such as the rheumatoid disorders. Similarly, the identification of activation antigens on platelets, particularly in coronary heart disease, has been shown to have clinical importance. Flow cytometric analysis of whole blood without cell isolation procedures offers the best method for detection and quantification of these molecules.

The identification of bacteria from various sources (water, sewage, food, blood) by flow cytometry has become possible as a result of the increased detection sensitivity of current bench-top flow cytometers. This has resulted in a dramatic increase in the use of flow cytometry in the field of microbiology, which is likely to lead to its increased use in routine clinical practice.

Originally, the ability to sort cells was developed so that immunologists could collect 'pure' populations of cells for functional analysis in *in vitro* culture systems. Today, the function of cells may be defined by cell surface or cytoplasmic molecular expression and multiparameter flow cytometric analysis. Cell sorting now has a role in the isolation of cells for subsequent use in assays such as the polymerase chain reaction. Chromosomes may also be sorted for karyotype studies or *in situ* hybridization. Thus flow cytometric cell sorting has now become a tool for the molecular biologist. All of these techniques and more are described in this book together with, where appropriate, their clinical applications.

M.G. Macey

List of Abbreviations

^{3}H-TdR	triated thymidine
AC	acid citrate
ACD	acid citrate dextrose
ACE	acetylcholine esterase
A-D	analogue-to-digital
ADP	adenosine diphosphate
AIN	autoimmune neutropenia
ALL	acute lymphoblastic leukaemia
AML	acute myeloid leukaemia
anti-MPO	anti-myeloperoxidase
AT	adenine-thymine
ATP	adenosine triphosphate
B-ALL	acute B-cell lymphoid/lymphoblastic leukaemia
B-PLL	B-cell prolymphocytic leukaemia
BMT	bone marrow transplantation
BrdUrd	bromodeoxyuridine
BSA	bovine serum albumin
bs MoAb	bi-specific MoAb
BSS	Bernard–Soulier syndrome
CA3	chromomycin A3
CCHE cells	Chinese hamster cells initiated from embryonic tissue
CDs	clusters of differentiation
c'FDA	carboxy-fluorescein diacetate
CGL	chronic granulocytic leukaemia
CLL	chronic lymphocytic leukaemia
CML	chronic myeloid leukaemia
CPB	cardiopulmonary bypass surgery
CTL	cytotoxic T lymphocytes
CV	coefficient of variation
DAB	diaminobenzidine
DAF	decay accelerating factor
DAPI	4',6-diamidino-2-phenylindole
DCFH-DA	2',7'-dichlorofluorescein diacetate
DEPC	di-ethyl-pyrocarbonate
DI	DNA index
DMS	dimethylsuberimidate
DVT	deep vein thrombosis
EB	ethidium bromide

ELISA	enzyme-linked immunosorbent assay
ET	essential thrombocythaemia
FAL(S)	forward angle light (scatter)
FBS	fetal bovine serum
FCS	fetal calf serum
FISH	fluorescence *in situ* hybridization
FITC	fluorescein isothiocyanate
FLM	fraction labelled mitosis (method)
F : P	fluorochrome : protein ratio
FSC	forward light scatter
G_0, G_1, G_2, etc.	phases of the cell cycle
GC	guanine-cytosine
GM-CSF	granulocyte macrophage colony-stimulating factor
GP	glycoprotein
GPI	glycosylphosphatydylinositol
GSH	glutathione
GT	Glanzmann's thrombasthenia
HBSS	Hank's balanced salt solution
HBSS-T	HBSS containing Tween-20
HCL	hairy cell leukaemia
HE	hydroethidine
HHBSS	Hepes-buffered Hank's balanced salt solution
HIV	human immunodeficiency virus
HPA	human platelet antigen
HRF	homologous restriction factor
HSR	homogeneously staining region
IL	interleukin
IL-2	interleukin-2
IMDM	Iscove's modified Dulbecco's medium
ITP	idiopathic thrombocytopenic purpura
IVIG	intravenous immunoglobulin
LAK	lymphokine-activated killer (cells)
LGL	large granular lymphocytic (leukaemia)
LIBS	ligand-induced binding sites
MAIPA	monoclonal antibody-specific immobilization of platelet antigens
LS MBCL	LS monochlorobimine (probe)
MDR	multidrug resistance
MEM	minimal essential medium
MESF	molecules equivalent standard fluorochrome
MFI	mean fluorescence intensity
MHC	major histocompatibility complex
MIRL	membrane inhibitor of reactive lysis
MMC	mithramycin
MoAb	monoclonal antibody
MPE	maximum permissible exposure
MRD	minimal residual disease

MTT	3-(4,5-dimethylthiazolyl-2-yl)-2,5-diphenyltetrazolium bromide
NADH	reduced nicotinamide adenine dinucleotide
NAIg	neutrophil-associated immunoglobulin
NHL	non-Hodgkin's lymphoma
NK	natural killer (cells)
PAIg	platelet-associated immunoglobulin
PBL	peripheral blood lymphocyte/leucocyte
PBMC	peripheral blood mononuclear cells
PBS	phosphate-buffered saline
PBSC	peripheral blood stem cells
PBSg	PBS containing gelatine and glucose
PCNA	proliferating cell nuclear antigen
PCR	polymerase chain reaction
PDIg	platelet-directed immunoglobulin
PE	phycoerythrin
PEG	polyethylene glycol
PI	propidium iodide
PIG	phosphatidyl-inositol glycan
PMA	phorbol myristate acetate
PMN	polymorphonuclear (granulocytes)
PMT	photomultiplier tube
PNH	paroxysmal nocturnal haemoglobinuria
PRINS	primer-initiated *in situ* hybridization
PRP	platelet-rich plasma
QA	quality assurance
QC	quality control
RBC	red blood cells
RCN	(fluorescence) relative channel number
RCV	red cell volume
RGD	peptide containing arg-gly-ala sequence of amino acids
RIBS	receptor-induced binding site
RT	room temperature
SCCA	single cell cytotoxicity assay
SCCS	surface connecting canalicular system
SDS	sodium dodecyl sulphate
SL	saturation level
SLE	systemic lupus erythematosus
SLVL	splenic lymphoma with circulating villous lymphocytes
SPD	storage pool disease
SPF	S-phase fraction
SSC	saline sodium citrate
SSC	side scatter
SSPE	saline−sodium phosphate − EDTA
ST-PE	streptavidin-phycoerythrin

T-ALL	acute T-cell lymphoid/lymphoblastic leukaemia
TBS	Tris-buffered saline
TCCA	total cell cytotoxicity assay
TdT	terminal deoxynucleotidyl transferase
TNF	tumour necrosis factor
TOF	time of flight
TSB	tryptic soya broth
vWF	von Willebrand factor
WBC	white blood cells
YAC	yeast artefactual chromosome

Chapter 1
Introduction

M. G. MACEY

History and development of flow cytometry

In 1956 Coulter described an instrument in which an electronic measurement for cell counting and sizing was made on cells flowing in a conductive liquid with one cell at a time passing a measuring point. This became the basis of the first viable flow analyser. Kamentsky *et al.* (1965) described a two-parameter flow cytometer that measured absorption and back-scattered illumination of unstained cells and this was used to determine cell nucleic acid content and size. This instrument represented the first multiparameter flow cytometer, and the first cell sorter was described that same year by Fulwyler (1965). Use of an electrostatic deflection ink-jet recording technique (Sweet, 1965) enabled the instrument to sort cells in volume at a rate of 1000 cells/s. By 1967 Van Dilla *et al.* exploited the real volume differences of cells to prepare suspensions of highly purified (>95%) human granulocytes and lymphocytes.

However, it is only comparatively recently that advances in technology, including availability of monoclonal antibodies and powerful but cheap computers, have brought flow cytometry into routine use. Previously, microscope-based static cytometry with cell-by-cell analysis had been the mainstay of most diagnostic work. However, with the increasing ability to measure up to five parameters on 20 000 cells in 1 s, cell surface antigen analysis has become almost routine and has not only enhanced the diagnosis and management of various disease states, but has also given new understanding of the pathogenesis of disease.

Principles of flow cytometry

Flow cytometry is a system for sensing cells or particles as they move in a liquid stream through a laser (light amplification by stimulated emission of radiation) or light beam past a sensing area. The relative light scattering

1

and colour-discriminated fluorescence of the microscopic particles is measured (Fig. 1.1). Analysis and differentiation of the cells is based on size and granularity, and whether the cell is carrying fluorescent molecules either in the form of antibodies or dyes (Fig. 1.2). As the cell passes through the laser beam, light is scattered in all directions and that scattered in the forward direction is proportional to the square of the radius of a sphere (Brunsting and Mullaney, 1974) and so to the size of the cell or particle. Light may enter the cell and be reflected and refracted by the nuclear contents of the cell, thus the 90° light (right-angled, side) scatter may be considered proportional to the granularity of the cell. The use of light scattering properties to distinguish cell morphology is discussed further in Chapter 3. The cells may be labelled with fluorochrome-linked antibodies or stained with fluorescent membrane, cytoplasmic or nuclear dyes. Thus differentiation of cell types, the presence of membrane receptors and antigens, membrane potential, pH, enzyme activity and DNA content may be facilitated.

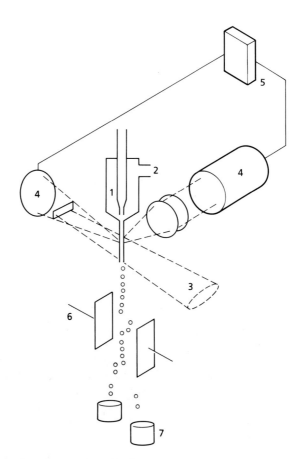

Fig. 1.1 Schematic representation of a flow cytometer. 1, flow cell; 2, sheath stream; 3, laser beam; 4, sensing system; 5, computer; 6, deflection plates; 7, droplet collection.

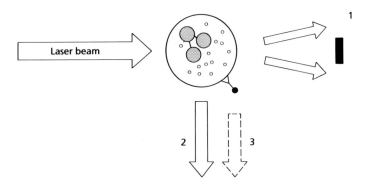

Fig. 1.2 The parameters of flow cytometric analysis. 1, FAL scatter; 2, 90°LS; 3, fluorescence.

Flow cytometers are multiparameter, recording several measurements on each cell, therefore it is possible to identify a cell population within a heterogeneous population. This is one of the most useful features of flow cytometers, and makes them preferable to other instruments such as spectrofluorimeters, in which measurements are based on analysis of the entire population.

Most commercial flow cytometers have the capacity to make four or more simultaneous measurements on every cell, but some specialized research instruments have considerably greater capacity. A typical flow cytometer consists of three functional units: (a) a light source or laser, and a sensing system which comprises the sample/flow chamber and optical assembly; (b) a hydraulic system which controls the passage of cells through the sensing system; and (c) a computer system which collects data and performs analytical routines on the electrical signals relayed from the sensing system.

Flow cytometers may utilize epifluorescent microscopy or dark-ground laser illumination; in both designs the flow chamber is instrumental in delivering the cells in suspension to the specific point that is intersected by the illuminating beam and the plane of focus of the optical assembly. Cells suspended in isotonic fluid are transported through the sensing system. Most instruments utilize a lamina/sheath flow technique (Crosland-Taylor, 1953) to confine cells to the centre of the flow stream, this also reduces blockage due to clumping. Cells enter the chamber under pressure through a small aperture which is surrounded by sheath fluid (Fig. 1.3a). The sheath fluid in the sample chamber creates a hydrodynamic focusing effect and draws the sample fluid into a stream (Fig. 1.3b). Accurate and precise positioning of the sample fluid within the sheath fluid is critical to efficient operation of the flow cytometer and adjustment of the relative sheath and sample pressures ensures that cells pass one by one through the detection point. This alignment may be performed manually on some machines, in others it is fixed.

FLOW CHAMBER

PNEUMATICS A

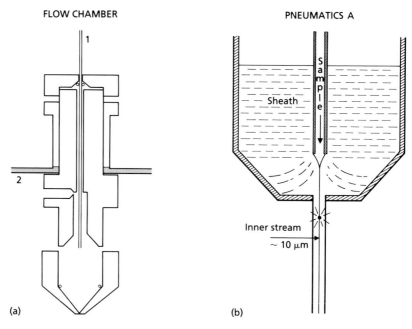

(a)   (b)

Fig. 1.3 (a) Example of a flow cell. 1, sample input; 2, sheath fluid input. (b) Illustration of the process of hydrodynamic focusing.

Chambers used in microscope-based flow systems (where fluorescence is measured in line with the optical system) are constrained by limitations. The chamber acts as the horizontal microscope stage (Fig. 1.4) and the top of the chamber is usually a glass coverslip. Scatter measurements are restricted to within the direct optical path of the immersion objectives. Some systems do not use an enclosed channel but simply squirt the hydrodynamically focused sample at a low angle across a microscope slide followed by vacuum aspiration to waste.

In laser-based flow cytometers, where fluorescence is measured at right angles to the illuminating beam, chambers may comprise flat-sided cuvettes to minimize unwanted light reflections (Fig. 1.5). Water-cooled laser sources in the range 50 mW to 5 W output power were used

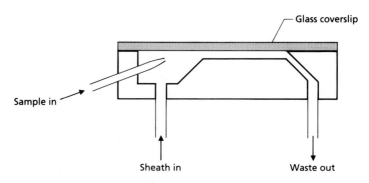

Fig. 1.4 Example of a chamber used in a microscope-based flow system.

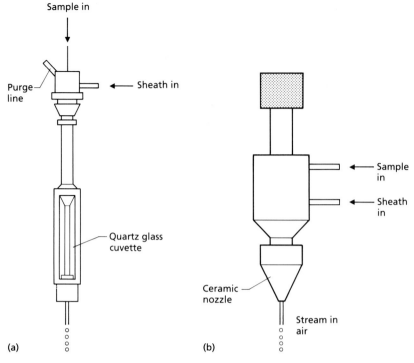

Fig. 1.5 (a) and (b) Example of a flat-sided cuvette system used in flow cytometers to minimize unwanted light reflections and increase sensitivity.

for fluorescence and light scatter measurements. Air-cooled lasers have a maximum 100 mW output and are now more commonly used in commercial instruments. Lasers have the advantage of producing an intense beam of monochromatic light which in some systems may be tuned to several different wavelengths. The most common lasers used in flow cytometry are: argon lasers, which produce light between wavelengths 351 and 528 nm; krypton lasers, which produce light between 350 and 799 nm; helium–neon lasers, which produce lines at 543, 594, 611 and 633 nm; and helium–cadmium lasers which produce lines at 325 and 441 nm.

Fluorescence analysis

Fluorescence is excited as cells traverse the laser excitation beam, and this fluorescence is collected by optics at 90° to the incident beam. A barrier filter blocks laser excitation illumination, while dichroic mirrors and appropriate filters (see Fig. 1.6) are used to select the required wavelengths of fluorescence for measurement. The photons of light falling upon the detectors are converted by photomultiplier tubes (PMTs) to an electrical impulse, and this signal is processed by an analogue-to-digital A-D converter, which changes the analogue impulse to a digital signal. The quantity and intensity of the fluorescence are recorded by the computer system and displayed on a visual display unit as a frequency distribution, which may be single, dual or multiparameter. Single parameter histograms usually convey information regarding the intensity of fluorescence and number of cells of a given fluorescence, so that weakly fluorescent cells are distinguished from those which are strongly fluorescent. Dual parameter histograms of forward angle scatter and 90° light scatter (90°LS) allow identification of the different cell types within the preparation, based on size and granularity. Right angle and side scatter are alternative names used for 90°LS.

Light scatter and detection

Filters

Light scattered by particles as they pass through a laser or light source must be efficiently detected and fluorescent light of a given wavelength requires specific identification. The amount of light scattered is generally high in comparison with the amount of fluorescent light. Photodiodes are therefore used as forward angle light (FAL) sensors that may be used with neutral density filters, which proportionally reduce the amount of light received by the detector. A beam absorber (diffuser or obscuration bar) is placed across the front of the detector to stop the laser beam itself and any diffracted light from entering the detector. The scattered light is focused by a collecting lens onto the photodiode(s), which converts the photons into voltage pulses proportional to the amount of light collected (integrated pulse). These pulses may be amplified by the operator. In some systems with multiple diodes upper and lower light may be collected, which may help separate populations of cells or particles.

Fluorescence detectors are usually placed at right angles to the laser beam and sample stream. Stray light is excluded by an obscuration bar in front of an asperic (objective) lens, which collects the light and refracts it into a parallel beam. To detect the components of the beam, filters and mirrors are used to remove unwanted wavelengths of light and direct light to the correct detector(s). Figure 1.6 describes some of the different types of lenses and filters used (see also Chapter 2) and Fig. 1.7 illustrates a possible lens configuration for detecting 90°LS, orange (phycoerythrin) and green (fluorescein) fluorescence.

Typically, the first filter used eliminates laser light that still may have passed through. This light may then be diverted to a beam splitter or a dichroic mirror. This mirror reflects light in one band of wavelengths (usually long) while allowing another band to pass through (usually short). It should be noted that there is no direct cut-off here between reflection and transmission. There is a middle band of wavelengths that will do both. For this reason, the colour components are passed through other filters before entering the detector. These filters remove the unwanted wavelengths and allow the desired wavelengths to pass through to the detector. These filters are called band-pass filters and are

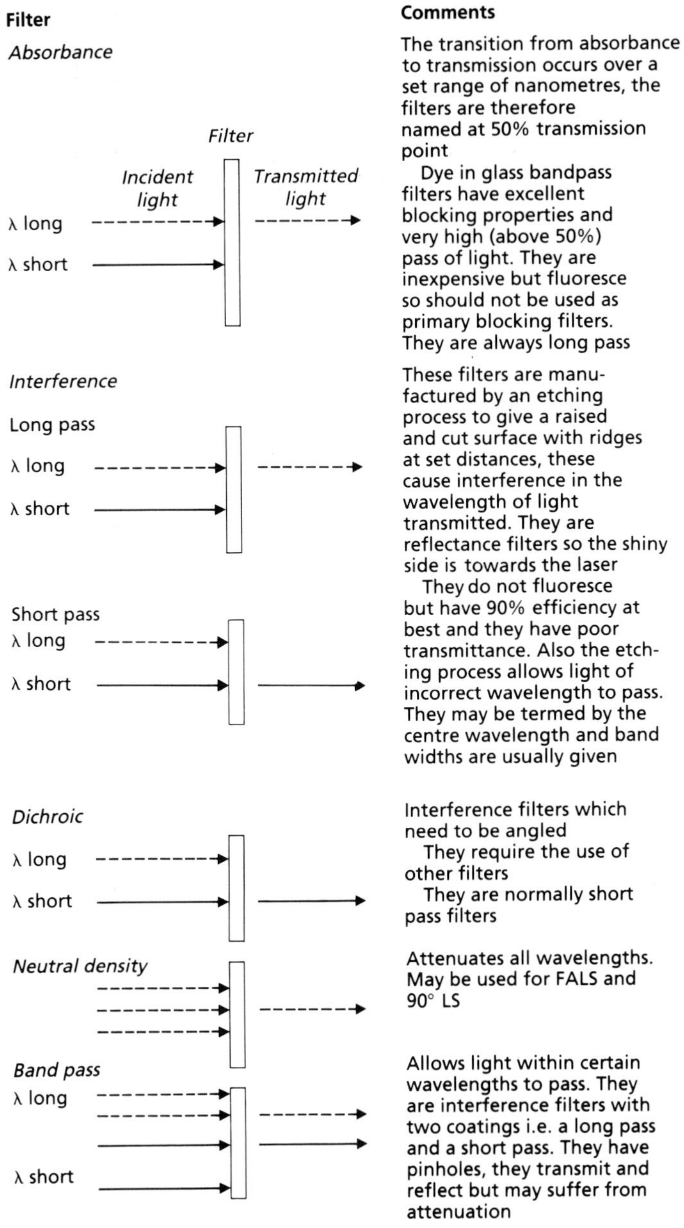

Filter

Absorbance

Filter

Incident light → Transmitted light

λ long

λ short

Comments

The transition from absorbance to transmission occurs over a set range of nanometres, the filters are therefore named at 50% transmission point

Dye in glass bandpass filters have excellent blocking properties and very high (above 50%) pass of light. They are inexpensive but fluoresce so should not be used as primary blocking filters. They are always long pass

Interference

Long pass

λ long

λ short

These filters are manu-factured by an etching process to give a raised and cut surface with ridges at set distances, these cause interference in the wavelength of light transmitted. They are reflectance filters so the shiny side is towards the laser

Short pass

λ long

λ short

They do not fluoresce but have 90% efficiency at best and they have poor transmittance. Also the etch-ing process allows light of incorrect wavelength to pass. They may be termed by the centre wavelength and band widths are usually given

Dichroic

λ long

λ short

Interference filters which need to be angled

They require the use of other filters

They are normally short pass filters

Neutral density

Attenuates all wavelengths. May be used for FALS and 90° LS

Band pass

λ long

λ short

Allows light within certain wavelengths to pass. They are interference filters with two coatings i.e. a long pass and a short pass. They have pinholes, they transmit and reflect but may suffer from attenuation

Fig. 1.6 Types of filters used in flow cytometers.

designated by whether they transmit long wavelengths (long pass) or shorter wavelengths (short pass). They may be termed by the centre wavelength and band widths are usually given (Fig. 1.8).

The sensors used are PMTs. These tubes serve as detectors and also amplifiers of the weak fluorescent signals. These tubes have their own high voltage power supplies, which provide the boost needed to amplify the signal internally within the PMT. The amount of high voltage and therefore the amplification is adjustable by the operator. A second

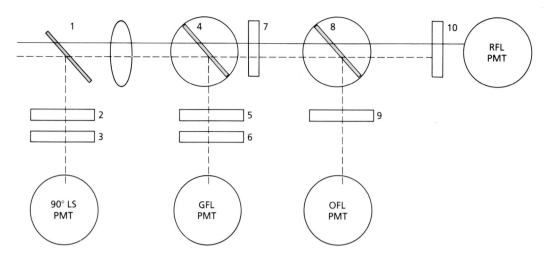

Fig. 1.7 Typical lens and mirror assembly for detection of 90°LS, fluorescein isothiocyanate and phycoerythrin fluorescence. 1, beam splitter, normal glass; 2, laser line filter 396–496 nm band pass; 3, diffuser; 4, dichroic mirror 570 nm long pass; 5, laser cut filter 490 nm short pass; 6, green filter 515–530 nm band pass; 7, orange filter 600 nm long pass; 8, dichroic mirror 610 nm long pass; 9, orange filter 565–592 nm band pass; 10, red filter 620 nm long pass. GFL, green fluorescence; OFL, orange fluorescence; RFL, red fluorescence.

amplification, also operator controlled, may be made on the PMT signal external to the PMT. PMTs are used only under weak light conditions as they may be damaged by high intensity light such as normal room light.

Filter sets. Filters are used in sets, usually pairs of band-pass filters with a dichroic mirror or beam splitter. Filter 1 is an excitation filter which is used to select a specific wavelength from the broad spectrum of light to produce a monochromatic illumination corresponding to the fluorophor's absorption band. Filter 2 is an emission filter which blocks the excitation wavelength and transmits the fluorescent emission. Light of any wavelength may pass through both the excitation and emission filters. Such light originating from the light source would either be erroneously observed as fluorescence or would make a coloured, rather than black, background. This is termed spectral overlap or filter crosstalk. This very low transmission may be measured spectrophotometrically and should not exceed 0.0001% or 10^{-6}. Examples of filter sets for a number of fluorochromes are given in Table 1.1.

Acquisition

Light scatter signals may be a measure of a combination of parameters: (a) the size (projected surface area) of the particle; (b) the surface topography (rough or smooth); (c) the optical density (light refracted through the particle); and (d) the internal structure of the particle

Table 1.1

(a) Examples of filter sets for use with commonly used dyes

Dye	Filter 1	Dichroic beam splitter	Filter 2
Cascade blue	355BP 40*	400LP	425BP 45
AMCA	355BP 40	400LP	450BP 65
Hoechst 33342	355BP 40	400LP	450BP 65
DAPI	355BP 40	400LP	450BP 65
FITC	485BP 22	505LP	530BP 30
FLUO 3	485BP 22	505LP	530BP 30
Acridine Orange	485BP 22	505LP	530BP 30
Propidium Iodide	535BP 23	565LP	625BP 38
Phycoerythrin	515BP 35	545LP	580BP 50
Rhodamine (TRITC)	540BP 23	565LP	605BP 55
Texas Red	560BP 40	595LP	635BP 60
Allophycocyanin	590BP 45	620LP	660BP 45

(b) Filter sets for fluorescent dyes with two excitation wavelengths

Dye	Filter 1	Filter 2	Dichroic beam splitter	Filter 3
Fura 2	340BP 10	380BP 13	400LP	510BP 40
BCECF	440BP 20	495BP 20	515LP	535BP 25
SNAFL-2	490BP 30	560BP 30	590LP	620BP 35

* Centre wavelength and bandwidth (nm) see Fig. 1.8.

(granular or uniform). Some of these components are present in all of the light scatter produced.

The purpose of analysing the light scatter or fluorescence signal is to determine the difference between particles in terms of voltage output from detectors. There are several methods of retrieving this information. A measure of the maximum voltage (or peak) level reached as the particle passes through the laser beam may be measured. The highest voltage level reached by the pulse (pulse height) may be a measure of the maximum fluorescence given off by a particle (Fig. 1.9a). Particles with different amounts of associated fluorescence have different pulse heights and so peak pulses. A particle with fluorescent molecules spread uniformly over the surface will produce a wide peak pulse compared with a particle with fluorescence concentrated at one point. The latter will produce a narrower and sharper peak pulse (Fig. 1.9b). However, the peak of the pulse may be the same for both particles and so they become indistinguishable on the basis of this parameter. The area under the two pulses will, however, be different. The area under the pulse allows generation of a second parameter referred to as the integrated pulse. A third parameter may also be used if the width or a portion or the peak or integrated pulse is measured. This is termed time of flight (TOF).

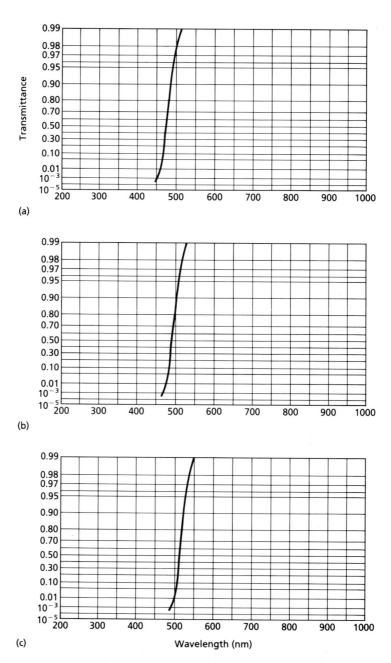

Fig. 1.8 (a)−(c) Example of transmittance profiles of filters.

Amplification

Some particles may also be better differentiated if the original peak or integrated pulse is amplified. Normal amplification accentuates the differences between pulses but in some cases this may not be sufficient to differentiate between small changes in pulse height. The use of logarithmic amplification makes small pulses much larger while amplifying

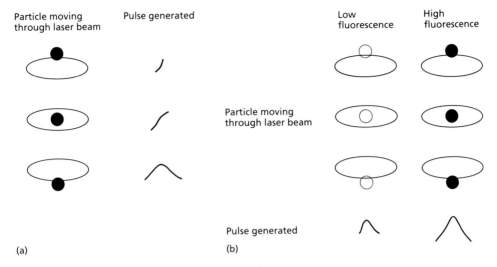

Fig. 1.9 (a) Illustration of the electronic pulse generated by a particle as it moves through a laser beam. (b) Illustration of the pulse generated by cells with high and low fluorescence intensities.

the larger pulses by a lesser amount. The result is that the differences in the smaller pulses are accentuated.

Histograms

Particles are analysed individually but interpreted collectively. The collective picture is represented as a histogram. These may be single, two or multiple parameter. Single parameter histograms are two-dimensional graphs in which the parameter to be interpreted is represented on the horizontal axis and the number of events is represented on the y-axis. The parameter could be the peak pulse height, TOF, or the integrated pulse height or a ratio based on the first three parameters. Light scatter or fluorescence pulses may also be used.

The production of a histogram relies on the measurement of pulses of a given value and their assignment to channels which represent different voltage levels. Each time a pulse falls into one of these channels a counter increments the channel. The process of counting each pulse in the appropriate channel is known as analogue-to-digital, A-D or conversion. Most systems have 256 or 1024 channels for single parameter histograms and may be generated based on fluorescence, FAL sensors or 90° light scatter. The pulses may be amplified; this may be linear or logarithmic. In some experiments the peak or integral pulses may vary widely in size. With linear amplification small pulses will be bunched up into a few channels making it difficult to distinguish differences between them. If the amplification is increased this helps to distinguish between the small pulses but the larger pulses become pushed off the scale of the histogram. In such cases the operator may elect to use pulses which have gone through a log amplification before plotting. The plot may include all pulses; however, the small pulses will be spread over more channels and the larger pulses over fewer channels. In this way all pulses are brought onto the scale of the histogram.

Coefficients of variation (CVs)

Ideally, the same particle passing repeatedly through the laser beam should produce identical light scatter or fluorescence pulses. Another particle might produce a consistent but different set of pulses. Practically, there are always some variations within the instrument, which causes some variation in the pulses even though the particles are the same. Any problems with the sample flow, the laser intensity, laser alignment, beam focusing and detection may result in variation of the pulses associated with a given particle. These variations lead to variation in histograms and it is important to determine whether the variation is due to instrument or particle variation or both. The operator can detect the severity of the instrument variations by calculating a CV on a good uniform test sample such as fluorescent beads (Coulter Electronics; Becton Dickinson; Polysciences). The basic equation for CV is:

$$CV = (s.d./mean) \times 100$$

where s.d. is the standard deviation and mean is the average value for the parameter measured for these particles (for a Gaussian distribution this would be the channel with the highest count). Most instruments calculate the CV for the operator. If the operator knows what the CV is normally, then any increase in CV will indicate that the instrument setting may be changing and result in broadening of histograms. However, if the beads have a good CV and a test sample has a broad histogram then it is a genuine phenomenon. Fluorescent beads may be added to the biological sample to be tested provided they do not interfere with the sample. The use of beads to count cells within a test sample and aspects of quality control are discussed further in Chapter 2.

Once a histogram has been produced the operator may now analyse it. The most common analysis is simply to determine what percentage a subpopulation is of the total population. This is possible if the populations are nicely separated, in practice this may not be the case. However, sophisticated computer programs are available to analyse overlapping populations. Computers can also be used to compare one histogram with another and determine if there are any significant differences.

All flow cytometry systems have the ability to analyse more than one signal simultaneously on particles and plot them as three-dimensional histograms. Many combinations of signals might be used. The histogram is like a chequerboard of channels. Each channel, like the single-parameter histogram, has a counter but now two pulse heights for a particle must fall within a channel to increment that channel. A three-dimensional histogram is therefore built up as the channels are incremented for a given sample (Fig. 1.10a). The two-parameter histogram

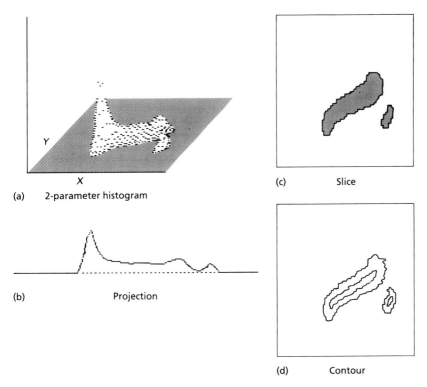

(a)   2-parameter histogram

(b)   Projection

(c)   Slice

(d)   Contour

Fig. 1.10 Examples of (a) a two-parameter three-dimensional histogram; (b) a projection histogram; (c) a slice; (d) a contour plot.

can be converted to a single-parameter histogram by viewing from the side (either axis x or y); this is called a projection (Fig. 1.10b). The two-parameter histogram may also be viewed from above and in this format it is referred to as a scattergram or dotplot. It is also possible to examine the distribution in all channels which have a certain operator selectable minimum count in the channels; Fig. 1.10c is termed a slice and an outline of a series of slices from the bottom to the top of a two-parameter histogram is termed a contour plot (Fig. 1.10d).

Safety aspects of lasers

Hazards from lasers can be summarized as follows:

1 Damage to the eye. The argon/krypton laser presents a possible hazard to the eye as 'stray' diffuse blue laser radiation can be focused by the eye on to the retina. Damage can occur due to either thermal or photochemical effects depending on exposure duration.

2 Skin burns. Interception of the beam by any part of the skin can possibly cause damage due to thermal effects.

3 Material combustion. Any unsuitable material in the vicinity of the beam can potentially cause fire, emission of toxic gases or explosion if irradiated.

Under normal operation of commercially available flow cytometers the laser requires covers to be installed and the laser output is interrupted if the cover is removed. Under these circumstances the laser is classified as a class 1 product, there is therefore no potential hazard. Safety standard BS EN 60825 (1992) applies. However, it is possible for the operator to defeat the interlock in the specimen irradiation area thus allowing the beam to be seen, although direct (intrabeam) viewing is impossible due to the equipment layout. A potential hazard exists from reflections. If the reflected beam is diffused in all directions this does not present a hazard. If the beam remains focused after reflection the maximum permissible exposure (MPE; intrabeam viewing) is $100\,J/m^2$. For a 60 second exposure, the MPE $= 1.67\,W/m^2$ and with a 2 W laser a safe viewing distance for such exposure would be 0.2 m. As a small source therefore an argon/krypton laser presents no hazard providing the operator does not view the beam reflection from any closer than 20 cm and for no longer than 60 seconds. Should prolonged viewing of the beam be necessary then the use of safety spectacles is recommended.

Cell sorting

An important function of flow cytometry is its ability to separate and collect a subpopulation of cells, identified by multiparameter analysis. Classically, this sorting of cells is accomplished as the cells exit from the sample chamber in a liquid jet. Savart (1833) showed that when a small jet of fluid was vibrated at the correct frequency the stream could be broken into a series of uniform droplets. In the flow cytometer the sheath stream is broken into a series of uniform droplets by vibrating the sample chamber with a piezoelectric crystal at a high frequency. Cells flowing through the flow cytometer are isolated in these tiny droplets. When the computer detects a cell that satisfies the parameters determined by the operator for sorting, an electrical charge is applied to the droplet (Thomson, 1967). The polarity of the charge — positive or negative — is determined by the sorting criteria. As the charged droplet passes an electrostatic field it is deflected to the right or left, carrying the sorted cell. Extremely pure populations of cells may be sorted at relatively rapid rates.

More recently an alternative technique has become available for sorting cells. The FACSort (Becton Dickinson) employs a system in which the required cell is removed from the sheath stream by a small rotating catcher tube. Up to 300 cells/s may be sorted but only one-way sorting is available at present. The technique is not dependent on droplet formation and takes place in an enclosed environment. Therefore, no aerosols are formed which is designed to eliminate the risk from biohazardous samples.

Commercial flow cytometers

There are three major manufacturers of flow cytometers, Coulter, Becton

Dickinson and Ortho. All originally introduced flow cytometers capable of sorting with water-cooled lasers. Coulter produced the EPICS™ (electronically programmable individual cell sorter) series, Becton Dickinson marketed the FACS™ (fluorescent activated cell sorter) while Ortho promoted Cytofluorographs. All manufacturers have moved toward production of clinically orientated analysers, employing air-cooled lasers and without the capacity to sort cells (Coulter Profile, Becton Dickinson FACScan, Ortho Orthocyte). Most recently Coulter have introduced the EPICs XL, which has an air-cooled argon laser and is capable of sorting; Ortho have marketed a flow cytometer capable of determining absolute counts on cell subpopulations; and Becton Dickinson have launched the FACSort and FACS Vantage. Table 1.2 illustrates the salient specifications of the currently available commercial flow cytometers.

Fluorochromes for use with flow cytometry

During the past few years there has been a rapid growth of interest in the application of fluorescent dyes to study physiological processes in single living cells. There are two factors which have facilitated this: first, the synthesis of a range of highly selective fluorochromes, each capable of physiologically detecting molecules and ions (Table 1.3); and second, the availability of low-cost commercial instruments capable of detecting and quantifying the weak signals emanating from single cells.

There are a number of requirements of any fluorochrome if it is to be used to monitor cell function. First, in experimentally used concentrations it should not be cytotoxic or, by itself modify the normal functioning of the cell. Second, it must be highly specific for the species to be detected. Third, it should be relatively easy to load a cell with the dye without causing damage or affecting cell function. Most of the dyes available fulfil the first two criteria. It should be considered a general principle that it is better to increase the sensitivity of the recording apparatus and to work with low dye concentrations and low levels of fluorescence rather than overload the cell with dye and risk modifying or killing the cell.

The active form of most fluorochromes is polyionic and hence does not cross the cell membrane easily. However, many fluorochromes are available in their esterified forms, which are lipophilic and can cross cell membranes easily. The ester forms of the dye are generally not fluorescent but, once inside the cell, the dye ester is converted, in principle, to the free form of the dye by non-specific intracellular esterases. Thus the active form of the dye, which is polar, can be trapped inside the cell. However, there is some evidence for incomplete hydrolysis of the esters and compartmentalization of the dye in intracellular organelles may occur, resulting in a complex and uninterpretable signal from the cell. It should also be pointed out that the reaction product from ester hydrolysis (acetic acid or formaldehyde, depending on the dye) may be cytotoxic. In many cell systems these problems can

Table 1.2 Specifications for commercial flow cytometers

Specification	Orthocyte	Cytoron absolute	FACScan	FACStar (Plus)
Light source				
Type	Xenon arc lamp mercury/xenon	Air-cooled argon laser	Air-cooled argon 15 mW laser	Water-cooled argon/krypton/dye lasers Air-cooled 100 mW argon available
Life-time	500–2000 h	—	>5000 h	Dependent on laser
Optics				
Usable spectrum	300 or 488 nm	488 nm	488 nm	300–488 nm
Fluorescence detectors	FITC/PE 3rd colour optional	FITC/PE/RED	FITC (488 nm) PE/PI (585 nm) RED (>650)	FITC/PE/PI/RED
Light scatter	Low/large angle	Forward/right-angle	Forward angle Side	Forward angle Side
Alignment	Pre-aligned, confocal epi-illumination	Pre-aligned laminar flow	Pre-aligned laminar flow	Manual alignment
Fluorescence sensitivity Molecules	<3000 FITC	300 FITC 1300 PE	<600 FITC 700 PE	800 FITC 1100 PE
Fluorescence CV	±2%	±2%	±2% full peak for PI-stained thymus nuclei	<2% full peak for PI-stained PBMNC
Light scattering sensitivity	0.2 nm particle	3.0 μm particle	0.1 μm	5.0 μm
Fluidics				
Flow cell	Jet on open surface	Hydrodynamic focusing	Quartz cuvette	Hydrodynamic focusing
Sample system	Hamilton syringe	Hamilton syringe	Continuous	Variable
Sheath flow	0.7 bar	—	60 or 12 μl/min	Variable
Analysing rate (cells/s)	Typical 2000	Maximum 20 000 Typical 2000	Maximum 20 000 Typical 2000	Typical 2000
Run cycle	40–60 s/sample	45 s/sample (50 Autosampler)	Operator controlled	Operator controlled
Additional options	—	—	Autosampler Air vent	Automatic cell deposition system FACS SortVIEW MacroSORT Camera accessory
Biosafety	—	—	Biosafety module	Biosafety module

FACSort	FACS Vantage	Profile	Elite	EPICS XL
Air-cooled argon 15 mW laser	Three laser assembly as for FACStar plus	Air-cooled argon 15 mW laser	Air-cooled argon Helium/neon 15 mW lasers	Air-cooled argon 15 mW laser
>5000 h	Dependent on lasers	>4000 h	>5000 h	>5000 h
488 nm	Five colour options Spectrum laser with variable lines	488 nm	300−488 nm	488 nm
FITC (488 nm) PE/PI (585 nm) RED (>650)	—	200−800 nm	200−800 nm	Up to 4 (from 200−800 nm)
Forward angle Side	Forward angle Side	Forward angle Side	Forward angle Side	Forward angle Side
Pre-aligned laminar flow	Operator controlled	Pre-aligned laminar flow	Manual alignment	Pre-aligned laminar flow
<600 FITC	<1000 FITC	<1000 FITC	<500 FITC	<500 FITC
700 PE	700 PE		<800 PE	<1000 PE
±2% full peak for PI-stained thymus nuclei	<2% full peak for PI-stained PBMNC	>1.5% half peak for PI-stained human lymphocytes	>1.5% with normal PI-stained human lymphocytes	<2.0% with normal PI-stained human lymphocytes
0.1 μm	1−2 μm	Forward scatter <1.5% half peak for 10 μm fluorospheres	0.5 μm particles over background with FALS	0.5 μm particles over background with FALS
Quartz cuvette	Hydrodynamic focusing FACS SortVIEW	BioSense cell	BioSense SortSense	250 μm BioSense flow cell quartz mounted
Continuous	Continuous	25−200 μl programmable in 1 μl increments	Continuous	Continuous
60 or 12 μl/min	Variable	Variable 10−100 μl in 1 μl steps	Variable	10, 30 or 60 μl/min
Maximum 20 000 Typical 2000	Typical 2000	Controlled variable Typical 2000	Maximum >35 000	Typical 3000
Operator controlled	Operator controlled Sorting by Lysis II	Operator controlled	Operator controlled	Operator controlled
FACSMate autosampler Air vent	—	Multi-Q-Prep	Autoclone sorting 5th PMT assembly Time delay facility	4th fluorescence detector Autoloader 650 megabyte optical storage
Enclosed module	Enclosed biosafe module for analysis	Closed biohazard wash station	Aerosol-free sort chamber	Aerosol-free sort chamber

Table 1.3 Reagents with fluorescent properties used in flow cytometry

Reagent	Ex	Em	Solvent storage	Additional applications	References
Cell viability					
CDDFA	490	520	DMSO, DMF, F, L, D	Intracellular pH Platelet labelling Preparation of lipophilic fluorescein derivatives	Babcock (1983) Horne et al. (1981) Altsteil et al. (1983)
DDFDA	505	530	DMF, AN, F, L, D	Quantitation of metabolic burst in neutrophils and monocytes Measurement of H_2O_2 production by neutrophils	Szejda et al. (1984) Hasui et al. (1989)
CDDFDA	505	530	DMF, AN, F, L, D	Quantitation of metabolic burst in neutrophils and monocytes Measurement of H_2O_2 production by neutrophils	Homan-Muller et al. (1975) Bass et al. (1983)
Dihydroethidium Dehydrogenated dihydroethedium	320 488	616	DMF, DMSO, F, A	Dehydrogenated by viable cells to ethidium which intercalates into DNA	Nishiwaki et al. (1974)
Propidium iodide	493	639	W, DMF	Live dead discrimination High resolution DNA analysis Reacts with RNA	Verhoef et al. (1986) Vindelov (1983)
7-AAD	523	647	DMF, DMSO, F, L	May be used with dual colour immunofluorescence Binds selectively to G-C regions of DNA	Schmidt et al. (1992) Rabinovitch et al. (1986) Zelenin et al. (1984)
EMA	488			Photoactivated form is excluded from viable cells and is distinguishable from fluorescein and phycoerythrin	Riedy et al. (1991)
RNA and DNA content					
Propidium iodide	493	639	W, DMF, F, L	Cell viability Reacts with RNA, DNA analysis requires RNA — see treatment	Papa et al. (1988) Orntoft et al. (1988)
Ethidium bromide	482	616	W, DMSO	Cell viability Liposome cell fusion	Poot (1990) Darzynkiewicz and Kapusciuski (1988) Aeschbacher et al. (1986) LePecq and Paoletti (1967)
DAPI	345	455	W, DMF	A-T selective DNA stain Does not bind RNA Identification of mycoplasma infection DNA-protein/antigen analysis	Stohr et al. (1978) Otto and Tsou (1986) Coleman et al. (1981) McCarthy and Hale (1988)
Acridine orange	487	510	W, E	Discrimination between DNA and RNA (DNA : green, RNA : orange, denatured DNA : red) Identification of viable pancreatic islet cells Neutrophil phagocytosis	Darzynkiewicz et al. (1980) Bank (1987) Rothe and Valet (1988) — —

Table 1.3 Continued

Reagent	Ex	Em	Solvent storage	Additional applications	References
7-AAD	523	647	DMF, DMSO	Cell viability Combined cell surface and DNA staining Efficiently discriminates between the G0 and G1 phases of the cell cycle	Schmidt *et al.* (1992) Schmidt *et al.* (1991b) Zelenin *et al.* (1984) Stokke *et al.* (1991)
Total protein					
SITS	351	465	W, F, L	Binds to outer components of plasma membrane Simultaneous DNA and protein analysis	Maddy (1964) Cornelius and Ploem (1976) Stohr *et al.* (1978)
DANS	351	525	E, F, L	Determination of lysine content	Rossilet and Ruch (1968)
SR101	488	615	W, F, L	Binds ionically rather than covalently so is reversible	Crissman and Steinkamp (1982)
TRITC	488	575	W, F, L	Dual fluorescent studies with FITC	Crissman and Steinkamp (1982)
FITC	488	560	W, F, L	Dual fluorescent studies with PI	Freeman and Crissman (1975) Crissman and Steinkamp (1973)
Sulphaflavin	488	575	W, F, L	Binds basic proteins at pH 8 and total protein at pH 2.8	Leeman and Ruch (1972)
Site specific					
NBD phallacidin	465	530	W, M, F, L	Identification, localization and quantitation of F-actin Study of cytoskeleton Labelled filaments remain functional	Barak *et al.* (1981) Runeberg *et al.* (1986) Keith *et al.* (1986)
MFDA Eosin diacetate	488 488			Halogenated dyes for cellular thiols that are excitable with visible light lasers	Poot *et al.* (1991)
NBD Colcemid	466	526	DMSO, DMF, F, L	The unbound form is non-fluorescent and permeant to cell membranes. NBD-colcemid has a fluorescein-like spectrum. It is specific for the colcemid binding site of tubulin and microtubules	Fecheimer and Zigmond (1983)
DPI	488	540	W	Labelling of lipoproteins	Corsetti *et al.* (1991)
Rhodamine 123	505	534	M, DMF, F, L, D	Cell permeant, sequestered by living mitochondria May be used for measurement of multidrug resistance in cells	Johnson *et al.* (1980) Tapiero *et al.* (1984) Verhoef *et al.* (1986)
Methotrexate, fluorescein, triammonium salt	496	520	DMF (pH 6)	Measurement of methotrexate resistance. Identification of dihydrofolate reductase production by cells	Kaufman *et al.* (1978) Gaudray *et al.* (1986)
Formyl-1 Nle-Leu Phe-Nle-Tyr-Lys fluorescein	491	518	DMF (pH 6) F, L	Study of chemotactic peptide receptor internalization by neutrophils	Sklar *et al.* (1984) Fay *et al.* (1991)

Continued on page 20

Table 1.3 Continued

Reagent	Ex	Em	Solvent storage	Additional applications	References
Dexamethasone fluorescein	491	520	DMF (pH 6) F, L	Analysis of steroid receptor internalization	Otto et al. (1987)
Naltrexone fluorescein	490	520	E, DMF, F, L, D	Analysis of opioid receptor function	Shipchandler (1987)
PLF	497	518	W, F, L	PLF is a fluorescein derivative of the lysine analogue of folic acid. It is used as a probe for the active site of dihydrofolate reductase	McAlinden et al. (1991)
FITC prolactin	488	530	W, F, L	Quantitation of luteinizing receptors	Lane and Chen (1991)
MCB				A glutathione-specific probe	Cook et al. (1991)
SAENTA-chi-2 fluorescein	488	530	W	Probe for the equilibrative inhibitor-sensitive nucleoside transporter	Wiley et al. (1991)
Membrane potential					
DiOC5 (3)	484	509	DMSO	Relatively toxic Accumulates in cells during hyperpolarization	Waggoner (1979)
DiOC6 (3)	484	510	DMSO, L	Measurement of membrane potential on single cells Mitochondrial probe Measurement of hyperpolarization	Rosenthal and Shapiro (1983) Bakeeva et al. (1970) Jenssen et al. (1986) McGinnes et al. (1988)
DiSC3 (5)	651	675	DMSO, L	Measurement of membrane potential on red cells Mitochondrial probe Platelet and neutrophil function	Tatham and Delves (1984) Castranova and Van Dyke (1984) Simons et al. (1982) Lazzari et al. (1986) Sims et al. (1974)
Trimethine oxonol	535	559	DMSO, E, F, L	Slow responding anions whose distribution across the membrane is potential dependent Less toxic than other membrane potential probes May be used in combination with intracellular Ca^{2+} measurement in single cells	Wilson and Chused (1985) Grinstein and Cohen (1987) Mohr and Fewtrell (1987) — —
W.W. 781 free acid	605	639	DMSO, E, F, L	Cell permeant due to high charge. Spectral response is faster than in other probes Decrease in fluorescence due to hyperpolarization	George (1988) Cohen and Lesher (1986) Gupta et al. (1981)
Rhodamine-123	505	543		Used for monitoring relative mitochondrial membrane potential	Johnson et al. (1981) Bernal et al. (1982) Myc et al. (1991)
Intracellular pH					
ADB	354	400	DMSO, F, L	Requires emission ratio measurement	Valet et al. (1981) Alabaster (1983)

Table 1.3 Continued

Reagent	Ex	Em	Solvent storage	Additional applications	References
4-MU	375	488	DMSO	Requires emission ratio measurement Tends to leak from cells	Gerson et al. (1982) Gerson and Kiefer (1983) —
COFDA	490	520	DMSO, DMF, F, L, D	Requires excitation at two wavelengths Does not enter mitochondria, is cytoplasmic specific Requires pH less than 7.0 to load cells	Musgrove et al. (1986)
BCECF	508	530	DMSO, DMF, F, L, D	Measurement of cytoplasmic pH only May be used at physiological pH Ratio emission at 520–550 nm obtained using two excitation wavelengths above and below 465	Grinstein et al. (1985) Simpson and Rink (1987) Rogers et al. (1983) —
SNARF, SNAFL	488/ 560	600	DMSO	Require dual excitation Are useful for measuring pH changes between 6.6 and 8.6 and are membrane permeant	Rijkers et al. (1990) Whitaker et al. (1988)
Cytoplasmic calcium					
Indo-1 High ion Low ion Cell impermeant	331 349	410 485	W, F, L	The fluorescence emission max. of Indo-1 shifts from 490 nm in Ca^{2+}-free medium to 405 nm when saturated with Ca^{2+}	Davies et al. (1988) June et al. (1987) Grynkiewics et al. (1985) Luckoff (1986) Ransom and DiGusto (1987)
Indo-1 AM Cell permeant	361	479	DMSO, DMF, F, L, D	Compartmentalization and esterase activity should be critically assessed	Rabinovitch et al. (1986) June et al. (1986)
Fura-2	335	510	DMSO	Requires ratiometric measurements using excitation at 340 and 380 nm	Tsein et al. (1985) Poenie et al. (1985) Williams et al. (1985)
Fluo-3	506	526	DMSO, DMF, F, L, D	To achieve minimal and maximal Ca^{2+}, calibration is required May be used in functional assay of multidrug resistance	Tsein (1985) Wall et al. (1991) —
Enzyme activity					
FDA	490	520	DMSO, DMF, AN, F, L, D	Measurement of cholinesterase and other esterases. Assay is non-specific and may require inhibitors and substrates to eliminate activity from other enzymes	Sengbusch et al. (1976) Wilder and Cram (1977)
Naphthol AS-B1 a-D-glucuronide	405	515	W, F, L	Used to measure glucuronidase activity	Dolbeare and Phares (1979)

Continued on page 22

Table 1.3 Continued

Reagent	Ex	Em	Solvent storage	Additional applications	References
Napthol AS phosphates	405	520	W, F, L	AS-B1 derivative may be used to measure phosphatase activity. However, the fluorescent product only remains in the cell for a brief period (8 min)	Dolbeare and Phares (1979)
NMA	345	430	W, F, L	Used to measure proteinase activity. Specific amino acid sequences may be attached to the aromatic amine group to facilitate analysis of enzymes such as Cathepsin B1 and dipeptidyl amino peptidase 1	Smith and Frank (1975) McDonald et al. (1975) Dolbeare and Smith (1977)
DDF	505	530	DMF, AN, F, L	Used to measure peroxidase activity and H_2O_2 production	Keston and Brandt (1965)
NAD/Resazurin	560	580	W, F, L, D	Lactic dehydrogenase and alcohol dehydrogenase assay. The NAD is reduced to NADH, which reduces resazurin to fluorescent resorufin. The reaction requires phenazine methosulphate	Guilbault and Kramer (1965) Dolbeare and Smith (1979)

Ex, optimum excitation wavelength; Em, optimum emission wavelength.

Reagents
7-AAD, 7-amino-actinomycin D; ADB, 1,4-diacetoxy-2,3-dicyanobenzene; BCECF-AM, 2',7'-bis-carboxyethyl-5(6)-carboxyfluoresceinacetoxymethyl-ester; BO, bis-(1,3-diethylthiobarbituric acid) thriethine oxonol; FDA, fluorescein diacetate; CDDFDA, 5',6'carboxy-2',7'-dichlorofluorescein diacetate; COFDA, carboxyfluorescein diacetate; DANS, dansyl chloride; DAPI, 4',6'-diamidino-2-phenylindole; FDA, fluorescein diacetate; DFDA, 2',7'-dichlorofluorescein diacetate; DiOC5(3), 3,3'-dipentyloxacarbocyanine iodide; DiOC3 (5), 3,3'-dipropylthiadicarbocyanine iodide; EMA, photoactivated ethidium monoazide; FITC, fluorescein isothiocyanate; MCB, monochlorobimane; MFDA, methylfluorescein-diacetate; 4-MU, 4-methylumbelliferone; NAD, nicotinamide adenine dinucleotide; NBD, N-(7-nitrobenzene-2-oxa-1,3-diazol-4-yl); NMA, 4-methyl-2-naphthylamine; PLF, N-α-pteroyl-N ε-(4'-fluoresceinisothiocarbamoyl)-L-lysine; SAENTA-χ' 2-fluorescein, 5-S-(2-aminoethyl)-N6-(4-nitrobenzyl)-5'-thioadenosine; SITS, 4-acetamido-4,4'-isothiocyanatostilbene-2',2'-disulphonic acid; SR101, sulphorhodamine 101; TRITC, tetramethylrhodamine isothiocyanate; XRITC, a sulphonyl chloride derivative of sulphorhodamine.

Solvents
AC, acetone; AN, acetonitrile; C, chloroform; D, dioxane; DMF, dimethylformamide; DMSO, dimethylsuphoxide; E, ethanol; EE, ethyl ether; H, hexane; M, methanol; T, toluene; THF, tetrahydrofuran; W, water.

Storage
A, protect from air; D, store desiccated; F, store frozen avoid freeze/thawing; L, light sensitive.

be evaluated with simple control experiments and the extent of possible artefacts assessed.

The protocols used for loading dye into cells are varied. In general cells are incubated with between 1 and 10 μmol/l of the esterified dye for times from a few minutes to several hours at temperatures ranging from 4 to 37°C. The ester form of dyes are prone to spontaneous hydrolysis and are thus rendered incapable of crossing the membrane and accumulating in the cell. Care must be taken when dissolving and aliquoting dyes. They may be sensitive to both light and aqueous environments. Polar, 'dry' solvents such as DMSO, ethanol or acetone should be used, aliquots should be screened from light and ideally stored desiccated at −80°C.

In general fluorochromes may be divided into three categories: single wavelength dyes; dual excitation dyes; and dual emission dyes. Once a dye is loaded into a cell the intensity of the fluorescence signal will be proportional to the concentration of the dye and the concentration of the molecule or ion to which the dye is sensitive. To derive quantitative information calibration is required. For dyes that have either their excitation or emission spectrum shifted when bound to their target molecule or ion, a ratio measurement is facilitated. By determining the position of the spectrum it is possible to obtain a measure of the target concentration. The position of the spectrum is independent of the dye concentration, so measurement of the spectrum position is directly proportional to the intracellular concentration of the species under analysis. The simplest way to determine the position of the spectrum is to measure the emitted light intensity at two wavelengths. The ratio of intensities, gives a measure of the intracellular dye concentration.

In principle, the dual excitation dyes may be used in the same way. The ratio of intensities, obtained by exciting at two wavelengths and measuring at a single emission wavelength, is used to obtain a signal which is independent of dye concentration and proportional to concentration of the molecule studied. Filter systems are readily available for dual excitation dyes and beam splitters are used to operate with dual emission dyes (see Table 1.1).

Monoclonal antibodies and clusters of differentiation (CDs)

Since 1975 when Kohler and Milstein introduced a method for generating clones of hybrid cells capable of producing monospecific immunoglobulins in high titres, a multitude of antibodies have been generated. To organize these antibodies into a classification there have been, to date, four international workshops, the aim of which has been to group antibodies into clusters based on their cellular reactivity. These clusters have been termed clusters of differentiation or CDs. After the fourth workshop 78 CDs were defined and these are shown in Table 1.4. The structure and function of the antigens for many of the CDs are now known. The clinical applications for these CDs are given in Table 1.5.

Note added in proof

The new CDs defined by and alterations to existing CD classifications made by the Vth International Workshop on Leucocyte Differentiation Antigens are shown in Appendix 2 on page 301.

Table 1.4 CD classification of leucocyte antigens

Antigens	Other names	Mol wt (kD)	Main cellular distribution	Comments
CD1a, b, c	T6	49, 45, 43	Cortical thymocytes, Langerhans cells	Similar to HLA-Class I (associated with β_2 microglobulin). 'Non-classical' antigen presenting? Hormone receptor?
CD2	T11	50	T cells	Receptor for sheep erythrocytes and LFA-3 (CD58). CD2R denotes an epitope expressed by activated T cells which is unrelated to LFA-3 binding
CD3	T3	16–29	T cells	Five chains linked to TCR involved in signal transduction
CD4	T4	59	T-cell subset, monocytes/macrophage	Receptor for HLA-Class II and HIV. Cytoplasmic part associated with p56-lck tyrosine kinase. Regulates function of CD3/TCR complex?
CD5	T1	67	T cells, B-cell subset	
CD6	T12	100	T cells, B-cell subset	
CD7		40	T cells	Similar to mouse Thy1. T-cell subset
CD8	T8	32	T-cell subset, splenic sinusoidal cells	Two chain molecule. (a/a or a/b) HLA-Class I receptor. Cytoplasmic part associated with p56-lck tyrosine kinase. Regulates function of CD3/TCR complex?
CD9	p24	24	Platelets, monocytes, pre-B cell, brain	? Protein kinase. No transmembrane moeity. Anti-CD9 aggregates platelets
CD10	CALLA	100	Stem cells, renal epithelium, ALL	Neutral endopeptidase cleaving peptides of the amino terminus of hydrophobic residues
CD11a	LFA-1 β_2-integrin	180	Many leucocytes	α-chain of LFA-1. Binds ICAM-1 (CD54). Mediates T-cell cytotoxicity and cell : cell adhesion. Epitope of CD18. Integrin supergene family
CD11b	Mac-1, CR3	165	Granulocytes, monocytes, NK cells	α-chain of Mac-1. Receptor for iC3b, fibrinogen, Factor X (see CD18). Integrin supergene family

CD	Name	MW	Cell distribution	Comments
CD11c	p150,95	150	Macrophages, granulocytes, NK cells, hairy cell leukaemia	α-chain of p150,95. ?C3bi receptor
CD12			Myeloid cells	
CD13	MY7, gp150	150	Granulocytes, monocytes, non-leucocytes, e.g. bile canaliculi, connective tissue	Aminopeptidase N. CD13 antibodies induce oxidative metabolic burst. Receptor for the enteropathogenic coronaviruses
CD14	gp55	55	Monocytes, Kupffer's cells, granulocytes, FDC	Receptor for the LPS: LPS binding protein complex. PIG-linked chain surface membrane glycoprotein
CD15	Hapten X	50–180	Granulocytes, epithelium, R-S cells	Gal1-4 (Fuc1–3)GlcNac. Some CD15 antibodies inhibit phagocytosis
CD16	FcRIII	50–65	Granulocytes, some macrophages, NK cells	Low affinity receptor for monomeric IgG, binds complexed IgG. Phosphoinositol glycan (PIG) linked on neutrophils. Transmembrane linked on NK cells
CDw17	Lactosyl-ceramide		Granulocytes, monocytes, platelets	Cer Glc, 1–4 Gal
CD18	LFA-1 Mo-1	95	Many leucocytes (CD11a,b and c)	β-chain of LFA/Mac-1 integrin family. Binds to ICAM-2 receptor
CD19	B4	90	Mature B cells	Belongs to immunoglobulin supergene family. Inhibition of B-cell activation
CD20	B1	35/37	B cells	? Involved in membrane ion transport
CD21	CR2	140	B cells, FDC	Receptor for C3d and EBV
CD22		135	B cells, Hairy cell leukaemia	Intracytoplasmic in early B cells. Surface expression in Hairy cell and prolymphocytic leukaemia. Belongs to Ig supergene family. Homologous to myelin-associated glycoprotein, NCAM and CD33
CD23	FcRII IgE	45–50	Activated B cells, some FDC	Low affinity receptor for IgE FcRII. Two forms: a and b. Soluble form has growth factor activity. Glycoprotein PI-linked on neutrophils

Continued on page 26

Table 1.4 Continued

Antigens	Other names	Mol wt (kD)	Main cellular distribution	Comments
CD24	BA1	38/41	Some B cells, granulocytes	
CD25	Tac	55	Activated cells, macrophages	Low affinity IL-2 receptor
CD26		120	Activated T and B cells, macrophages	Dipeptylpeptidase IV. Serine type exopeptidase
CD27		55	T cells, plasma cells	Present on cell surface as a disulphide-linked homodimer (110 kD)
CD28		44	T-cell subset	Present on cell surface as a homodimer (88 kD). Belongs to immunoglobulin supergene family. Regulation of lymphokine mRNA stability
CD29	gpI1a VLA-chain	130	T-cell subset, platelets many non-leucocytes	Forms heterodimer with at least six different VLA-chains. Mediation of cell adhesion to cells
CD30	Ki-1	105	Activated lymphocytes, R-S cells, ALCL	
CD31	gpIIa'	140	Granulocytes, monocytes, platelets, B cells, endothelium	Carcinoembryonic antigen-like molecule. Belongs to immunoglobulin supergene family. Induces integrin-mediated adhesion. Present on naive T cells
CDw32	FcIgGRII	40	Granulocytes, B cells, monocytes macrophages, platelets	IgG receptor for aggregated IgG. Several isoforms with differing distribution have been identified. Functional role in cell activation
CD33	My9	67	Myeloid progenitors, monocytes	
CD34		120–150	Haemopoietic progenitors, capillary endothelium	Putative stem cell
CD35	CR1	160, 190, 220, 250	FDC, red cells, granulocytes, some NK cells, glomeruli	C3b receptor. Four allotypes differ in molecular weight. Function in processing of immune complexes, promotion of binding and phagocytosis of C3b-coated particles
CD36	gpIV	90	Monocytes/macrophages, platelets	Endothelial cell receptor for *Plasmodium faciparum* infected red blood cells. Platelet and monocyte receptor for thrombospondin. May also be a platelet collagen adhesion receptor

CD	Other names	MW (kD)	Cellular distribution	Comments
CD37		40–52	B cells, macrophages, T cells	
CD38	T10	45	Germinal centre cells, plasma cells, activated T cells, thymocytes	
CD39		70–100	B cells, macrophages, endothelium, other cells	
CD40		44–48, 50	B cells, interdigitating reticulum cells, carcinomas	? Receptor for growth factor promoting B-cell proliferation. Homologous to NGFR
CD41	gpIIbIIIa	155 + 110	Megakaryocytes, platelets	Ca^{2+}-dependent complex of gpIIb (120 kD α-chain + 33 kD β-chain) and gpIIIa (CD61 110 kD). Deficient in Glanzmann's thrombasthenia. Binds fibrinogen, fibronectin and vWF
CD42a	gpIX	23	Megakaryocytes, platelets	Complexes with gp1b (CD42b) to form receptor for vWF. Deficient in Bernard–Soulier syndrome
CD42b	gp1b	135 + 25	Megakaryocytes, platelets	Function as for CD42a. Two-chain molecule comprising 135 kD α-chain and 25 kD β-chain
CD43	Leucosialin, sialophorin	95	Leucocytes, red cells, brain	Defective in Wiskott–Aldrich syndrome. Involved in activation of T cells, B cells, NK cells and monocytes
CD44	HERMES, Pgp-1 ECMRIII	80–95	Leucocytes, red cells	Cell homing receptor. Binds to hyaluronic acid. Carries I^{na}/In^b blood group antigens. Cartilage link protein
CD45	LCA	180–220	Most leucocytes	Tyrosine phosphatase active in signal transduction. Four different isoforms produced via alternative splicing
CD45RA		220	B cells, T-cell subset, monocytes/macrophages	Epitope encoded by exon A. Identifies naive T cells
CD45RB		190, 205, 220	B cells, T-cell subset, monocyte/macrophages, granulocytes	Epitope encoded by exon B, detected by antibody PD7/26
CD45RO		180	T cells, B-cell subset, monocytes/macrophages, myeloid cells	Epitope detected by antibody UCHL1. Not encoded by exon A, B or C. Identifies memory T cells

Continued on page 28

Table 1.4 Continued

Antigens	Other names	Mol wt (kD)	Main cellular distribution	Comments
CD46	MCP	56/60	Many cell types	Membrane co-factor protein MCP. Co-factor for I mediated cleavage of C3b/C4b. Structure similar to DAF
CD47		47–52	Pan reactive	Associated with rhesus blood groups
CD48		?41	Monocytes and neutrophils	PIG linked may be used in diagnosis of PNH
CDw49	VLA-chain	120–170	Platelets, lymphocytes, monocytes	Three chains (b, d, f) which complex to CD29 (VLA-chains) to produce gpIa/IIa, a lymphocyte homing and laminin receptor, respectively. CD49b is a collagen receptor. CD49d is a Peyer's patch-specific lymphocyte homing receptor. CD49f is a laminin receptor
CDw50		108/140?	Leucocytes	
CD51	VNR-chain	125 + 25	Platelets, non-leucocytes	Complexes with VNR-chain (CD61/gpIIIa) to form vitronectin receptor
CDw52	Campath-1	21–28?	Leucocytes	Antibody used in preventing GVH disease
CD53		32–40	Leucocytes	Stimulation of the oxidative metabolic burst
CD54	ICAM-1	90	Endothelial cells, activated T cells, epithelial cells	Ligand for LFA-1 (CD11a). Receptor for rhinovirus
CD55	DAF	70	Many cell types	Limits complement activation. Absent from PNH red cells
CD56	NKH-1	135/220	NK cells, neuroectodermal cells	Isoform of neural cell adhesion molecule
CD57	HNK-1	110	NK cells, T-cell subset	
CD58	LFA-3	40–65	Many cell types	Ligand for CD2 (sheep red blood cell receptor). PI-linked
CD59	MAC inhibitor, protectin	18–20	Many cell types	Inhibits complement-mediated activation. Homologous to mouse Ly-6
CDw60		Carbohydrate	T-cell subset, platelets	Neu-Ac-Neu-Ac-Gal sequence on gangliosides
CD61	gpIIIa, VNRb-chain	110	Platelets, megakaryocytes	Associates with gpIIb (in CD41) or with VNR α-chain (CD51) to form receptors for fibrinogen, vitronectin, vWF

CD	Name	MW (kD)	Expression	Comments
CD62	PADGEM GMP-140 P-selectin	140	Activated platelets, endothelium	Present in platelet α-granules and endothelial Weibel palade bodies. Expressed on surface after activation
CD63	gp53	53	Activated platelets, monocytes, endothelium	Present in lysosomal granules in platelets. Expressed on surface after activation
CD64	Fc RI	75	Monocytes	High affinity receptor for monomeric IgG. Transduces activation signals
CDw65		Carbohydrate	Granulocytes, monocytes	Type II chain fucoganglioside
CD66		180–200	Granulocytes	
CD67		100	Granulocytes	
CD68		110	Monocytes/macrophages	
CD69	AIM	28/34	Activated cells, NK cells	Involved in early lymphocyte activation
CDw70	Ki-24	?	Activated lymphocytes, R-S cells	
CD71	T9	95	Activated cells, macrophages, proliferating cells	Homodimer. Transferrin receptor
CD72		39/43	B cells, some macrophage, epithelium	
CD73		69	B cells and T-cell subset	Ecto-5' nucleotidase. PI-linked. Catalyses the dephosphorylation of purine/pyrimidine ribo/deoxyribonucleotide monophosphates. Regulates uptake of nucleotides
CD74	LN2	35/33/41	B cells, monocytes/macrophages, epithelial cells	Invariant chain of HLA-Class II. Putative involvement in intracellular transport of MHC class II and processing of antigen
CDw75	LN1	53	Mature B cells, epithelial cells	
CD76		67/85	Mature B cells, T-cell subset, epithelial cells	Sialylated glycosphingolipid
CD77	BLA	Carbohydrate	Follicle centre B cells	Neutral glycosphingolipid. Equivalent to P^k blood group
CD78	Ba	?	B cells	

ALCL, anaplastic large cell lymphoma; ALL, acute lymphocytic leukaemia; CD, cluster of differentiation; DAF, decay accelerating factor; FDC, follicular dendritic cells; GVH, graft-*vs*-host; IL, interleukin; NK, natural killer (cells); PI, phosphoinositol; PIG, PI glycan; PNH, paroxysmal nocturnal haemoglobinuria; R-S, Reed-Sternberg; TCR, T-cell receptor; vWF, von Willebrand's factor.

Table 1.5 Clinical applications for CDs

CD	Clinical application	Reference
CD1a, b, c	Characterization of leukaemia and lymphoma	Calabi *et al.* (1989) Freedman and Nadler (1991)
CD2	Evaluation of immunodeficiency, chronic inflammatory diseases. Characterization of leukaemia and lymphoma. T cell depletion in BMT	Plunkett *et al.* (1987) Illum *et al.* (1991)
CD3	Immunosuppressive therapy in organ and BMT, immunoregulation in auto-aggressive diseases, characterization of immunodeficiencies (Omenn's syndrome), leukaemias and lymphomas	Clevers *et al.* (1988) Le Deist *et al.* (1991) Weiner and Hillstrom (1991)
CD4	Evaluation of T-cell subpopulations, immunosuppressive therapy	Viellette *et al.* (1989) Haynes *et al.* (1981) Rudd *et al.* (1991)
CD5	Bone marrow purging in allogeneic BMT. Characterization of CLL	Ledbetter *et al.* (1986) Weisdorf *et al.* (1991) Antin *et al.* (1991) Geisler *et al.* (1991)
CD6	Immunosuppressive therapy. T-cell depletion in bone marrow purging. Member of new gene superfamily	Reinherz *et al.* (1982) Aruffo *et al.* (1991a)
CD7	Characterization of leukaemias and immunodeficiencies	Ware *et al.* (1989) Yumura *et al.* (1991) Schanberg *et al.* (1991)
CD8	Evaluation of T-cell subpopulations. Diagnosis of immunodeficiency virus infection	Barber *et al.* (1989) Melnick *et al.* (1991) Smith *et al.* (1991)
CD9	Bone marrow purging in autologous transplantation	Higashihara *et al.* (1985) Weisdorf *et al.* (1991)
CD10	Immunophenotype for acute lymphoblastic leukaemia (ALL) with relatively good prognosis. Identification of Burkitt's lymphoma	Letarte *et al.* (1988) Barker *et al.* (1989) Freedman and Nadler (1991)
CD11a	Monoclonal antibodies used for prevention of GVHD in BMT. Characterization of LFA-1 immunodeficiency	Larson *et al.* (1989) Zimmerman *et al.* (1992) Hogg (1991)
CD11b	Characterization of LFA-1 immunodeficiency	Corbi *et al.* (1988) Hogg (1991)
CD11c	Characterization of leukaemias and lymphomas	Myanes *et al.* (1988)
CD13	Phenotyping myeloid leukaemias	Look *et al.* (1989) Favaloro *et al.* (1988) Delmas *et al.* (1992)
CD14	Identification of monocytes and macrophage. Identification of monocytic and bilineal leukaemias	Goyert *et al.* (1988) Wright *et al.* (1990) Akashi *et al.* (1991)

Table 1.5 Continued

31

CHAPTER 1
Introduction

CD	Clinical application	Reference
CD15	Identification of Hodgkin and Reed–Sternberg cells except in the lymphocyte-predominant form of disease. Non-Hodgkin lymphomas are usually unreactive with CD15	Stein *et al.* (1986) Schmidt *et al.* (1991a) Ball *et al.* (1991)
CD16	Identification of immature neutrophils. Measurement of platelet functional ability	Rosenfeld *et al.* (1987) Fanger *et al.* (1989)
CD18	Antibodies used for GVHD prevention in transplantation. Molecule lacking in LFA-1 immunodeficiency. Inflammation induced	Fischer (1991) Shimizu *et al.* (1992)
CD19	Leukaemia and lymphoma typing. CD19-CR2 complex involved in humoral immunosuppression	De Rie *et al.* (1989) Hebell *et al.* (1991)
CD20	Enumeration of B cells, leukaemia and typing	Clark and Lane (1991) Geisler *et al.* (1991)
CD21	Typing of mature leukaemias and lymphomas	Geisler *et al.* (1991)
CD22	Typing of mature leukaemias	Schwartz *et al.* (1991)
CD23	Typing of mature leukaemias and lymphomas, analysis of IgE responses. Regulation by soluble IgE	Richards and Katz (1991)
CD24	Identification of activated granulocytes	Feldmann *et al.* (1991)
CD25	Serum IL-2 receptor in transplantation, inflammatory and malignant disorders, typing lymphomas and leukaemias. Antibodies used for suppression of transplantation and autoimmunity	Hofmann *et al.* (1991) Raziuddin *et al.* (1991) Blaise *et al.* (1991) Engert *et al.* (1991)
CD26	Identification of maturation and activation in T cells	Torimoto *et al.* (1991) Dang *et al.* (1991)
CD27	Measurement of T cell activation by antigens	Camarini *et al.* (1991)
CD28	Involved in IL-2 production by CD4$^+$ T cells. Antibodies used in tumour immunotherapy	Jenkins *et al.* (1991) Jung *et al.* (1991)
CD29	B cell activation. Involved in T cell lymphoma metastasis	Postigo *et al.* (1991) Roos (1991)
CD30	Typing of lymphomas and leukaemias, detection of CD30 antigen in infectious mononucleosis, Hodgkin's disease, anaplastic large cell lymphoma and T cell leukaemia	Schwarting *et al.* (1989) Gianotti *et al.* (1991)
CD31	Identification of lymphomas	Roos (1991)
CDw32	Diagnosis of autoimmune neutropenia. Measurement of neutrophil phagocytic ability. Bi-specific antibodies used for targeting tumour cell lysis	Veys *et al.* (1989) Huizinga *et al.* (1989) Greenman *et al.* (1991)

Continued on page 32

Table 1.5 Continued

CD	Clinical application	Reference
CD33	Phenotyping of leukaemias	Favaloro *et al.* (1988) Cantu *et al.* (1991)
CD34	Identification of stem cells, characterization of leukaemias	Sutherland *et al.* (1988)
CD35	Studies of complement receptors in autoimmune and immune complex diseases; characterization of leukaemias and lymphomas	Hogg *et al.* (1984) Loken *et al.* (1988)
CD36	Involved in haemostasis and apoptotic cell phagocytosis	Shattil and Brugge (1991) Savill *et al.* (1990)
CD37	Lymphoma typing	Wyatt and Dawson (1991)
CD38	Leukaemia and lymphoma typing, detection of plasma cells	Raziuddin *et al.* (1991)
CD39	B lymphoma typing	Valentine *et al.* (1988) Mielke and Moller (1991)
CD40	Role in survival of activated B cells	Camerini *et al.* (1991)
CD41	Diagnosis of Glanzmann's thrombasthenia (CD41−) and megakaryoblastic/cytic leukaemias (CD41+). Detection of human alloantibodies (anti-Zw^{a,b}, and anti-Yuk^{a,b}) against GpIIbIIIa (MAIPA assay)	Matolcsy *et al.* (1991) Keifel *et al.* (1987) Keifel *et al.* (1991)
CD42a	Detection of human auto-antibodies against Gp1b, diagnosis of Bernard−Soulier syndrome (CD42a−) and megakaryocytic/blastic leukaemia	Fox *et al.* (1988)
CD42b	Detection of Bernard−Soulier syndrome	Vincente *et al.* (1988) Keifel *et al.* (1991)
CD43	Involved in the C1q-mediated enhancement of phagocytosis	Guan *et al.* (1991)
CD44	Measurement of inflammatory disease. Involved in lymphoid ontogeny. Affects tumour growth *in vivo*. Anti-CD44 inhibits T cell activation by OKT3	Haynes *et al.* (1991) Collado *et al.* (1991) Sy *et al.* (1991) Rothman *et al.* (1991)
CD45	Typing of leukaemias and lymphomas. Discrimination of non-Hodgkin's lymphoma from carcinoma and non-lymphoid leukaemia	Maddy *et al.* (1991) Trowbridge *et al.* (1991)
CD46	Member of the regulators of complement activation gene cluster	Liszewski *et al.* (1991)
CD48	Required for γ/δ T-cell receptor recognition. Diagnosis of PNH	Mami *et al.* (1991) Stefanova *et al.* (1991)
CDw49b	Detection of human alloantibodies against VLA-2	Pesando *et al.* (1986)
CDw49d	Required for cell aggregation. Involved in haemopoiesis	Pulido *et al.* (1991) Williams *et al.* (1991)

Table 1.5 Continued

33

CHAPTER 1

Introduction

CD	Clinical application	Reference
CDw49f	Laminin receptor adhesion to arg-gly-arp containing sequences in vitronectin, von Willebrand factor, fibrinogen and thrombospondin	Sonnenberg *et al.* (1988)
CD51	VNR mediates cell adhesion to arg-gly-arp containing sequences in vitronectin, von Willebrand factor, fibrinogen and thrombospondin	Quinn *et al.* (1991)
CDw52	The Campath-1 antibody has been used for prevention of GVHD in allogeneic BMT	Hale *et al.* (1983) Friend *et al.* (1991)
CD53	Discrimination of haematopoietic neoplasms from sarcomas and melanomas	Horejsi and Vlcek (1991) Amiot (1991)
CD54	Important in leucocyte endothelial cell interactions	Hogg (1992)
CD55	Diagnosis of PNH	Rosse *et al.* (1991)
CD56	Identification of NK cell subpopulations	Acevedo *et al.* (1991) Mechtersheimer *et al.* (1991)
CD57	Identification of NK cell subpopulations particularly following BMT and in HIV-1 infection	Aotsuka *et al.* (1991) Prince and Jensen (1991)
CD58	Diagnosis of PNH. Involved in the inhibition of T cells in Hodgkin's disease	Roux *et al.* (1991)
CD59	Diagnosis of PNH. Reduced expression in HIV infected lymphocytes	Shichishima *et al.* (1991) Weiss *et al.* (1992)
CDw60	Antibodies provide costimulatory signals for T cells	Fox *et al.* (1990)
CD61	Identification of megakaryoblastic/cytic leukaemias and idiopathic thrombocytopenic purpura	Matolcsy *et al.* (1991)
CD62	Detection of activated platelets	Aruffo *et al.* (1991b)
CD63	Detection of activated platelets. Identical to the stage-specific melanoma-associated antigen ME491	Metzelaar *et al.* (1991) Azorsa *et al.* (1991)
CD64	Expression on neutrophils is modulated by interferon-γ	Cassatella *et al.* (1991)
CD65	Characterization of leukaemias	Macher *et al.* (1988)
CD66	Neutrophil activation	Hundt *et al.* (1991)
CD67	Neutrophil activation	Kuijpers *et al.* (1991)
CD68	Identification of macrophages	Betjes *et al.* (1991)
CD69	Involved in T-cell inactivation	Hommel *et al.* (1991)
CDw70	Typing of lymphomas	Fend *et al.* (1991)
CD71	Typing of lymphomas and leukaemias	Raziuddin *et al.* (1991) Freedman and Nadler (1991)
CD72	Typing of acute leukaemias	Fend *et al.* (1991)

Continued on page 34

Table 1.5 Continued

CD	Clinical application	Reference
CD73	Reduced endo-5'-NT activity in some immunodeficiency diseases	Johnson (1991) Clark and Lane (1991)
CD74	Associated with MHC class II and processing of antigen	Koch *et al.* (1991)
CDw75	Leukaemia and lymphoma typing	Wyatt and Dawson (1991) Stamenkovic *et al.* (1991) Schmidt *et al.* (1991a)
CD76	Leukaemia and lymphoma typing	Wyatt and Dawson (1991) Fend *et al.* (1991)
CD77	Lymphoma typing	Wyatt and Dawson (1991)
CDw78	Lymphoma typing	Kikutani *et al.* (1991)

GVHD, graft-*vs*-host disease; IL, interleukin; PNH, paroxysmal nocturnal haemoglobinuria; NK, natural killer (cells); BMT, bone marrow transplantation; MHC, major histocompatibility complex.

References

Acevedo A, Arambura J, Lopez J, Fernandez HJ, Fernandez RJ, Lopez BM (1991) Identification of natural killer (NK) cells in lesions of human cutaneous graft-versus-host disease: expression of a novel NK-associated surface antigen (Kp43) in mononuclear infiltrates. *J. Invest. Dermatol.* **97**: 659–666.

Aeschbacher M, Reinhardt CA, Zbinden G (1986) A rapid cell membrane permeability test. *Cell Biol. Toxicol.* **2**: 247–251.

Akashi K, Harada M, Shibuya T *et al.* (1991) Simultaneous occurrence of myelomonocytic leukaemia and multiple myeloma: involvement of common leukaemic progenitors, and their developmental abnormality of 'lineage infidelity'. *J. Cell Physiol.* **148**: 446–456.

Alabaster O (1983) Tumor cell metabolic heterogeneity: An adaptive survival response. *Proc. Am. Assoc. Cancer Res.* **24**: 6–12.

Altsteil L, Branton D (1983) Fusion of coated vesicles with lysosomes: measurement with a fluorescence assay. *Cell* **32**: 921–926.

Amiot M (1991) Identification and analysis of cDNA clones encoding CD53. A panleukocyte antigen related to membrane transport proteins. *J. Immunol.* **145**: 4322–4325.

Antin JH, Bierer BE, Smith BR *et al.* (1991) Selective depletion of bone marrow T lymphocytes with anti-CD5 monoclonal antibodies: effective prophylaxis for graft-versus-host-disease in patients with haematological malignancies. *Blood* **78**: 2139–2149.

Aotsuka N, Asai T, Oh H, Toshida S (1991) Lymphocyte subset reconstitution following human allogeneic bone marrow transplantation. *Rinsho Ketsueki* **32**: 844–850.

Aruffo A, Melnik MB, Linsley PS, Seed B (1991a) The lymphocyte glycoprotein CD6 contains a repeated domain structure characteristic of a new family of cell surface and secreted proteins. *J. Exp. Med.* **174**: 949–952.

Aruffo A, Kolanus W, Walz G, Fredman P, Seed B (1991b) CD62/P-selectin recognition of myeloid and tumor cell sulfatides. *Cell* **67**: 35–44.

Azorsa DO, Hyman JA, Hildreth JE (1991) CD63/Pltgp140: a platelet activation antigen identical to the stage specific, melanoma-associated antigen ME491. *Blood* **78**: 280–284.

Babcock DF (1983) Examination of the intracellular ionic environment and of ionophore action by null point measurements employing the fluorescein chromophore. *J. Biol. Chem.* **258**: 6380–6388.

Bakeeva LE, Grinius LL, Jasaitis AA (1970) Conversion of biomembrane-produced energy into electric form. Intact mitochondria. *Biochim. Biophys. Acta* **216**: 13–21.

Ball ED, Schwartz LM, Bloomfield CD (1991) Expression of CD15 antigen on normal and leukaemic myeloid cells: effect of neuraminidase and variable detection with a panel of monoclonal antibodies. *Mol. Immunol.* **28**: 951–958.

Bank HL (1987) Assessment of islet cell viability using fluorescent dyes. *Diabetologia* **30**: 812–820.

Barak LS, Yocum RR, Webb WW (1981) *In vivo* staining of cytoskeletal actin by autointernalization of nontoxic concentrations of nitrobenzoxaziadole-phallacidin. *J. Cell Biol.* **89**: 368–372.

Barber EK, Dev Dasgupta J, Schlossman SF, Trevillyan JM, Rudd CE (1989) The CD4 and CD8 antigens are coupled to a protein-tyrosine kinase (p56-lck) that phosphorylates the CD3 complex. *Proc. Natl. Acad. Sci. USA* **86**: 3277–3281.

Barker PE, Shipp MA, D'Aarmio L, Masteller EL, Reinhertz EL (1989) The common acute lymphoblastic leukaemia antigen gene maps to chromosomal region 3 (q21–27). *J. Immunol.* **142**: 283–287.

Bass DA, Parce JW, Dechatelet LR, Szejda P, Seeds MC, Thomas M (1983) Flow cytometric studies of oxidative product formation by neutrophils: a graded response to membrane stimulation. *J. Immunol.* **130**: 1910–1917.

Bernal SD, Shapiro HM, Chen LB (1982) Monitoring the effect of anti-cancer drugs on L1210 cells by a mitochondrial probe, rhodamine 123. *Int. J. Cancer* **30**: 219–224.

Betjes MG, Haks MC, Tuk CW, Beelen RH (1991) Monoclonal antibody EBM11 (anti-CD68) discriminates between dendritic cells and macrophages after short term culture. *Immunobiology* **183**: 79–87.

Blaise D, Olive D, Hirn M *et al.* (1991) Prevention of acute GVHD by *in vivo* use of anti-interleukin-2 receptor monoclonal antibody (33B3.1): a feasibility trial in 15 patients. *Bone Marrow Transplant.* **8**: 105–111.

British Standard BS EN 60825 (1992) Radiation safety of laser products equipment classification. Requirements and user's guide. BSI, Linford Wood, Milton Keynes.

Brunsting A, Mullaney PF (1974) Differential light scattering from mammalian cells. *Biophys. J.* **14**: 439–453.

Calabi F, Jarvis JH, Martin L, Milstein C (1989) Two classes of CD1 genes. *Eur. J. Immunol.* **19**: 285–292.

Camarini D, Walz G, Loenen WA, Borst J, Seed B (1991) The T cell activation antigen CD27 is a member of the nerve growth factor/tumor necrosis factor receptor gene family. *J. Immunol.* **147**: 3165–3169.

Cantu RA, Putti C, Saitta M *et al.* (1991) Co-expression of myeloid antigens in childhood acute lymphoblastic leukaemia: relationship with the stage of differentiation and clinical significance. *Br. J. Haematol.* **79**: 40–43.

Cassatella MA, Bazzoni F, Calzetti F, Guasparri T, Rossi F, Trinchieri G (1991) Interferon-gamma transcriptionally modulates the expression of the genes for the high affinity IgG-Fc receptor and the 47-kDa cytosolic component of NADPH oxidase in human polymorphonuclear leukocytes. *J. Biol. Chem.* **266**: 22079–22082.

Castranova V, Van Dyke K (1984) Analysis of oxidation of membrane potential probe Di-S-C3 (5) during granulocyte activation. *J. Microchem.* **29**: 151–159.

Clark EA, Lane PJ (1991) Regulation of human B-cell activation and adhesion. *Annu. Rev. Immunol.* **9**: 97–127.

Clevers H, Alarcon B, Wileman T, Terhorst C (1988) The T cell receptor/CD3 complex: a dynamic protein ensemble. *Annu. Rev. Immunol.* **6**: 629–662.

Cohen LB, Lesher S (1986) Optical monitoring of membrane potential: methods of multisite optical measurement. *Soc. Gen. Physiol. Ser.* **40**: 71–99.

Coleman AW, Maguire MJ, Coleman JR (1981) Mithramycin- and 4'-6-diamidino-2-phenylindole (DAPI)-DNA staining for fluorescence microspectrophometric measurement of DNA in nuclei, plasmids and virus particles. *J. Histochem. Cytochem.* **29**: 959–968.

Collado A, Canadas E, Ruiz CF, Gomez O, Pedrinaci S, Garrido F (1991) Characterisation of CD44 during lymphoid ontogeny. *Immunobiology* **183**: 1–11.

Cook JA, Iype SN, Mitcell JB (1991) Differential specificity of monochlorobimane for isozymes of human and rodent glutathione S-transferases. *Cancer Res.* **51**: 1606–1612.

Corbi AL, Larson RS, Kishimoto TK, Springer TA, Morton CC (1988) Chromosomal location of the genes encoding the leukocyte adhesion receptors LFA-1, Mac-1 and p150,95. *J. Exp. Med.* **167**: 1597–1607.

Cornelius CJ, Ploem JS (1976) A new type of two colour fluorescence staining for cytology specimens. *J. Histochem. Cytochem.* **24**: 72–81.

Corsetti JP, Weidner CH, Cianci J, Sparks CE (1991) The labeling of lipoproteins for studies of cellular binding with a fluorescent lipophilic dye. *Anal. Biochem.* **195**: 122–128.

Coulter WH (1956) High speed automatic blood cell counter and cell analyzer. *Proc. Natl. Elec. Conf.* **12**: 1034–1035.

Crissman HA, Steinkamp JA (1973) Rapid simultaneous measurement of DNA, and protein and cell volume from large mammalian cell populations. *J. Cell Biol.* **59**: 766–771.

Crissman HA, Steinkamp JA (1982) Rapid one step staining procedure for analysis of cellular DNA and protein by single and dual laser flow cytometry. *Cytometry* **3**: 84–89.

Crosland-Taylor PJ (1953) A device for counting small particles suspended in a fluid through a tube. *Nature* **171**: 37–38.

Dang NH, Torimoto Y, Shimamara K *et al.* (1991) IF7 (CD26): a marker of thymic maturation involved in the differential regulation of CD3 and CD2 pathways of human thymocyte activation. *J. Immunol.* **147**: 2825–2832.

Darzynkiewicz Z, Kapusciuski J (1988) Condensation of DNA *in situ* in metaphase chromosomes induced by intercalating ligands and its relationship to chromosome banding. *Cytometry* **9**: 7–18.

Darzynkiewicz Z, Taganos F, Melamed MR (1980) New cell compartments identified by multiparameter flow cytometry. *Cytometry* **1**: 98–103.

Davies TA, Drotts D, Weil GJ, Simons ER (1988) Flow cytometric measurement of cytoplasmic calcium changes in human platelets. *Cytometry* **9**: 138–142.

Delmas B, Gelfi J, L'Haridon R *et al.* (1992) Aminopeptidase N is a major receptor for enteropathogenic coronavirus TGEV. *Nature* **357**: 417–422.

De Rie MA, Schumacher TN, Van Lier RA, Meidema F (1989) Regulatory role of CD19 molecules in B cell activation and differentiation. *Cell Immunol.* **118**: 368–381.

Dolbeare FA, Phares WF (1979) Biochemical and flow cytometric assay of acid naphthol AS-BI phosphatase and beta-glucuronidase in Chinese hamster ovary cells. *J. Histochem. Cytochem.* **27**: 120–124.

Dolbeare FA, Smith RE (1977) Flow cytometric measurement of peptidase with use of 5-nitrosalicylaldehyde and 4-methoxy-naphthylamine derivatives. *J. Clin. Chem.* **23**: 1485–1491.

Dolbeare FA, Smith RE (1979) Flow cytoenzymology: Rapid enzyme analysis of single cells. In: Melamed MR, Mullaney PF, Mendelsohn ML, eds, *Flow Cytometry and Cell Sorting.* Wiley, New York, pp. 317–333.

Engert A, Martin G, Amlot P, Wijdenes J, Diehl V, Thorpe P (1991) Immunotoxin constructed with anti-CD25 monoclonal antibodies and deglycosylated ricin A-chain have potent anti-tumour effects against human Hodgkin cells *in vitro* and solid Hodgkin tumours in mice. *Int. J. Cancer* **49**: 450–456.

Fanger MW, Shen L, Graziano RF, Guyre PM (1989) Cytotoxicity mediated by human Fc receptors for IgG. *Immunol. Today* **10**: 92–99.

Favaloro EJ, Bradstock KF, Kabral A, Grimsley P, Zowtyj H, Zola H (1988) Further characterisation of human myeloid antigens (gp160,95; gp150; gp67): investigation of epitopic heterogeneity and non-haemopoietic distribution using panels of antibodies belonging to CD11b, CD13, CD33. *Br. J. Haematol.* **69**: 163–171.

Fay SP, Posner RG, Swann WN, Sklar LA (1991) Real time analysis of the assembly of ligand, receptor and G-protein by quantitative fluorescence flow cytometry. *Biochemistry* **30**: 5066–5075.

Fecheimer M, Zigmond SH (1983) Changes in cytoskeletal proteins of polymorphonuclear leukocytes induced by chemotactic peptides. *Cell Motility* **3**: 349–354.

Feldmann T, Gadd S, Majdic S *et al.* (1991) Analysis of function-associated receptor molecules on peripheral blood and synovial fluid granulocytes from patients with rheumatoid and reactive arthritis. *J. Clin. Immunol.* **11**: 205–212.

Fend F, Nachbaur D, Oberwasserlechner F, Kreczy A, Huber H, Muller HHK (1991)

Phenotype and topography of human thymic B cells. An immunohistologic study. *Virchows Arch. B. Cell. Pathol.* **60**: 381–388.

Fischer A (1991) Anti LFA-1 antibodies as immunosuppressive reagent in transplantation. *Chem. Immunol.* **50**: 89–95.

Fox DA, Millard JA, Kan L *et al.* (1990) Activation pathways of synovial T lymphocytes. Expression and function of the UM4D4/CDw60 antigen. *J. Clin. Invest.* **86**: 1124–1236.

Fox JE, Aggerbeck LP, Berndt MC (1988) Structure of 1b.IX complex from platelet membranes. *J. Biol. Chem.* **263**: 4882–4890.

Freedman AS, Nadler LM (1991) Immunological markers in non-Hodgkin's lymphomas. *Hematol. Oncol. Clin. North Am.* **5**: 871–889.

Freeman DA, Crissman HA (1975) Evaluation of six fluorescent protein stains for use in flow microfluorimetry. *Stain Technol.* **50**: 279–289.

Friend PJ, Waldmann H, Hale G *et al.* (1991) Reversal of allograft rejection using the monoclonal antibody, Cammpath-1G. *Transplant. Proc.* **23**: 2253–2254.

Fulwyler MJ (1965) Electronic separation of biological cells by volume. *Science* **36**: 131–132.

Gaudray P, Trotter J, Wahl GM (1986) Fluorescent methotrexate labelling and flow cytometric analysis of cells containing low levels of dihydrofolate reductase. *J. Biol. Chem.* **261**: 6285–6292.

Geisler CH, Larsen JK, Hansen NE *et al.* (1991) Prognostic importance of flow cytometric immunophenotyping of 540 consecutive patients with B-cell chronic leukaemia. *Blood* **78**: 1795–1802.

George EB (1988) Impermeant potential sensitive oxonol dyes: evidence for an On–Off mechanism. *J. Membrane Biol.* **103**: 245–252.

Gerson DF, Kiefer H (1983) Intracellular pH and the cell cycle of mitogen-stimulated murine lymphocytes. *J. Cell Physiol.* **114**: 132–136.

Gerson DF, Kiefer H, Eufe W (1982) Intracellular pH of mitogen stimulated lymphocytes. *Science* **216**: 1009–1010.

Gianotti R, Alessi E, Cavicchini S, Berti E (1991) Primary cutaneous pleomorphic lymphoma expressing CD30 antigen. *Am. J. Dermatopathol.* **13**: 503–508.

Goyert SM, Ferrero EM, Rettig WJ, Yenamandra AK, Obata F, Le Beau MM (1988) CD14 monocyte differentiation antigen maps to a region encoding growth factors and receptors. *Science* **239**: 497–500.

Greenman J, Tutt AL, George AJ, Pulford KA, Stevenson GT, Glennie MJ (1991) Characterisation of a new monoclonal anti-Fc gamma RII antibody, AT10, and its incorporation into a bi-specific F(ab')2 derivative of cytotoxic effectors. *Mol. Immunol.* **28**: 1243–1254.

Grinstein J, Goetz E, Grinstein S, Cohen J (1985) Control of free cytoplasmic calcium by intracellular pH in T lymphocytes. *Biochim. Biophys. Acta* **819**: 267–272.

Grinstein S, Cohen S (1987) Cytoplasmic Ca^{2+} and intracellular pH in lymphocytes. *J. Gen. Physiol.* **89**: 185–192.

Grynkiewics G, Poenie M, Tsien RY (1985) A new generation of Ca^{2+} indicators with greatly improved fluorescence properties. *J. Biol. Chem.* **260**: 3440–3450.

Guan EN, Burgess WH, Robinson SL, Goodman EB, McTigue KJ, Tenner AJ (1991) Phagocytic cell molecules that bind to the collagen like region of C1q. *J. Biol. Chem.* **266**: 20345–20455.

Guilbault GG, Kramer DN (1965) Fluorometric procedure for measuring the activity of dehydrogenases. *Anal. Chem.* **37**: 1219–1221.

Gupta RK (1981) Improvements in optical methods for measuring rapid changes in membrane potential. *J. Membr. Biol.* **58**: 123–130.

Hale G, Bright S, Chumbley G *et al.* (1983) Removal of T cells from bone marrow for transplantation; a monoclonal anti-lymphocyte antibody that fixes human complement. *Blood* **62**: 873–882.

Hasui M, Hirabayashi Y, Kobayashi Y (1989) Simultaneous measurement by flow cytometry of phagocytosis and hydrogen peroxide production of neutrophils in whole blood. *J. Immunol. Methods* **117**: 53–58.

Haynes BF, Metzzgar RS, Minna JD, Bunn PA (1981) Phenotypic characterisation of cutaneous T cell lymphoma. Use of monoclonal antibodies to compare with other malignant T cells. *N. Engl. J. Med.* **304**: 1319–1323.

Haynes BF, Hale LP, Patton KL, Martin ME, McCallum RM (1991) Measurement of an adhesion molecule as an indicator of inflammatory disease activity. Up regulation of the receptor for hyaluronate (CD44) in rheumatoid arthritis. *Arthritis Rheum.* **34**: 1434–1443.

Hebell T, Ahearn JM, Fearon DT (1991) Suppression of the immune response by a soluble complement receptor of B lymphocytes. *Science* **254**: 102–105.

Higashihara M, Maeda H, Shibata Y, Kume S, Ohashi T (1985) A monoclonal anti-human platelet antibody; a new platelet aggregating substance. *Blood* **65**: 382–391.

Hofmann B, Nishanian P, Fahey JL *et al.* (1991) Serum increases and lymphoid cell surface losses of IL-2 receptor CD25 in HIV infection: distinctive parameters of HIV-induced change. *Clin. Immunol. Immunopathol.* **61**: 212–224.

Hogg N (1991) Integrins and ICAM-1 in immune responses. *Chem. Immunol.* **50**: 89–95.

Hogg N (1992) Roll, roll, roll, your leukocyte gently down the vein. *Immunol. Today* **13**: 113–115.

Hogg N, Ross GD, Slusarenko M, Walport MJ, Lachmann P (1984) Identification of an anti-monocyte mononuclear antibody that is specific for membrane complement receptor type one (CR1). *Eur. J. Immunol.* **14**: 236–243.

Homan-Muller JW, Weening RS, Roos D (1975) Production of hydrogen peroxide by phagocytosing human granulocytes. *J. Lab. Clin. Med.* **85**: 198–207.

Hommel BGA, Shenoy AM, Brahmi Z (1991) Receptor modulation and early signal transduction events in cytotoxic T lymphocytes inactivated by sensitive target cells. *J. Immunol.* **147**: 3237–3243.

Horejsi V, Vlcek C (1991) Novel structurally distinct family of leukocyte surface glycoproteins including CD9, CD37, CD53 and CD63. *FEBS Lett.* **288**: 1–4.

Horne WC, Normann NE, Schwartz DB, Simons DF (1981) Changes in cytoplasmic pH and in membrane potential in thrombin stimulated human platelets. *Eur. J. Biochem.* **120**: 295–302.

Huizinga TW, van-Kemenade F, Koederman L *et al.* (1989) The 40kDa Fc gamma receptor (FcRII) on human neutrophils is essential for the IgG induced respiratory burst and IgG induced phagocytosis. *J. Immunol.* **142**: 2365–2369.

Hundt M, Zielinska SM, Schmidt RE (1991) Severe vasculitis in cryoglobulinemia-mechanisms of Fc gamma receptor activation of granulocytes. *Immunol. Infekts.* **19**: 87–88.

Illum N, Ralfiaekiaer E, Pallesen G, Geisler C (1991) Phenotypic and functional characterisation of double negative (CD4 CD8) alpha beta T cell receptor positive cells from an immunodeficient patient. *Scand. J. Immunol.* **34**: 635–645.

Jenkins MK, Taylor PS, Norton SD, Urdahl KB (1991) CD28 delivers a costimulatory signal involved in antigen-specific IL-2 production by human T cells. *J. Immunol.* **147**: 2461–2466.

Jenssen HL, Redman K, Mix E (1986) Flow cytometric estimation of transmembrane potential of macrophages — a comparison with microelectrode measurements. *Cytometry* **7**: 339–346.

Johnson LV, Walsh ML, Chen LB (1980) Localisation of mitochondria in living cells with rhodamine 123. *Proc. Natl. Acad. Sci. USA* **77**: 990–998.

Johnson LV, Walsh ML, Bockus BJ (1981) Monitoring the relative mitochondrial membrane potential of living cells by fluorescence microscopy. *J. Cell Biol.* **88**: 526–535.

Johnson SM (1991) The effect of interferon-alpha on the 5'-nucleotidase of human lymphoblastoid B cell lines depends on the class of immunoglobulin secreted. *Immunology* **74**: 44–49.

June CH, Ledbetter JA, Rabinovitch PS, Martin PI, Beatty PG, Hansen JA (1986) Distinct patterns of transmembrane calcium mobilization after differentiation antigen cluster 2 (E rosette receptor) or 3 (T3) stimulation of human lymphocytes. *J. Clin. Invest.* **77**: 1224–1232.

June CH, Rabinovitch PS, Ledbetter JA (1987) CD5 antibodies increase intracellular ionized calcium concentration in T cells. *J. Immunol.* **138**: 2782–2792.

Jung G, Freiman U, Von-Marschall Z, Reisfield RA, Wilmanns W (1991) Target cell induced T cell activation with bi- and tri-specific antibody fragments. *Eur. J. Immunol.* **21**: 2431–2435.

Kamentsky LA, Melamed MR, Derman H (1965) Spectrophotometer: new instrument for ultrarapid cell analysis. *Science* **150**: 630–631.

Kaufman RL, Bertino RT, Schimke RT (1978) Quantitation of dihydrofolate reductase in individual parental and methotrexate resistant murine cells. Use of a fluorescent activated cell sorter. *J. Biol. Chem.* **253**: 5852–5860.

Keifel V, Santosa S, Weisheit M, Mueller-Eckhardt C (1987) Monoclonal antibody-specific immobilization of platelet antigens (MAIPA): a new tool for the identification of platelet-reactive antibodies. *Blood* **70**: 1722–1726.

Keifel V, Santosa S, Kaufman E, Mueller-Eckhardt C (1991) Autoantibodies against platelet glycoprotein 1b/IX: a frequent finding in autoimmune thrombocytopenic purpura. *Br. J. Haematol.* **79**: 256–262.

Keith CH, Bajer AS, Ratan R, Maxfield FR, Shelanski ML (1986) Calcium and calmodulin in the regulation of the microtubular cytoskeleton. *Ann. N. Y. Acad. Sci.* **466**: 375–391.

Keston AS, Brandt R (1965) The fluorometric analysis of ultramicro quantities of hydrogen peroxide. *Anal. Biochem.* **11**: 1–5.

Kikutani H, Nakamura H, Sato R *et al.* (1991) Delineation and characterisation of human B-cell subpopulations at various stages of activation using a B-cell specific monoclonal antibody. *J. Immunol.* **136**: 4027–4034.

Koch N, Moldenhauer G, Hofmann WJ, Moller P (1991) Rapid intracellular pathway gives rise to cell surface expression of the MHC class II-associated invariant chain (CD74). *J. Immunol.* **147**: 2643–2651.

Kohler G, Milstein C (1975) Continuous cultures of fused cells secreting antibody of predefined specificity. *Nature* **256**: 495–497.

Kuijpers TW, Tool AT, van-der-Schoot CE *et al.* (1991) Membrane surface antigen expression on neutrophils: a reappraisal of the use of surface markers for neutrophil activation. *Blood* **78**: 1105–1101.

Lane TA, Chen TT (1991) Heterologous down-modulation of luteinizing receptors by prolactin: a flow cytometry study. *Endocrinology* **128**: 1833–1840.

Larson RS, Corbi AL, Berman L, Springer TA (1989) Primary structure of the leukocyte function-associated molecule-1 alpha subunit: an integrin with an embedded domain defining a protein superfamily. *J. Cell Biol.* **108**: 703–712.

Lazzari KG, Proto PJ, Simons ER (1986) Simultaneous measurement of stimulus induced changes in cytoplasmic calcium and in membrane potential of human neutrophils. *J. Biol. Chem.* **261**: 9710–9713.

Ledbetter JA, Parsons M, Martin PJ, Rabinovitch PS (1986) Antibody binding to CD5 (Tp67) and Tp44 T cell surface molecules: effects on cyclic nucleotides, cytoplasmic free calcium, and cAMP mediated suppression. *J. Immunol.* **137**: 3299–3305.

Le Deist F, de Saint Bastile G, Mazerolles F *et al.* (1991) Primary membrane T cell immunodeficiencies. *Clin. Immunol. Immunopathol.* **61**: 56–60.

Leeman U, Ruch M (1972) Cytofluorometric demonstration of basic and total proteins with sulfaflavins. *J. Histochem. Cytochem.* **20**: 659–665.

LePecq JB, Paoletti C (1967) A fluorescent complex between ethidium bromide and nucleic acids. Physical–chemical characterization. *J. Mol. Biol.* **27**: 87–106.

Letarte M, Vera S *et al.* (1988) Common acute lymphoblastic leukaemia antigen is identical to neural endopeptidase. *J. Exp. Med.* **168**: 1247–1253.

Liszewski MK, Post TW, Atkinson JP (1991) Membrane cofactor protein (MCP or CD46): newest member of the regulators of complement activation gene. *Annu. Rev. Immunol.* **9**: 431–455.

Loken MR, Shah VO, Hollander Z, Civin CI (1988) Flow cytometric analysis of normal B lymphoid development. *Pathol. Immunopathol. Res.* **7**: 357–370.

Look AT, Ashmun RA, Shapiro LH, Peiper SC (1989) Human myeloid plasma membrane glycoprotein CD13 (gp150) is identical to aminopeptidase. *J. Clin. Invest.* **83**: 1299–1307.

Luckoff A (1986) Measuring cytosolic free calcium concentration in endothelial cells with Indo-1: The pitfall of using the ratio of two fluorescence intensities recorded at different wavelengths. *Cell Calcium* **7**: 233–240.

Macher BA, Bucher J, Scudder P, Knapp W, Feizi T (1988) A novel carbohydrate antigen on fucogangliosides of human myeloid cells recognised by monoclonal antibody VIM-2. *J. Biol. Chem.* **263**: 10186–10191.

Maddy AH (1964) A fluorescent label for the outer components of the plasma membrane. *Biochim. Biophys. Acta* **88**: 390–406.

Maddy A, Lyons AB, Wu ZW, Taylor H, Sanderson A, Mackie M (1991) Discrete subpopulations defined by CD45 isoforms, coexist within leukaemic cells of B-chronic lymphocytic leukaemia patients. *Leuk. Res.* **15**: 791–799.

Mami CF, Del-Porto P, Delorme D, Hercend T (1991) Further evidence for a gamma/delta T cell receptor-mediated TCT.I/CD48 recognition. *J. Immunol.* **147**: 2864–2867.

Matolcsy A, Kalman E, Pajor L, Konya T, Weber E (1991) Morphologic and flow cytometric analysis of circulating megakaryoblasts in myeloid leukaemia. *Leuk. Res.* **15**: 887–897.

McAlinden TP, Hynes JB, Patil SA *et al.* (1991) Synthesis and biological evaluation of a fluorescent analogue of folic acid. *Biochemistry* **30**: 5674–5681.

McCarthy KF, Hale ML (1988) Flow cytometric techniques in radiation biology. *Toxicol. Lett.* **43**: 219–233.

McDonald JK, Callahan PX, Ellis S, Smith RE (1975) Polypeptide degradation by dipeptidyl amino peptidase I (Cathepsin C) and related peptidases. In: Barrett AJ, Dingle JT, eds, *Tissue Proteinases*. North-Holland Publishing, Amsterdam, pp. 69–99.

McGinnes K, Chapman G, Penny P (1988) Effects of interferon on natural killer (NK) cells assessed by fluorescent probes and flow cytometry. *J. Immunol. Methods* **107**: 129–136.

Mechtersheimer G, Staudter M, Moller P (1991) Expression of the natural killer cell-associated antigens CD56 and CD57 in human neural and striated muscle cells and in their tumors. *Cancer Res.* **51**: 1300–1307.

Melnick SL, Hannan P, Decher L *et al.* (1991) Increasing CD8$^+$ T lymphocytes predict subsequent development of intraoral lesions among individuals in the early stages of infection by the human immunodeficiency virus. *J. AIDS* **4**: 1199–1207.

Metzelaar MJ, Wijngaard PL, Peters PJ, Sixma JJ, Nieuwenhuis HK, Clevers HC (1991) CD63 antigen. A novel lysosomal membrane glycoprotein, cloned by a screening procedure for intracellular antigens in eukaryotic cells. *J. Biol. Chem.* **266**: 3239–3245.

Mielke B, Moller P (1991) Histomorphologic and immunophenotypic spectrum of primary gastro-intestinal B-cell lymphomas. *Int. J. Cancer* **47**: 334–343.

Mohr FC, Fewtrell C (1987) IgE receptor-mediated depolarization of rat basophilic leukaemia cells measured with the fluorescent probe Bis-oxonol. *J. Immunol.* **138**: 1564–1570.

Musgrove E, Rugg C, Hedley D (1986) Flow cytometric measurement of cytoplasmic pH: A critical evaluation of available fluorochromes. *Cytometry* **7**: 347–355.

Myanes BL, Dalzell JG, Hogg N, Ross GD (1988) Neutrophil and monocyte cell surface p150,95 has iC3b-receptor (CR4) activity resembling CR3. *J. Clin. Invest.* **82**: 640–651.

Myc A, DeAngelis P, Kimmel M, Melamed MR, Darzynkiewicz Z (1991) Retention of the mitochondrial probe rhodamine 123 in normal lymphocytes and leukaemic cells in relation to the cell cycle. *Exp. Cell Res.* **192**: 198–202.

Nishiwaki H, Miura M, Imai K (1974) Experimental studies on the antitumor effect of ethidium bromide and related substances. *Cancer Res.* **34**: 2966–2703.

Orntoft FT, Perterson SA, Wolf H (1988) Dual-parameter flow cytometry of transitional cell carcinomas. *Cancer* **61**: 963–970.

Otto F, Tsou KC (1985) A comparative study of DAPI, DIPI, and Hoechst 33258 and 33342 as chromosomal DNA stains. *Stain Technol.* **60**: 7–11.

Otto JM, Grenett HE, Fuller GM (1987) The coordinated regulation of fibrinogen gene transcription by hepatocyte stimulating factor and dexamethasone. *J. Cell Biol.* **105**: 1067–1072.

Papa S, Vitale M, Mariani AR, Roda P, Facchini A, Manzoli FA (1988) Natural killer function in flow cytometry, evaluation of NK cell lines. *J. Immunol. Methods* **107**: 73–78.

Pesando JM, Hoffman P, Abded MJ (1986) Antibody-induced antigenic modulation is antigen dependent: characterisation of 22 proteins on a malignant human B-cell line. *J. Immunol.* **137**: 3689–3695.

Plunkett ML, Sanders ME, Selvaraj P, Dustin ML, Springer TA (1987) Rosetting of activated human T lymphocytes with autologous erythrocytes: definition of receptor and ligand molecules as CD2 and lymphocyte function-associated 3 (LFA-3). *J. Exp. Med.* **165**: 664−766.

Poenie M, Alderton M, Tsein RY, Steinhardt RA (1985) Changes of free calcium levels with stages of cell division cycle. *Nature* **315**: 147−149.

Poot M (1990) Cell kinetic analysis using continuous BrdU labelling and bivariate hoechst 33358/ethidium bromide flow cytometry. In: Ormerod MG, ed., *Flow Cytometry. A Practical Approach.* IRL Press, Oxford, pp. 105−112.

Poot M, Kavanagh TJ, Kang HC, Haugland RP, Rabinovitch PS (1991) Flow cytometric analysis of cell cycle-dependent changes in cell thiol levels by combining a new laser dye with Hoechst 33342. *Cytometry* **12**: 184−187.

Postigo AA, Pulido R, Campanero MR *et al.* (1991) Differential expression of VLA-4 integrin by resident and peripheral blood B lymphocytes. Acquisition of functionally active alpha 4 beta 1-fibronectin receptor upon B cell activation. *Eur. J. Immunol.* **21**: 2437−2445.

Prince HE, Jensen ER (1991) Three-color cytofluorometric analysis of CD8 subsets in HIV-1 infection. *J. AIDS* **4**: 1227−1232.

Pulido R, Caampanero MR, Garcia Pardo A, Sanchez MF (1991) Structure−function analysis of the human integrin VLA-4 (alpha 4/beta 1). Correlation of proteolytic alpha 4 peptides with alpha 4 epitopes and sites of ligand interaction. *FEBS Lett.* **294**: 121−124.

Quinn JM, Athanasou NA, McGee JO (1991) Extracellular matrix receptor and platelet antigens on osteoclasts and foreign body giant cells. *Histochemistry* **96**: 169−176.

Rabinovitch PS, June CH, Grossmann A, Ledbetter JA (1986) Heterogeneity among T cells in intracellular free calcium responses after mitogenic stimulation with PHA or anti CD3. Simultaneous use of Indo-1 and immunofluorescence with flow cytometry. *J. Immunol.* **137**: 952−961.

Ransom JT, DiGusto DL (1987) Flow cytometric analysis of intracellular calcium mobilization. *Methods Enzymol.* **141**: 53−63.

Raziuddin S, Malatani T, al Sediary S, al Saigh AH (1991) Peripheral T-cell lymphomas. Immunophenotype, lymphokine production, and immunological functional characteristics of the lymph-node malignant T cells. *Am. J. Pathol.* **139**: 1181−1189.

Reinherz EL, Geha R, Rappeport JM *et al.* (1982) Reconstitution after transplantation with T-lymphocyte-depleted HLA haplotype-mismatched bone marrow for severe combined immunodeficiency. *Proc. Natl. Acad. Sci. USA* **79**: 6047−6051.

Richards ML, Katz DH (1991) Biology and chemistry of low affinity IgE receptor (Fc epsilon RII/CD23). *Crit. Rev. Immunol.* **11**: 65−86.

Riedy MC, Muirhead KA, Jensen CP, Stewart CC (1991) Use of photolabeling technique to identify nonviable cells in fixed homologous or heterologous cell populations. *Cytometry* **12**: 133−139.

Rijkers GT, Justement LB, Griffioen AW, Cambier JC (1990) Improved method for measuring intracellular Ca^{++} with Flou-3. *Cytometry* **11**: 923−927.

Rogers J, Hesketh TR, Smith GA, Metcalfe JC (1983) Intracellular pH of stimulated lymphocytes measured with a new fluorescent indicator. *J. Biol. Chem.* **258**: 5994−5997.

Roos E (1991) Adhesion molecules in lymphoma metastasis. *Cancer Metastasis Rev.* **10**: 33−48.

Rosenfeld SI, Ryan DH, Looney RJ, Anderson CL, Abraham GN, Leddy JP (1987) Human platelet Fc receptors: Quantitative expression correlates with functional responses. *J. Immunol.* **138**: 2869−2873.

Rosenthal KS, Shapiro (1983) Cell membrane potential changes following Epstein−Barr virus binding. *J. Cell Physiol.* **117**: 39−44.

Rosse WF, Hoffman S, Campbell M, Borowitz M, Moore JO, Parker CJ (1991) The erythrocytes in paroxysomal nocturnal haemoglobinuria of intermediate sensitivity to complement lysis. *Br. J. Haematol.* **79**: 99−107.

Rossilet A, Ruch F (1968) Cytofluorometric determination of lysine with dansylchloride. *J. Histochem. Cytochem.* **16**: 459−466.

Rothe G, Valet G (1988) Phagocytosis, intracellular pH, and cell volume in the multifactorial analysis of granulocytes by flow cytometry. *Cytometry* **9**: 316−324.

Rothman BL, Blue ML, Kelley KA, Wunderlich D, Mierz DV, Aune TM (1991) Human T cell activation by OKT3 is inhibited by a monoclonal antibody to CD44. *J. Immunol.* **147**: 2493−2499.

Roux M, Schraven B, Roux A, Gamm H, Mertelsmann R, Meuer S (1991) Natural inhibitors of T-cell activation in Hodgkin's disease. *Blood* **78**: 2365–2371.

Rudd CE, Barber EK, Burgess KE *et al.* (1991) Molecular analysis of the interaction of p56lkc with the CD4 and CD8 antigens. *Adv. Exp. Med. Biol.* **292**: 85–96.

Runeberg M, Raudaskoski M, Virtanen I (1986) Cytoskeletal elements in the hyphae of the homobasidiomycete with indirect immunofluorescence and NBD-phallacidin. *Eur. J. Cell Biol.* **41**: 25–30.

Savart F (1833) Mémoire sur la constitution des veines liquides lancées par des orifices circulaires en mince paroi. *Ann. Clin. Phys.* **53**: 337–386.

Savill J, Dransfield I, Hogg N, Haslett C (1990) Vitronectin receptor-mediated phago-cytosis of cells undergoing apoptosis. *Nature* **343**: 170–173.

Schanberg LE, Fleenor DE, Kurtzberg J, Haynes BF, Kaufman RE (1991) Isolation and characterisation of the genomic human CD7 gene: Structural similarity with murine Thy-1 gene. *Proc. Natl. Acad. Sci. USA* **88**: 603–607.

Schmidt C, Pan L, Diss T, Isaacson PG (1991a) Expression of B-cell antigens by Hodgkin's and Reed-Sternberg cells. *Am. J. Pathol.* **139**: 701–707.

Schmidt I, Uittenbogaart CH, Giorgi JV (1991b) A gentle fixation and permeabilization method for combined cell surface and intracellular staining with improved precision in DNA quantification. *Cytometry* **12**: 279–285.

Schmidt I, Krall WJ, Uittenbogaart, Braun J, Giorgi JV (1992) Dead cell discrimination with 7-amino-actinomycin D in combination with dual color immunofluorescence in single laser flow cytometry. *Cytometry* **13**: 204–208.

Schwarting R, Gerdes J, Durkop H, Falini B, Pileri S, Stein H (1989) BER-H2: a new anti-Ki-1 (CD30) monoclonal antibody directed at a formol-resistant epitope. *Blood* **74**: 1678–1698.

Schwartz AR, Dorken B, Monner DA, Moldenhauer G (1991) CD22 antigen: bio-synthesis, glycosylation and surface expression of a B lymphocyte protein involved in B cell activation and adhesion. *Int. Immunol.* **3**: 623–633.

Sengbusch CV, Couwenbergs C, Kuhner J, Muller U (1976) Fluorogenic substrate in single living cells. *Histochem. J.* **8**: 341–350.

Shattil SJ, Brugge JS (1991) Protein tyrosine phosphorylation and the adhesive function of platelets. *Curr. Opin. Cell Biol.* **3**: 869–879.

Shichishima T, Terasawa T, Hashimoto C, Ohto H, Uchida T, Maruyama Y (1991) Heterogeneous expression of decay accelerating factor and CD59/membrane attack complex inhibition factor on paroxysmal nocturnal haemoglobinuria (PNH) erythrocytes. *Br. J. Haematol.* **78**: 545–550.

Shimizu Y, Newman W, Tanaka Y, Shaw S. (1992) Lymphocyte interactions with endothelial cells. *Immunol. Today* **13**: 106–112.

Shipchandler MT (1987) 4-{Aminomethyl} fluorescein and its N-alkyl derivatives: useful reagents in immunodiagnostic techniques. *Anal. Biochem.* **162**: 89–101.

Simons ER, Schwartz DB, Norman NE (1982) Stimulus response coupling in human platelets: Thrombin-induced changes in pH. In: Nuccitelli R, Deamer DW, eds, *Intracellular pH; Its Measurement, Regulation and Utilization in Cellular Functions.* AR Liss, New York, pp. 463–483.

Simpson AWM, Rink TJ (1987) Elevation of pH is not an essential step in calcium mobilisation in Fura-2-loaded human platelets. *FEBS Lett.* **222**: 144–150.

Sims PJ, Waggoner AS, Wang CH (1974) Studies on the mechanism by which cyanine dyes measure membrane potential in red blood cells and phosphotidylcholine vesicles. *Biochemistry* **13**: 3315–3330.

Sklar LA, Finnan DA, Painter RG, Cochrane CG (1984) Ligand/receptor internalization; A kinetic flow cytometric analysis of the internalization of N-formly peptides by human neutrophils. *J. Biol. Chem.* **259**: 5661–5669.

Smith GM, Forbes MA, Cooper J *et al.* (1991) Prognostic indicators for the development of AIDS in HIV antibody positive haemophiliac patients: results of a three-year longitudinal study. *Clin. Lab. Haematol.* **13**: 115–125.

Smith RE, Frank RM (1975) The use of amino acid derivatives of 4-methoxy-naphthylamine for the assay and subcellular localization of tissue proteinases. In: Dingle JT, Dean RT, eds, *Lysosomes in Biology and Pathology*, Vol. 4. North-Holland Publishing, Amsterdam, pp. 193–249.

Sonnenberg A, Modderman PW, Hogerworst F (1988) Laminin receptor on platelets is the integrin VLA-6. *Nature* **336**: 487–489.

Stamenkovic I, Sgroi D, Aruffo A, Sy MS, Anderson T (1991) The B lymphocyte adhesion molecule CD22 interacts with leukocyte common antigen CD45RO on T cells and alpha 2-6 sialyltransferase, CD75, on B cells. *Cell* **66**: 1133–1144.

Stefanova T, Horejsi V, Ansotegui IJ, Knapp W, Stockinger H (1991) GPI-anchored cell surface molecules complexed to protein tyrosine kinases. *Science* **254**: 1016–1019.

Stein H, Hansmann M, Lennert K (1986) Reed-Steinberg and Hodgkin cells in lymphocyte predominant Hodgkin's disease of nodular subtype contain J chain. *Am. J. Clin. Pathol.* **86**: 292–297.

Stohr M, Vogt-Schaden M, Knobloch M, Vogel G, Futterman G (1978) Evaluation of eight fluorochrome combinations for simultaneous DNA-protein flow analysis. *Stain Technol.* **53**: 205–215.

Stokke T, Holte H, Erikstein H, Davies CL, Funnderud S, Steen HB (1991) Simultaneous assessment of chromatin structure, DNA content and antigen expression by dual wavelength excitation flow cytometry. *Cytometry* **12**: 172–178.

Sutherland DR, Watt SM, Dowden G *et al.* (1988) Structural and partial amino-acid sequence analysis of the human hemopoietic progenitor cell antigen CD34. *Leukemia* **2**: 793–803.

Sweet RG (1965) High frequency recording with electrostatically deflected ink-jets. *Rev. Sci. Instrum.* **36**: 131–132.

Sy MS, Guo YJ, Stamenkovic I (1991) Distinct effects of two CD44 isoforms on tumour growth *in vivo*. *J. Exp. Med.* **174**: 859–866.

Szejda P, Pearce JW, Seeds MS, Bass DA (1984) Flow cytometric quantitation of oxidative product formation by polymorphonuclear leukocytes during phagocytosis. *J. Immunol.* **133**: 3303–3307.

Tapiero H, Munck JN, Fourcade A, Lampidis TJ (1984) Cross resistance to rhodamine 123 in adriamycin and daunorubicin resistant Friend leukaemia cell variants. *Cancer Res.* **44**: 5544–5549.

Tatham PER, Delves PJ (1984) Flow cytometric detection of membrane potential changes in murine lymphocytes induced by concanavalin A. *Biochem. J.* **221**: 137–146.

Thomson W (1967) On a self-acting apparatus for multiplying and maintaining electric charges, with applications to illustrate the voltaic theory. *Proc. Roy. Soc. London* **16**: 67–72.

Torimoto Y, Dang NH, Vivier E, Tanaka T, Schlossman SF, Morimoto C (1991) Coassociation of CD26 (dipeptidyl peptidase IV) with CD45 on the surface of human T lymphocytes. *J. Immunol.* **147**: 2514–2517.

Trowbridge IS, Ostergaard HL, Johnson P (1991) CD45: a leukocyte-specific member of the protein tyrosine phosphatase family. *Biochim. Biophys. Acta* **1095**: 46–56.

Tsein RY, Rink TL, Poenie M (1985) Measurement of cytosolic Ca^{2+} in individual small cells using fluorescence microscopy with dual excitation wavelengths. *Cell Calcium* **6**: 145–150.

Valentine MA, Clark EA, Shu GL, Norris NA, Ledbetter JA (1988) Antibody to a novel 95-KDa surface glycoprotein on human B-cells induces calcium mobilisation and B-cell activation. *J. Immunol.* **140**: 4071–4078.

Valet G, Raffael A, Moroder L (1981) Fast intracellular pH determination in single cells by flow cytometry. *Naturwissenschaften* **68**: 265–272.

Van Dilla MA, Fulwyler MJ, Boone IV (1967) Volume distribution and separation of normal human leukocytes. *Proc. Soc. Exp. Biol. Med.* **125**: 367–370.

Verhoef V, Ashmun R, Fridland A (1986) Rhodamine 123 and flow cytometry to monitor the cytotoxic actions of nucleoside analogs in non-dividing human lymphocytes. *Anticancer Res.* **6**: 1117–1123.

Veys PA, Macey MG, Gutteridge CN, Ord J, Newland AC (1989) Detection of granulocyte antibodies using flow cytometric analysis of leukocyte immunofluorescence. *Vox Sang.* 42–47.

Viellette A, Bookman MA, Horak EM, Samelson LE, Bolen JB (1989) Signal transduction through the CD4 receptor involves activation of the internal membrane tyrosine-protein kinase p56. *Nature* **338**: 257–259.

Vincente VV, Kostel PJ, Ruggeri ZM (1988) Isolation and functional characterisation of von Willebrand factor-binding domain located between residues His[1]-Arg[293] of the alpha-chain of glycoprotein 1b. *J. Biol. Chem.* **263**: 18473–18479.

Vindelov LL, Christensen IJ, Jensen G, Nissen NI (1983) Limits of detection of nuclear DNA abnormalities by flow cytometric DNA analysis. Results obtained by a set of methods for sample storage, staining and internal standardisation. *Cytometry* **3**: 337–339.

Waggoner AS (1979) Dye indicators of membrane potential. *Annu. Rev. Biophys. Bioeng.* **8**: 47–53.

Wall DM, Hu XF, Zalcberg JR, Parkin JD (1991) Rapid functional assay for multidrug resistance in human tumour cell lines using the fluorescent indicator fluo-3. *J. Natl. Cancer Inst.* **83**: 206–207.

Ware RE, Scearce RM, Dietz MA, Starmer CF, Palker TJ, Haynes BF (1989) Characterisation of the surface topography and putative tertiary structure of the human CD7 molecule. *J. Immunol.* **143**: 3632–3640.

Weiner GJ, Hillstrom JR (1991) Bispecific anti-idiotype/anti CD3 antibody therapy of murine B cell lymphoma. *J. Immunol.* **147**: 4035–4044.

Weisdorf DJ, Haake R, Miller WJ *et al.* (1991) Autologous bone marrow transplantation for progressive non-Hodgkin's lymphoma: clinical impact of immunophenotyping and *in vitro* purging. *Bone Marrow Transplant.* **8**: 135–142.

Weiss L, Okada H, Haeffner-Cavaillon N *et al.* (1992) Decreased expression of the membrane inhibitor of complement-mediated cytolysis CD59 on T-lymphocytes of HIV-infected patients. *AIDS* **6**: 379–385.

Whitaker JE, Haugland FG, Prendergast FG (1988) Seminaphtho-fluoresceins and rhodafluors: dual fluorescence pH indicators. *Biophys. J.* **53**: 197a (Abstr. M-Pos369).

Wilder ME, Cram LS (1977) Differential fluorochromasis of human lymphocytes as measured by flow cytometry. *J. Histochem. Cytochem.* **25**: 288–291.

Wiley JS, Brocklebank AM, Snook MB *et al.* (1991) A new fluorescent probe for the equilibrative inhibitor sensitive nucleoside transporter. 5'-S-(2-aminoethyl)-N6-(4-nitrobenzyl)-5'-thioadenosine (SAENTA)-chi-2-fluorescein. *Biochem. J.* **273**: 667–672.

Williams DA, Fogarty KE, Tsien RY, Fay FF (1985) Calcium gradients in single smooth muscle cells revealed by digital imaging microscope using Fura-2. *Nature* **318**: 558–561.

Williams DA, Rois M, Stephens C, Patel VP (1991) Fibronectin and VLA-4 in haematopoietic stem cell–microenvironment interactions. *Nature* **352**: 438–441.

Wilson HA, Chused TM (1985) Lymphocyte membrane potential and Ca^{2+} sensitive potassium channels described by oxonol dye fluorescence measurements. *J. Cell Physiol.* **125**: 72–81.

Wright SD, Ramos RA, Tobias PS, Ulevitch RJ, Mathison JC (1990) CD14, a receptor for complexes of lipopolysaccharide (LPS) and LPS binding protein. *Science* **249**: 1431–1440.

Wyatt RM, Dawson JR (1991) Characterisation of a subset of human B lymphocytes interacting with natural killer cells. *J. Immunol.* **147**: 3381–3388.

Yumura YK, Hara J, Kurahashi H *et al.* (1991) Clinical significance of CD7 positive stem cell leukaemia. A distinct subtype of mixed lineage leukaemia. *Cancer* **68**: 2273–2280.

Zelenin AV, Poletaev AI, Stepanova NG *et al.* (1984) α-amino-actinomycin D as a specific fluorophore for DNA content analysis by laser flow cytometry. *Cytometry* **5**: 348–354.

Zimmerman AG, Prescott SM, McIntyre TM (1992) Endothelial cell interactions: tethering and signaling molecules. *Immunol. Today* **13**: 93–100.

Chapter 2
Quality Control in Clinical Flow Cytometry

M. W. LOWDELL AND J. LAWRY

Introduction

The need for internal and external quality control (QC) in clinical laboratories has been recognized for many years. Every laboratory, regardless of its discipline, employs a variety of internal QCs and is exhorted to participate in external schemes as part of an overall quality assurance programme. In this chapter a variety of systems are presented that can be used for internal QC and an outline of the external QC schemes that are currently available is given.

Whether the cytometer is used for routine clinical support or front-line scientific research, it is essential that all operators can be confident of the validity of the results obtained. For research purposes it is generally sufficient that an instrument is stable and that results obtained on different occasions are comparable. In the case of clinical results used for patient diagnosis or management there is the additional requirement that a result obtained in one laboratory should be comparable with the result of the same investigation performed elsewhere. This difference between research and routine clinical laboratories may seem obvious but it serves to illustrate the point that the quality assurance programme adopted by individual laboratories must be appropriate for the laboratory concerned. It is necessary to select the particular controls which best regulate the tasks performed with a given cytometer.

Every laboratory should develop a quality assurance programme to encompass internal and external QC of instruments, reagents and operators. Standard operating procedures for each technique performed in the laboratory should be drawn up. Adherence to these methods must be confirmed regularly by the laboratory manager to ensure that all members of staff are working to the agreed methods. There have been few publications on QC/quality assurance in flow cytometry but Giorgi *et al*. (1990) and Parker *et al*. (1990) are recommended reading. Finally, the quality assurance programme should confirm a commitment to continued training. Like all QC measures, this seems obvious, but the inclusion of a commitment to further training in a quality assurance programme may be used as a means to plan funding for study leave in the departmental budget.

Internal QC

An internal QC programme should be designed to address instrument stability, instrument sensitivity, reproducibility of technique and inter-operator variability (when the cytometer has multiple users). Assessment of stability and sensitivity can be considered as general requirements irrespective of the use of the cytometer. QC of techniques and operator competence is application dependent. Some measures will be described that are appropriate to immunophenotyping and the analysis of DNA which are considered to be the most common applications of cytometers at the moment; there are many more, including cell sorting. It is hoped that the examples given will stimulate derivation of QC measures for applications not covered here.

Instrument stability

All manufacturers of flow cytometers provide a variety of beads for checking optical alignment, calibration and compensation settings and linearity of signal. Beads conjugated with a greater range of fluorochromes and of different sizes may be purchased from specialist suppliers such as Flow Cytometry Standards Corporation (FCSC) (marketed in the UK by Becton Dickinson) or PolySciences.

Beads for checking optical alignment

The size of bead used for this task should approximate the maximum width of the focused laser beam. This ensures that even a slight drift out of the centre of the beam will lead to a reduction in the degree of illumination of the bead and a subsequent reduction in excitation of the fluorochrome. This will be apparent as a reduction in emitted fluorescent signal and will broaden the coefficient of variation (CV) of the fluorescence histogram. Small beads are less sensitive indicators of misalignment (see Fig. 2.1). This will be true for any fluorochrome studied but it is usually sufficient to perform the task with only one fluorochrome. Analysis should be limited to single bead suspensions so it may be necessary to exclude clumped beads and/or debris by electronic gating on forward light scatter (FALS or FSC) and 90° light scatter (90° LS or SSC). At least 5000 events should be acquired in the gate and the

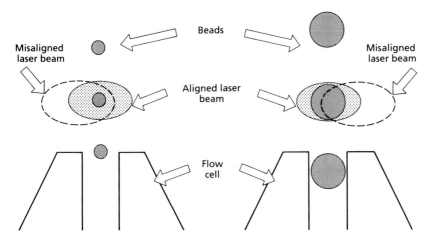

Fig. 2.1 Choice of optimum bead size for laser alignment. Misalignment of the laser will lead to a partial illumination of the large beads, while small beads will be fully illuminated.

peak, mean or median channel fluorescence and CV recorded. Whether the data are provided as peak, mean or median channel will depend upon the flow cytometer and software available. Becton Dickinson cytometers, for example, will provide mean, median and mode data in the more recent software programs but only mean and mode data in older packages. Mean or median data may be used, but it is necessary to ensure that the same parameter is recorded each time. The mean/median channel fluorescence and the CV should fall within 2 s.d. of their calculated mean. If one or both parameters are outside the range the laser will require realignment; this procedure will be described in the instrument manual.

The question of what the mean and s.d. of beads should be must be addressed. If it is possible to adjust the alignment of the laser on the cytometer this should be done so as to achieve the best mean channel fluorescence with the smallest CV. If the cytometer has a fixed flow cell and laser as in the case of Becton Dickinson machines, the alignment is checked using proprietary 'Calibrite' beads and 'Autocomp' software. If beads supplied by another manufacturer are used, the alignment is confirmed with the proprietary beads and then the following procedures are undertaken. Five to 10 identical samples of beads are run through the cytometer; the results are then recorded. This is performed each day for 5 consecutive days and the data are used to calculate the mean 'mean channel' and mean 'CV' and the s.d. for these distributions. Fortunately, this should need to be done only once, since whenever a new batch of beads is introduced it can be compared with the previous set of results. If the instrument is producing acceptable CVs with the current beads but failing with a new batch then the new beads are at fault and should be returned. If the only available replacement beads are of the inferior quality then it will be necessary to repeat the standardization procedure described above.

The next question to consider is, what to do if the cytometer fails the alignment test. The answer depends upon a number of variables. First, fluidics should be cleaned as detailed in the manufacturer's instructions. Routine use of the instrument will lead to the build-up of protein deposits in the fluid lines and flow cell, which should be cleaned regularly. If this deposit becomes severe it will lead to a total blockage but long before then it will cause erratic fluctuations in sheath fluid pressure. This will affect the hydrodynamic focusing and although the laser may be aligned with the nominal centre of the sheath fluid, the centre of the sheath will be moving erratically with respect to the laser beam. Cleaning of the instrument fluid system will cure this problem. An example of the effect of a dirty flow cell is demonstrated in Fig. 2.2. Figure 2.3 shows the same beads after the instrument has been cleaned.

If the problem persists and if the laser can be realigned, do so. Becton Dickinson FACScan or FACStrak cytometer lasers cannot be realigned but the stability of these instruments means that laser non-alignment is very unlikely.

The beads used for alignment may deteriorate upon refrigeration. If any different beads which are used for other control purposes such as linearity checking are available these may be run to confirm the alignment. If no other beads are available then fixed stained cells may be used to check the compensation (see below). If neither of these are available it will necessary to assume that the beads are satisfactory.

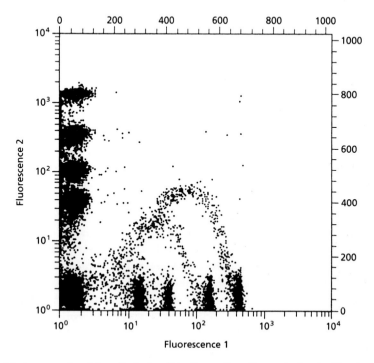

Fig. 2.2 An example of the effect of a dirty flow cell on the analysis of calibration beads.

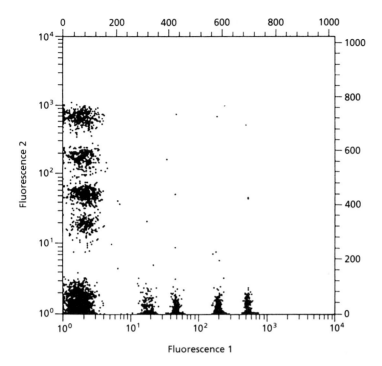

Fig. 2.3 The same analysis of calibration beads after the instrument has been cleaned.

If cleaning and realignment has failed or is not possible and the beads are confirmed as satisfactory then a visit from the cytometer engineer is required.

Beads for colour compensation setting

Those interested in using more than one fluorochrome simultaneously will need to come to terms with the concept of spectral overlap. This is the phenomenon where two fluorochromes excited at the same wavelength have emission spectra which are not mutually exclusive. The common example is fluorescein isothiocyanate (FITC) and phycoerythrin (PE) (reviewed in Shapiro, 1988). The amount of spectral overlap is corrected in all cytometers by an electronic compensation network. This is called fluorescence subtraction in some older Coulter instrument software. Many flow cytometers have software to calculate the compensation on the basis of red and green bead populations. When using mixtures of unlabelled and fluorescent beads for compensation setting it is advisable that these only approximate the biological system and small adjustments may be required when dual- or triple-stained cell populations are analysed. Indeed, many cytometrists use normal peripheral blood lymphocytes labelled with mutually exclusive antigen/antibody complexes as a biological control for compensation setting; for example, CD4 and CD8 have been used as appropriate cell populations for such a control. However, the ability of some normal CD4 cells to co-express CD8 may add a degree of confusion. The use of T-cell antibodies such as CD4 or CD8 with CD19 or CD20, that label only B-cells will provide a biological reagent which consists of distinct green, red and unlabelled subpopulations. It is often inconvenient to obtain normal peripheral blood so many cytometrists prepare a stained sample of peripheral blood lymphocytes and fix the cells as detailed below:

Preparation of fixed cells for QC

1 Peripheral blood mononuclear cells are separated on Ficoll-Paque or equivalent.
2 The cells are resuspended in phosphate-buffered saline (PBS; pH 7.2) 0.02% sodium azide to a concentration of 10^6/ml.
3 Cells (1 ml) are incubated with the manufacturer's recommended amount of FITC- and PE-conjugated monoclonal antibodies to T- and B-cell determinants (CD4 or CD8 and CD19 or CD20) for 10–15 min at room temperature in the dark.
4 The cells are washed twice with 1 ml PBS/azide and resuspended in 5 ml ice-cold 2% paraformaldehyde in PBS/azide.
5 After overnight incubation at 4°C these cells are ready for use and should be stable for up to 3 months refrigerated.

Unfortunately, lysed whole blood preparations are not as stable after fixation as separated peripheral blood lymphocytes. Within 3 or 4 days at 4°C a high degree of autofluorescence develops, which makes the preparations unsuitable for analysis.

Beads for measurement of absolute cell number by internal standard

The majority of cytometers, with a few notable exceptions, are unable to calculate the absolute number of cells, although, in clinical use, particularly in the monitoring of HIV infection, this is a measurement of prime importance. Cell counts can be determined by using the leucocyte count and differential from a separate haematology analyser. But external QC exercises have shown that this expedient is generally rather unsatisfactory.

'Bead loading' has been used as a simple approach to the problem, since many cytometers lack the ability to include 'time' as a parameter and the flow rate of most cytometers is highly variable. The principle is to add a known number of microbeads to a known volume of a sample of cells in suspension. When the mixed suspension is analysed by the flow cytometer the relative proportion of cells : beads can be determined. Given that the absolute number of beads added to the cell suspension is known, the absolute number of cells can be readily calculated.

The technique depends upon certain assumptions: First, the beads and cells must have comparable but different light scatter characteristics to ensure that they can be analysed with the same gain settings as the cells of interest. Second, the bead concentration in suspension must be

51

CHAPTER 2

Quality Control

stable over time. Third, changes in the number of beads added to a given population of cells must give rise to proportional changes in the estimate of cell numbers.

Diluted beads are unstable and should be made fresh before use. Estimates of absolute lymphocyte count obtained by 'bead loading' and

Procedure

1 Latex microbead particles are employed, 5.8 µm particles (100 µl) (Polysciences) diluted 1:10 in PBS are used and added to a lysed whole blood sample (500 µl).

2 Ten thousand events are collected with an analysis gate, drawn to exclude all red cell ghosts and other debris.

3 The proportion of beads and of lymphocytes is recorded for each sample. The results are used to calculate the absolute lymphocyte count as follows: Suppose,

the bead (B) concentration $= X$ particles/ml

the lymphocyte (L) concentration $= Y$ particles/ml

then in an assay containing 100 µl beads + 500 µl lysed whole blood the total concentration of $B + L$ particles is:

$100X + 500Y$ particles suspended in 600 µl.

The proportion of beads to beads plus lymphocytes in the mixture, which is measured by the flow cytometer is:

$$\frac{B}{B + L} = \frac{100X}{100X + 500Y}$$

and thus Y, the absolute count is given by

$$Y = \frac{100\,L}{500\,BX}$$

where X, the bead concentration is known. Here 100 in the expressions represents the volume of beads (V) added to the mixture. So, when V changes:

$$Y = V\,\frac{L}{500\,BX}$$

X, the bead concentration is in fact unknown; but since it is unchanging, the following expression may be used:

$$Y = V\,\frac{L}{500\,B}$$

FACScan analysis give good correlation ($r = 0.942$; $P = 0.00015$) when compared with those provided directly by a Technicon H-2 (Fig. 2.3).

Bead suspensions of known concentration will soon be available commercially from the major cytometer manufacturers.

Instrument sensitivity

The degree of sensitivity which is required from the instrument will be determined by the applications for which it is used. For example, in the study of DNA analysis a small beam width and a high degree of sensitivity on the forward scatter detector to discriminate between doublets (two nuclei passing the detector simultaneously) and true multiploid cells will be required. The detection of cell surface or cyto-plasmic antigens will have different requirements. Cytometers can oper-ate over a very broad range of cell sizes and densities. The fluorescence detectors (photomultiplier tubes (PMTs)) can be adjusted to detect weak or strongly expressed antigens. For routine immunophenotyping only a fraction of the range of the instrument may be used on a daily basis. However, it is important to be aware of the limitations of the machine at each end of its operational range.

In terms of fluorescent signals it is important to know the linear range of the laser and the minimum level of detection of the PMTs at different voltage (or gain) settings. This is easily achieved using calibrated beads and an example using Quantum 1000 beads from Flow Cytometry Standards Corporation is shown in Fig. 2.4.

The Quantum 1000 kit used in this example contains nine bead populations in separate dropper bottles. Four contain beads labelled with differing quantities of FITC. The number of molecules of the fluorochrome per bead is expressed in terms of 'molecules equivalent standard fluorochrome' (MESF) and the value is given on the individual bottle labels. A further four contain beads labelled with PE. The final

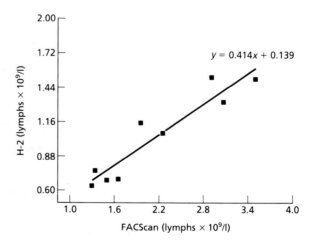

Fig. 2.4 Graph of the correlation between absolute counts determined by FACScan analysis and Technicon H-2 differential counts.

bottle contains blank beads. After shaking the bottles to reduce clumping of beads, half a drop from each bottle is added to a tube containing 2 ml of sheath fluid. The cytometer is set up as for the study of human lymphocytes with the FSC and SSC in linear mode and the two fluorescence detectors in logarithmic mode. The beads should appear on the FSC/SSC display with a low FSC and high SSC signal. Clumped beads will have a slightly higher FSC and SSC signal and should be excluded by electronic gating. Ten thousand events are acquired and the median, mean or peak channel value for each bead population is recorded. The figure recorded will be dependent upon the cytometer and software used but it is best to use the peak channel value from a Coulter cytometer and the median channel figure from a Becton Dickinson cytometer when available. On older Becton Dickinson machines only the peak channel and mean channel values may be available, in which case it is best to use the mean channel. Having recorded the values, a record of the gain or voltage settings of the two PMTs should be made. Both PMT settings should be reduced by 10% and the appropriate fluorescence value recorded. The compensation settings may have to be adjusted to achieve this. This exercise is repeated until only three bead populations can be visualized on each of the two fluorescent channels. The PMT voltages are then returned to the starting values and the exercise repeated but with voltages increased by 10% each time.

Graphs of the FITC and PE data with the MESF values on the x-axes and the channel values on the y-axes should be constructed. Lines are drawn through the points relating to a single PMT setting. As the PMT voltage decreases, the line moves towards the lower margin but the slope of the lines should remain the same. Eventually the bead population with the lowest MESF level is undetectable (Figs 2.5 and 2.6). The slope

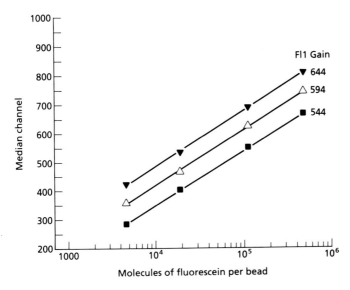

Fig. 2.5 Graph of the PMT gain related FITC data with MESF values on the x-axis and the fluorescence channel values on the y-axis.

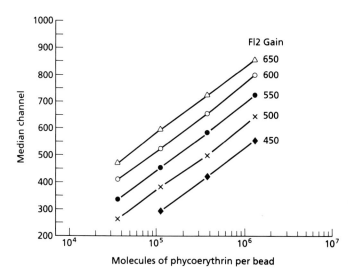

Fig. 2.6 Graph of the PMT gain related PE data with MESF values on the *x*-axis and the fluorescence channel values on the *y*-axis.

of the line may change when the PMT setting falls below a certain level. At this stage analysis is outside the linear range of the amplifier. The voltage setting producing the first parallel line is at the lowest level at which samples can be studied. This should be recorded.

If a computerized graphics program is available it may be able to calculate the formula of the lines. By entering the value of the blank bead for each PMT setting it is possible to calculate the minimum detection limit (sensitivity) of the cytometer for each fluorochrome at each PMT setting. The same result can be achieved with a ruler and pencil if graphs are drawn by hand by checking the MESF value where the blank bead channel value intercepts the line. The sensitivity of PE detection is greater than that of FITC. This is why most monoclonal antibody manufacturers conjugate antibodies with antigens which have low cell surface expression, with PE.

The Quantum 1000 beads can also be used to standardize the cytometer against other machines by calculating the 'relative channel number' (RCN) associated with a particular standardized bead. The RCN relates the instrument settings used and the resulting median or peak channel number so that any two channel numbers can be directly related to one another. The equation is provided by FCSC and is dependent upon whether you acquire fluorescence data with a linear or logarithmic amplifier. For a linear amplifier the equation is given by:

$$RCN = \frac{(p) \times (g) \times 10^{nd}}{G}$$

and for a logarithmic amplifier:

$$RCN = \frac{(p) \times 10^{nd}}{G}$$

where (p) = peak or median channel fluorescence, (g) = maximum instrument settings, nd = power of the neutral density filter, G = actual gain settings.

Once the RCN of each calibrated bead has been calculated, a calibration curve can be constructed and subsequent data can be converted to MESF rapidly and reproducibly. Conversion of flow cytometry results to MESF allows comparison of data from different machines.

Internal quality assurance in immunophenotyping

Reproducibility of technique

Determining the sensitivity of the cytometer is not something that requires a regular weekly exercise, whereas confirming the reproducibility of operator technique is. This is easily achieved by selecting a couple of routine samples each week and removing a small quantity of blood (for analysing cell subsets) into two fresh tubes labelled 'A' and 'B'. Members of staff may then process them blindly. The laboratory manager can compare the 'blind' results with those obtained from the original two samples. What is an acceptable deviation may be determined by carrying out the same exercise on 20 or so matched pairs.

Operator competence

General operator competence is checked by the blind internal QC detailed above but it is important to ensure that adequate care has been taken with every specimen. It is impossible to cover all eventualities but careful design of the monoclonal antibody panels used is a simple internal control which is used widely. For example, an appropriate monoclonal antibody panel used for monitoring human immunodeficiency virus (HIV) patients might be as follows: (a) tube 1 — CD3 FITC, CD19 PE; (b) tube 2 — CD3 FITC, CD4 PE; and (c) tube 3 — CD8 FITC, CD16 PE.

1 Tube 1 will identify T and B cells.
2 The unlabelled cells will be natural killer cells.
3 The total $CD3^+$ T cells from tube 2 should equal that in tube 1.
4 The $CD8^+/16^-$ cells in tube 3 will be $CD3^+$ and this should equal the $CD3^+/4^-$ cells from tube 2.
5 The total $CD16^+$ from tube 3 should equal the $CD3^-/19^-$ from tube 1.

This simple exercise ensures that adequate mixing of cells and antibodies has been done and that all cell types are adequately labelled. This internal QC method is not so readily applicable when studying leukaemic cells but similar panels can be developed.

External QC

External QC schemes in immunology and clinical chemistry have operated since the 1970s and have addressed detection and semi-quantitation of many auto-antibodies as well as the measurement of most serum proteins. The need for such schemes was driven by the increasing clinical importance placed upon these measurements. With the recent advent of flow cytometers designed for routine clinical use and the need for highly accurate enumeration of specific lymphocyte subsets in the diagnosis and management of HIV positive subjects, the requirement for external QC of immunophenotyping has become apparent. Indeed, the organizers of the recent Medical Research Council/Inserm Concorde trial of Zidovudine foresaw this need and established a QC programme for those laboratories responsible for monitoring patients enrolled in the trial. This trial ended in the summer of 1991 but the national QC programme which had been established has continued as a preliminary National External Quality Assurance Scheme (NEQAS) for immuno-phenotyping and is organized by the Department of Haematology at the Northern General Hospital, Sheffield. A second scheme for leukaemia phenotyping has also been established. Both are traditional QC schemes in which a single specimen is despatched by the organizers to each participant who then analyses it and returns the results.

Since 1990, two external QC schemes have been co-ordinated from the Department of Immunology at The Royal London Hospital, White-chapel. The original scheme was aimed at laboratories involved in monitoring HIV patients. After a successful first year a second scheme for leukaemia phenotyping was also established. Both programmes approach external QC in the same, novel manner. A consistent problem in any traditional external QC programme is the provision of sufficient material for circulation. This is particularly apparent in immunopheno-typing because of the relatively large quantities of blood required. This has led to the use of normal blood samples in the past and has restricted the frequency of distributions. Both schemes co-ordinated from the Royal London Hospital rely upon each participant despatching aliquots of a single clinical sample by post to a number of fellow participants at a predetermined time each month. Each sample is analysed by at least four laboratories and each laboratory analyses at least four samples each month. This provides a wealth of different clinical material to each participant. The results are analysed by the co-ordinators and deviations from the mean results are reported to the participants.

There has been a single distribution of samples for immunopheno-typing on a European basis (Martini *et al.*, 1989). The results of this study were encouraging but it is noteworthy that the greatest number of outlier results were found in the group of cytometrists involved in 'basic research' rather than in 'clinical' work. This implies that experience in immunophenotyping is an important parameter since the participants who were most familiar with clinical samples were more consistent. This highlights the need for training in flow cytometry and immuno-phenotyping.

QC in DNA analysis

Flow cytometry has a wide acceptance not only in the area of cell phenotyping by monoclonal antibody analysis, but also in the measurement of DNA ploidy and cell cycle. To date, very few QC studies have emerged to address the latter. DNA flow cytometry has been proven to be of value in the detection and classification of neoplasms, and in the prediction of survival for a wide range of tumours including breast (Visscher *et al.*, 1990), colon (Jones *et al.*, 1988), prostate (Visakorpi *et al.*, 1991), cervix (Tsou *et al.*, 1984), renal (Dekernion *et al.*, 1989), uveal melanoma (Rennie *et al.*, 1989), meningioma (Ironside *et al.*, 1987) and Hodgkin's disease (Joensuu *et al.*, 1988). However, it is still not the general practice to request DNA flow cytometric analysis when a patient first presents at a clinic or hospital. In contrast to this the flow cytometric immunofluorescent analysis of HIV patients, leukaemias, bone marrow and organ transplants and other haematology patient groups, has become routine.

QC of DNA analysis is perhaps even more difficult to address than that of immunophenotyping. Cell sources may be more variable. Tissue or cell processing prior to analysis may be extensive, subject to individual preferences and will vary from laboratory to laboratory and will affect cytometric features (Thunnissen *et al.*, 1992). For example, samples from solid tumours or paraffin-embedded tissue may require extensive processing (see Chapters 8 and 9). The choice of fluorochrome may be limited by the laser available. Analysis may be complicated by the need for a DNA ploidy control or the inclusion of internal standards and the nature of the data presentation. The data acquired are often complicated: more than one ploidy population may be present and this can lead to misinterpretation of the data. Some of these issues are discussed below.

Fluorochromes

It is important to understand a little about the nature of DNA staining in order to appreciate potential problems, especially if fixed cells or nuclei are used. Propidium iodide (PI) is the fluorochrome of choice, being relatively cheap, easy to use and having a good storage life if kept at 4°C and protected from light. Propidium iodide and a comparable fluorochrome, ethidium bromide (EB), both intercalate non-specifically with double-stranded nucleic acid and fluoresce in the red spectrum. Both are capable of binding to fold back single-stranded RNA. Samples of actively dividing cells will produce elevated levels of fluorescence because both DNA and RNA are stained, resulting in poorer quality peaks on the DNA histogram. This is easily resolved by incubating the cell sample with 50 μl RNAse (1 mg/ml) for 30 min at room temperature prior to staining with PI (50 μg/ml).

Other fluorochromes are DNA base-pair specific, such as mithramycin (MMC) which binds to G-C regions of DNA with peak excitation at 421 nm and emission at 575 nm. Benzimides such as Hoechst 33342 bind preferentially to A-T rich regions in the small groove of DNA and have peak excitation at 395 nm with peak emission at 450 nm. A similar dye is 4',6-diamidino-2-phenylindole (DAPI) with peak excitation at 372 nm and emission at 456 nm. 3',6-bis(dimethylamino) acridine or acridine orange has dual binding, with green fluorescence when intercalated with double-stranded nucleic acid and red fluorescence when stacked on charged phosphates of single-stranded nucleic acid. This dye has peak excitation at 503 nm with emission at 530 nm for DNA and 640 nm for RNA.

It is clear that fluorochrome penetration into the nucleus, as well as its ability to associate and bind to the nucleic acid, is a major consideration in the choice of use of either fresh permeabilized or fixed cells. Extensive fixation with formaldehyde, as used in paraffin-embedded tissue, is known to result in an overall reduction in the fluorescent intensity of stained cells when compared with fresh, unfixed cells (Lawry et al., 1987). Also, in a sample of extracted nuclei from a paraffin-block of tumour, there is likely to be variation in fluorochrome penetration and thus staining intensity; this is an area that has not been fully studied.

Methodology considerations

All stains except the Hoechst dyes require membrane permeabilization to allow entry to the nucleus, so protocols will recommend the use of either a detergent (Triton-X-100, Tween or Nonidet-P) or a lipid solubilizing fixation stage incorporating an alcohol such as 70% methanol. Care must be taken with either process, as detergents can make cells extremely delicate and prone to clumping if left at room temperature for more than an hour. Alcohol fixation can also result in severe aggregation. Two cells stuck together will appear as a 'G$_2$-phase peak' unless steps are taken to eliminate them, such as filtration through 50 μm gauze, the use of a 21- or 25-gauge needle and syringe and some process of doublet discrimination.

Single parameter DNA analysis has a disadvantage; it does not allow normal and aneuploid cells within the population to be distinguished. Many so-called tumour samples contain high numbers of normal cells. Dual parameter analysis employing PI to stain DNA and FITC-labelled monoclonal antibodies, can be successfully used to resolve tumour populations from any other cells present (Lawry et al., 1988).

The choice of controls is an important consideration in that most tumour samples require the calculation of the DNA ploidy index, as a measure of total (abnormal) DNA content, compared with a normal diploid control. It may be assumed that there will always be a proportion of normal stromal or infiltrative cells present as an internal control: but in a leukaemia sample this may not be the case. Samples of known normal lymphocytes, for example, should be run in parallel if external controls are required. Alternatively, the test sample may be 'spiked' with chick or trout red blood cells which have a DNA content approximately one-third that of humans.

Since the development of techniques to extract nuclei from paraffin-wax embedded tissue blocks by Hedley *et al.* (1983), many DNA studies have been reported on prognostic correlations of the DNA ploidy index and S-phase fraction, yet few have considered issues of QC. Possible fixation artefacts cannot be ignored. With extensive aldehyde bond cross-links between the DNA and histones, DNA fluorochromes cannot be expected to intercalate as effectively as in fresh tissue, even with the enzymatic action of pepsin. Diploid controls may be difficult to obtain, as normal tissue samples of the same age, processed in the same way, cannot always be found. In this case, the internal control of infiltrating and stromal cells has to be used. However, the particular problem in this case is the inability to identify hypo-diploid cells, as the peak with the lowest fluorescence intensity has to be assumed to be the diploid peak.

An additional problem associated with nuclear preparations, especially those taken as thick sections, is the presence of variable amounts of nuclear debris caused by slicing through cells. This can swamp the true DNA peaks of a sample and lead to an overcalculation of the S-phase fraction. Computer models have been developed to subtract background noise (debris) from the histogram (Bagwell *et al.*, 1991) but it is preferable to reduce the problem prior to analysis by selecting an optimal section thickness (Stephenson *et al.*, 1986).

Finally, it would seem to be common sense to state that, as for all flow cytometric procedures, sample and reagent sterility should be ensured: cell cultures should be mycoplasma-free upon screening; fluorochromes should be held frozen or in a refrigerator, and always protected from light. Stained samples should be stored in capped tubes at 4°C until analysed, with thorough mixing and filtration immediately prior to analysis to minimize cell aggregation. All DNA fluorochromes are at least poisonous, at worst carcinogenic, mutagenic and teratogenic and should be handled with extreme care.

Cytometer considerations

In many cytometers enclosed fluidic systems, fixed optics and the lack of laser realignment may make the cytometrist complacent about what may go wrong and what to look for when things do go wrong. DNA analysis is one of the most demanding technologies applied to flow cytometry and requires the most precise running conditions. Samples must be as free as possible from cell clumps and be run slowly through the cytometer to ensure maximal excitation of any fluorochrome bound to the cell. In addition, thought must be given to the quality and choice of optics, the elimination of cell doublets and also to the nature of amplification and final presentation of the fluorescence signal. Data should always include the CV of the G_0/G_1 peak, as a measure of the width of the peak and hence the apparent uniformity of staining of cells and thus an overall measure of the quality of staining and alignment of the cytometer.

Linearity and offset

The simple check for linearity is to run fluorescent beads and measure the peak location for single beads, doublets and triplets which should be located equidistantly along a linear scale. If the peak separation increases (or decreases), then the scale is non-linear and the amplifier should be serviced or replaced. If the peak separation does not double from singles to doublets to quadruplet bead clusters, yet the error seems to be constant, then the fault is most likely to be in the offset setting or zero location of the fluorescence scale. On some cytometers this can be corrected by the operator, while on others a service engineer will be required. Assuming the number of channels this error causes is known, any peak data can be manually corrected by adding on the appropriate offset.

A third technique for checking the accuracy of amplifiers (both linear and logarithmic) is to run beads and measure peak locations and separations, then insert a 50% neutral density filter into the optical pathway of the appropriate detector. A positive offset will result in peaks higher than the calculated 50% value, while a negative offset will cause peaks to fall below this level. This can only be carried out on cytometers with removable filter blocks.

The reason for carrying out these linearity checks is that true DNA analysis can only be made on a linear fluorescence scale. The use of DNA fluorochromes is based on the assumption that the resultant fluorescence will be proportional to the DNA content of the cell. A normal resting cell in G_0/G_1 ($2n$) will increase its relative DNA content and hence fluorescence intensity, by a factor of two by the time it has progressed to the G_2/M-phase of the cell cycle ($4n$). Thus, the analysis of single and doublet beads mimics those peaks seen in the DNA histogram in that the latter should peak at a channel number twice that of the former and any amplification offsets can be noted prior to ploidy measurements being made.

Optical considerations

Typical sources of filters include Ealing optics (Ealing Beck) and Schott filters (H.V. Scan). All filters should be handled with care, held by the outer edges only and polished with at least a double thickness of lens tissue. They should be checked for signs of damage (scratches, pitting of the surface, cracks or chips) and should be stored in a suitable protective container.

Filters may be of a simple coloured glass type, with various transmission qualities or general neutral density properties or have interference properties. Long-pass, short-pass and band-pass filters are also available. A third type are the polarizing filters capable of allowing light to pass through only in a specific linear plane of polarization, but these are not used for DNA measurement (see also Chapter 1).

Coloured glass filters are usually of low cost and hence not always of the highest quality. However, they are generally adequate for light filtering with the advantage of an extensive range being available to suit most fluorochromes. It should be noted that glass can cause some fluorescence of its own under certain conditions. Neutral density filters have the property of being able to attenuate an incident light beam, without altering its spectral distribution. Hence, they can be used to decrease the overall intensity of light before it reaches the detector.

Interference filters may be either constructive or destructive, allowing light to pass through or be reflected back. Carefully controlled thicknesses of vacuum deposited chemical layers are arranged so that wavelengths outside the pass-band combine to cancel each other (destructive interference which prevents light passage), whereas those within the pass-band combine to reinforce each other and are transmitted (constructive interference).

Band-pass filters only transmit a single discrete wavelength band over a given spectral range. Long-pass filters only transmit light equal to or longer than the stated wavelength. Short-pass (edge) filters only transmit light equal to or shorter than the stated wavelength.

The mirrored plane should always be positioned towards the light source to minimize heating effects, as the optimal operating temperature is 23°C.

Spherical *vs* elliptical optics

Spherical optics are used to focus the laser light source to a fine point on the sample stream. However, there are limitations as to how this can be achieved. The usual minimum is 10 μm. Elliptical focusing uses crossed cylindrical paired lenses to focus the light source to an elliptical plane. A cell crossing this is thus illuminated by a very even light source, with a slight loss in overall intensity compared with spherical optics. Typically the ellipse of illumination may be 60 × 15 μm, so large cells, especially binucleate cells are not totally illuminated. Hence peak height measurements may be inaccurate, the integrated peak value should be used instead. Spherical optics enable the full illumination of a large cell so peak height can be used for doublet discrimination.

The old Ortho range of flow cytometers (Ortho Cytofluorograph) focused the laser via a crossed cylindrical pair of lenses to a beam width of about 6 μm and the Ortho Cytoron Absolute bench-top cytometer focuses to a beam width of 7–8 μm. This prevents the analysis of doublets of nuclei since it can illuminate a single nucleus at a time. However, such a narrow beam width may not be optimum for the analysis of lymphocyte surface antigens. The Coulter Profile II and the Becton Dickinson FACScan, for example, employ a focused beam width of 14.3 and 20 μm, respectively. This is ideal for analysis of lymphocytes but will not discriminate between single nuclei and doublets. The problem has been addressed by the introduction of an electronic doublet discriminator on later versions of the FACScan, although there remains much debate as to the reliability of such a system.

Pulse analysis

The electrical impulse produced by the fluorescent detector on receiving fluorescence emitted from the cell as it crosses the excitation source, can be analysed to measure both fluorescence intensity and also its duration. Thus a single cell emits a predicted amount of fluorescence over a limited time period as it crosses the light source. This signal will have a zero phase, a rise phase, a peak and then a fall back to zero. A larger cell would be expected to emit more light over a slightly longer period, yet have the same peak characteristics of rise and fall. However, two small cells stuck together would emit light as the first cell passes the light source and then emit a second time as the second part of the cell clump is excited. A bimodal peak will be produced with no return to the zero baseline between cells. This is the principle used in flow cytometers for doublet discrimination. Not only is the peak height and width (duration) measured but the peak area is calculated. These parameters are then plotted as dual parameter displays together with the real fluorescence emission of the cell sample to enable exclusion gates to be made around the single cell population only.

Sample data analysis

The cell cycle

The normal cycle of division of a cell starts in the quiescent or resting phase (G_0) and with an appropriate stimulus (cytokine, growth factor or mitogen) the cell enters the division cycle at G_{1a}/G_{1b}. At this stage there is no net increase in DNA content, so by flow cytometry, all cells in these phases will fluoresce equally brightly. However, there will be an increase in RNA content, possibly detected by the non-base pair specificity of PI staining. Cells then enter the stage during which DNA is synthesized (S-phase), and this is seen by an increase in the relative level of fluorescence. Cells then proceed to G_2-phase and then to M-phase, during which they undergo mitosis and cytokinesis, with no further net increase in DNA content and fluorescence. The G_0/G_1, S and G_2/M-phase can therefore be resolved as individual peaks within the total population.

DNA ploidy index

The overall level of DNA of a cell can be expressed as a DNA ploidy index. Normal diploid cells ($2n$) give a characteristic peak on the fluorescence axis, while DNA aneuploid cells contain higher levels of DNA and have a peak further along the axis. The ratio of this (abnormal) peak channel, divided by that of the diploid control peak channel, provides the DNA ploidy index. Diploidy is thus denoted by an index of 1.0, tetraploidy of 2.0 and those peaks between 1.1 and 1.9 are termed DNA aneuploid (not to be confused with the cytogenic use of the word aneuploid). Peaks below the diploid channel are termed hypo-diploid and those greater than the tetraploid channel are hyper-tetraploid.

Determination of tetraploidy

A serious problem occurs in the determination of tetraploid populations compared with an enlarged G_2/M diploid peak. In considering the correct identification of such peaks, the presence or absence of tetraploid S/G_2/M-phases must be noted, together with the possible presence of cell clumps. These will enlarge the diploid G_2/M-phase peak, but will also produce a peak in the 'triploid' region of the axis. If seen, the possibility of tetraploidy is minimal, with all peaks above the G_0/G_1 being attributed to cell aggregation. In general, true tetraploidy can only be guaranteed if the population exceeds 15% of the total.

S-phase determination

S-phase determination may present difficulties. For example, rapidly dividing cell cultures will have a high proportion of cells in S-phase, and the degree of overlap of peaks will be considerably increased, as in G_0/G_1 and S-phase and late S-phase with G_2/M. The presence of aneuploidy will also make S-phase calculation particularly difficult, with populations from different phases of the cell cycle overlapping. Software packages fit Gaussian curves into the G_0/G_1 and G_2/M-phase peaks and then approximate the proportion of cells in S-phase by linear regression of the area between the mid-points of the G_1 and G_2 peaks. S-phase overlap can usually be accounted for, except in synchronous cultures or samples with elevated levels of cycling cells, where modification in the programs take into consideration these effects and recalculate the proportion of S-phase cells. Dean (1980) reported a simple calculation technique for synchronously growing cells by fitting a second degree polynomial to the mid-S-phase part of the histogram in order to avoid any major influence from the G_1 and G_2 peaks in the S-phase measurement.

Commercial packages are now available and usually offer a range of software options to suit the sample under analysis. Multicycle[TM] (Phoenix Flow Systems) is one such package allowing curve fitting to single, multiple and overlapping cell cycle data and is illustrated in Fig. 2.7 for cells undergoing cell cycle arrest.

DNA QC studies reported to date

The first is a report of the National Cancer Institute's flow cytometry network experiences sending archival bladder sections between its five institutions for DNA analysis. The report concludes that there was a

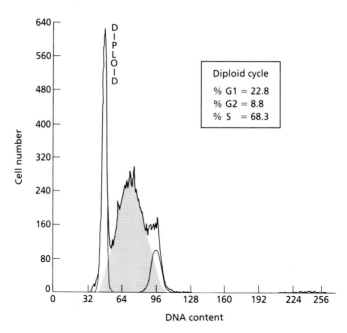

Fig. 2.7 Example of the Multicycle DNA histogram analysis package on a sample of cultured A375 melanoma cells, incubated with IGF-II causing the induction of an S-phase accumulation.

substantial agreement in actual data generated (Coon *et al.*, 1988).

The College of American Pathologists have reported on the introduction of inter-laboratory proficiency testing (Homburger *et al.*, 1989). A third report summarizes the findings of the Bladder Flow Cytometry Network of the National Cancer Institute of a QC study involving mixtures of lymphocytes and DNA aneuploid cell lines, with reference to standards. Six laboratories participated, with findings of intra- and inter-laboratory variability (Wheeless *et al.*, 1991). Lawry (1992) reported on a QC study in which stained lymphocyte/DNA aneuploid cells were analysed by 20 laboratories. Data collected indicated that the most accurate measurement made was that for the DNA ploidy index.

Further reading

Hiddemann *et al.* (1984) gave the first short report produced from the committee on nomenclature of the Society for Analytical Cytology on guide-lines for DNA staining, terminology and standards. A review article covering many aspects of quality assurance but focusing on pre-analytical considerations affecting results both in immunophenotyping and DNA analysis may be found in McCarthy and Fetterhoff (1988). Hedley (1989) provides an overview of the clinical applications of DNA flow cytometry using archival material, new developments and improvements including areas for future work and increased understanding.

Conclusion

Quality control and assurance is an issue for every laboratory irrespective of its discipline. A laboratory in one of the major teaching hospitals in the UK recently replied to a questionnaire on flow cytometry QC, 'We are a clinical research department and do not feel that quality control/ assurance is an issue for us'. In the same post-bag a letter from a pharmaceutical company whose drug trial was being monitored by one of our laboratories requested, 'detail of your laboratory practices regarding internal and external quality control together with an outline of your quality assurance programme for immunophenotyping'. The advent of clinical laboratory accreditation and the obvious demands of the pharmaceutical industry will motivate a greater awareness of QC/ quality assurance. It is hoped that this chapter has outlined some of the measures which should be employed in a comprehensive quality assurance programme and that it has stimulated interest to discover more about the correct functioning of cytometers.

References

Bagwell CB, Majo SW, Whetstone SD *et al.* (1991) DNA histogram debris theory and compensation. *Cytometry* **12**: 107–118.

Coon JS, Deitch AD, De Vere RW *et al.* (1988) Interinstitutional variability in DNA flow cytometric analysis of tumours. *Cancer* **61**: 126–130.

Dean PN (1980) A simplified method of DNA distribution analysis. *Cell Tissue Kinet.* **13**: 299–308.

Dekernion JB, Mukel E, Ritchie AWS, Blyth B, Hannah J, Bohman R (1989) Prognostic significance of the DNA content of renal carcinoma. *Cancer* **64**: 1669–1673.

Giorgi JV, Cheng H-L, Margolick JB *et al.* (1990) Quality control in the flow cytometric measurement of T-lymphocyte subsets: The Multicentre AIDS Cohort Study experience. *Clin. Immunol. Immunopathol.* **55**: 173–186.

Hedley DW (1989) Flow cytometry using paraffin-emdedded tissue: five years on. *Cytometry* **10**: 229–241.

Hedley DW, Friedlander ML, Taylor IW, Rugg CA, Musgrove EA (1983) Methods for analysis of cellular DNA content of paraffin-embedded pathological material using flow cytometry. *J. Histochem. Cytochem.* **31**: 1333–1355.

Hiddemann W, Schuman J, Andreef M *et al.* (1984) Convention on nomenclature for DNA cytometry. *Cancer Genet. Cytogenet.* **13**: 181–183.

Homburger HA, MacCarthy R, Deodhar S (1989) Assessment of interlaboratory variability in analytical cytology. *Arch. Pathol. Lab. Med.* **113**: 667–672.

Ironside JW, Battersby RDE, Lawry J, Loomes RS, Day CA, Timperley WR (1987) DNA in meningioma tissues and explant cell cultures. *J. Neurosurg.* **66**: 588–594.

Joensuu H, Klemi PJ, Korkeila E (1988) Prognostic value of DNA ploidy and proliferative activity in Hodgkin's disease. *Am. J. Clin. Pathol.* **90**: 670–673.

Jones DJ, Moore M, Schofield PF (1988) Refining the prognostic significance of DNA ploidy status in colorectal cancer: a prospective flow cytometric study. *Int. J. Cancer* **41**: 206–210.

Lawry J (1992) Clinical applications of bench-top flow cytometers — report of the quality control study. *Proc. Royal. Mic. Soc.* **27**: 16–17.

Lawry J, Rogers K, Percival RC, Day CW, Potter CW, Underwood JCE (1987) Flow cytometric DNA analysis of breast carcinomas: a comparative study of fresh, frozen and fixed embedded breast. *Surg. Res. Commun.* **2**: 27–37.

Lawry J, Rogers K, Duncan JL (1988) Simultaneous measurement of DNA cycle and monoclonal antibody binding of breast carcinoma by flow cytometry. *Surg. Res. Commun.* **3**: 61–70.

Martini E, D'Hautcourt JL, Brando B, Lawry J, O'Connor JE, Sansonetty F (1989) *First European Quality Control of Cellular Phenotyping by Flow Cytometry*. Publ. Editions Frison-Roche, Paris.

McCarthy RC, Fetterhoff TJ (1989) Issues of quality assurance in clinical flow cytometry. *Arch. Pathol. Lab. Med.* **113**: 658–666.

Parker JW, Adelsberg B, Azen SP *et al.* (1990) Leukocyte immunophenotyping by flow cytometry in a multisite study: Standardisation, Quality Control and Normal values in the Transfusion Safety Study. *Clin. Immunol. Immunophatol.* **55**: 187–220.

Rennie IG, Rees RC, Parsons MA, Lawry J, Cottam D (1989) Estimation of DNA content in uveal melanoma by flow cytometry. *Eye* **3**: 611–617.

Shapiro HM (1988) *Practical Flow Cytometry*, 2nd edn. Alan R Liss Inc., New York.

Stephenson RA, Gay H, Fair WR, Melamed MR (1986) Effect of section thickness on quality of flow cytometric DNA content determinations in paraffin-embedded tissues. *Cytometry* **7**: 41–44.

Thunnissen FBJM, Perdaen H, Forrest J (1992) Influence of different cell extraction methods on cytometric features. *Cytometry* **13**: 485–489.

Tsou KC, Hong DH, Varello M *et al.* (1984) Flow cytometric DNA analysis as a diagnostic aid for cervical condyloma and cancer. *Cancer* **54**: 1778–1787.

Visakorpi T, Kallioniemi OP, Paronen IYI, Isola JJ, Heikkinen AI, Kiovula TA (1991) Flow cytometric analysis of DNA ploidy and S-phase fraction from prostatic carcinomas: implications for prognosis and response to endocrine therapy. *Br. J. Cancer* **64**: 578–582.

Visscher DW, Zarbo RJ, Greenawald KA, Crissman JD (1990) Prognostic significance of morphological parameters and flow cytometric DNA analysis in carcinoma of the breast. *Pathol. Ann.* **25**: 171–210.

Wheeless LL, Coon JS, Cox C *et al.* (1991) Precision of DNA flow cytometry in inter-institutional analysis. *Cytometry* **12**: 405–412.

Chapter 3
Immunophenotypic Analysis of Lymphocytes and Leukaemias

M. G. MACEY

Introduction

Flow cytometric analysis enables the researcher and clinician to enumerate lymphocyte subsets within the peripheral blood mononuclear cells (PBMC). Often blood samples are collected at one site and then shipped to another for analysis. Many options for storage, preparation and staining of PBMC for flow cytometric analysis exist. Changes that occur due to the preparatory process and due to a delay in preparation have been shown to result in inaccurate T-cell percentages and T-cell subset ratios (Weiblen *et al.*, 1983; Paoli *et al.*, 1984; Fletcher *et al.*, 1987; Ashmore *et al.*, 1989).

Preparation techniques include the conventional Ficoll-Paque density gradient centrifugation (Boyum, 1968).

Ficoll-Paque method

1 Blood either diluted 1:2 (in phosphate-buffered saline, PBS) or undiluted is layered over an equal volume of density gradient medium (Ficoll-Paque, Pharmacia; Lymphoprep, Nyegaard; His-

Continued on page 68

67

topaque, Sigma) and centrifuged at 400–450 g at room temperature for 20–30 min.
2 Cells at the interface between the Ficoll and plasma are removed and washed in balanced salt solution or medium and resuspended.
3 Cells are then labelled either directly or indirectly with fluorochrome-conjugated antisera.

This technique, however, has been criticized in a number of studies which have suggested that density gradient centrifugation: (a) increased the relative proportion of B cells (Brown and Greaves, 1974); (b) results in non-viable cells being lost to the red cell pellet (Adri *et al.*, 1980); and (c) causes selective loss of CD8$^+$CD57$^+$ cells to the red cell pellet (Paoli *et al.*, 1984). This has led to the development of whole blood techniques in which red cells are lysed prior to or after fixation and labelling of the white blood cells (WBC). Whole blood methods also have their failings mainly due to the effect of: fixatives on antigenic epitopes and lysing agents on cell membrane integrity (Carter *et al.*, 1992). However, whichever method is used, analysis should be performed on fresh blood (within 2–4 hours) without storage, particularly if anticoagulated with EDTA (Behnken *et al.*, 1984; Carter *et al.*, 1992).

Lyse, fix, label method

1 Freshly drawn whole blood (1 ml) without anticoagulant is mixed with an equal volume of 0.4% formaldehyde in Hepes-buffered (0.01 mol/l) Hank's balanced salt solution (HHBSS) for 4 min at 37°C.
2 The red blood cells (RBC) are then lysed by the addition of 40 ml 0.01 mol/l Hepes-buffered ammonium chloride (0.155 mol/l).
3 After incubation at 37°C for up to 30 min the cells are washed twice in HHBSS by centrifugation at 300 g and resuspended to 1 ml in HHBSS.
4 Aliquots are then labelled at room temperature, either directly or indirectly with fluorescein isothiocyanate (FITC)-conjugated antisera (Hamblin *et al.*, 1991).

Label, lyse, fix method

1 Freshly drawn blood anticoagulated with EDTA K$_3$ (0.17 mol/l) or acid citrate (AC; 0.105 mol/l) is aliquoted (100 µl) into tubes containing antisera.
2 After 10 min incubation with antisera at room temperature, in the dark, the RBC are lysed with distilled water (FACS-Lyse, Becton Dickinson) or formic acid (Q-Prep, Coulter).
3 The WBC are then fixed with formaldehyde (0.1–1.5%).

4 After washing in PBS the cells are usually resuspended in 1%
formaldehyde and stored at 4°C in the dark until analysed.

Preparation of tissue infiltrating lymphocytes

Many cells of the immune system are situated in tissues; analysis of
these cells requires their isolation from the surrounding tissue. A number
of techniques have been described (Rudberg *et al.*, 1986; Ritson and
Bulmer, 1987); two are presented here.

Procedure 1

1 Fresh tissue samples are sliced thinly and incubated for 1 hour
at room temperature in RPMI1640 (Gibco) containing 0.1% collagenase type II (Sigma) and 0.1% deoxyribonuclease (Sigma) with
occasional agitation.
2 The cell digest is sieved through a 100 μm nylon filter, washed
twice in RPMI, resuspended, then layered over an equal volume of
Ficoll-Paque.
3 After 20 min centrifugation at 650 g the cells at the sample gradient
interface are collected and washed prior to analysis.

Procedure 2

1 Fresh lymphoid tissue is collected into 5 ml cold (4°C) RPMI1640
containing 10% fetal calf serum in a Petri dish.
2 The tissue is gently teased between the blades of two scalpels to
release the cells.
3 The suspended cells are placed in a conical tube on ice for
1–2 min to allow aggregates to settle.
4 The supernatant may then be layered over Ficoll-Paque and
treated as above.

Use of light scattering

Ideally the process of lymphocyte gating should result in the inclusion
of all lymphocytes and exclusion of all other mononuclear cells. The
presence of contaminating monocytes is a problem for the purposes of
studying lymphocytes. Monocytes phagocytose 'foreign' particles
including fluorochrome-labelled antibodies causing false-positive results
(Cline and Lehrer, 1968). Monocytes also cause significant background
reactivity with antibodies due to Fc-receptor mediated binding of
antisera (Slease *et al.*, 1979).

Forward and 90° light scatter parameters are used to distinguish between lymphocytes, monocytes and neutrophils in mononuclear and whole blood preparations. In spite of the lack of a clear understanding of what precisely governs 90° light scatter, it has been proposed to correlate with nuclear shape and to measure internal cellular structure (Brunsting and Mullaney, 1974). Forward light scatter is more clearly understood and has been shown to be proportional to the square of the radius of a sphere (Mullaney and Dean, 1970). The combination of forward and 90° light scatter has been employed in a multiparametric approach to distinguish the various haemopoietic subpopulations found in bone marrow and peripheral blood (Loken *et al.*, 1987). Use of 90° scatter alone, forward scatter alone and forward and 90° light scatter simultaneously to identify lymphoid cells has been shown to result in exclusion of 12, 17 and 23% of lymphocytes, respectively (Thompson *et al.*, 1985). This suggests that 90° light scatter alone is the optimal method to eliminate monocytes electronically from mononuclear cell populations in which lymphocytes are being studied.

Under some conditions the intensity of light scattering from cells is a non-linear function of cell volume. McMann *et al.* (1988) have shown that the intensity of 90° light scatter varied inversely with cell volume in hypertonic and hypotonic solutions but cell damage induced by freezing and thawing resulted in significant reduction in the intensity of forward angle light scatter with little change in cell volume. These observations show that light scatter and cell volume can vary independently and that care should be taken when interpreting the phenomenon of light scattering from living cells.

Quantitation of cell surface fluorescence intensity

Flow cytometry allows analysis of the level of antigen expression by individual cells. However, cellular fluorescence intensities measured by flow cytometry are generally expressed in arbitrary units such that the absolute numbers of the respective cell surface determinants per antibody remain unknown. Fluorescence quantitation may be achieved using calibrated fluorescent standard beads (Flow Cytometry Standards Corporation). Fluorescent standards matched to dyes used in the test sample, allow the direct conversion of fluorescence intensity of a sample into the number of molecules of equivalent soluble fluorochrome (MESF). Five calibration standards with different known levels of fluorescence are analysed using log fluorescence. The peak channel for each of the five standards is recorded together with the instrument settings (Fig. 3.1).

The fluorescence relative channel number (RCN) for each standard is calculated from the following equation:

1   For a linear amplifier:

$$RCN = \frac{\text{peak channel} \times \text{max. gain} \times 10^{nd}}{\text{actual gain}}$$

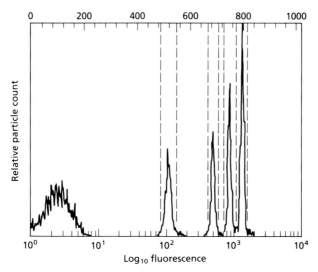

Fig. 3.1 Histogram showing the peak channel distribution for each of five fluorescent calibration bead standards.

2 For a log amplifier:

$$RCN = \text{peak channel} \times 10^{nd}$$

nd is the power of the neutral density filter; if no filter is used *nd* = 0.

A plot of MESF (*y*-axis) *vs* RCN (*x*-axis) of the standards on a semi-log graph provides a calibration curve which may be used to determine the MESF value that corresponds to any RCN at the recorded instrument settings (Fig. 3.2). Conversion of flow cytometry results to MESF allows comparison of data from different machines and enables inter-laboratory quality control (see Chapter 2).

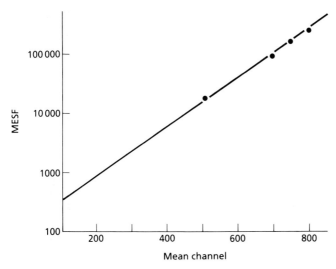

Fig. 3.2 A plot of molecules of equivalent soluble fluorochrome (MESF) and mean channel fluorescence (MCF) of standards.

Quantitation of antibody binding to cells

The above method allows the quantitation of the mean number of fluorescence equivalents associated with a given cell within a population, but it does not provide the number of antibodies bound to antigens or receptors on the cell. This may be calculated by:

$$\text{Number of antibodies} = \frac{\text{The average MESF}}{\text{F}:\text{P}}$$

where (F:P) is the fluorochrome:protein ratio for the antibody used to identify the antigen. This F:P may be determined by absorption spectroscopy at the absorption wavelength of the fluorochrome (492 nm for fluorescein) and antibody (280 for protein), the ratio of the two absorptions provides the F:P ratio. However, the F:P ratio determined by this method does not translate directly to the fluorescence intensity associated with the cell because of environmental conditions. Also, if there are more than three fluorochrome molecules per antibody, quenching may occur and if the fluorochrome is ionizable then pH and diluent may influence the fluorescence intensity. To overcome this, the average fluorescence intensity per antibody (effective fluorescence F:P) is determined, instead of the number of fluorochrome molecules per antibody.

Determination of the effective fluorescence F:P ratio

Calibrated beads coated with covalently bound goat–anti mouse are available commercially (Becton Dickinson; Polysciences). The beads are incubated with the antibody under saturating conditions, either directly or indirectly labelled with fluorochrome. The fluorescence intensity of the saturated beads is determined from the calibration curve of MESF (y-axis) *vs* RCN (x-axis) as described above. The effective fluorescence F:P ratio is calculated by:

$$\text{F}:\text{P} = \frac{\text{Saturated fluorescence intensity of beads}}{\text{Number of calibrated antibody binding sites on beads}}$$

To determine the number of available antibody binding sites per cell, the fluorescence intensity per cell labelled with the antibody is divided by the effective F:P ratio.

Further considerations

The calculation above assumes a 1:1 ratio of antibody to antigen. The fact that antibody molecules are divalent and that even under saturating conditions an antibody may bind to two antigens should be taken into consideration (Roe *et al.*, 1985). The affinity of antibodies for antigens may also be influenced by the concentration of the antigen as demonstrated by the sigmoidal curve obtained if antibody concentration is plotted against the fluorescence of bound antibody.

Before determining the mean number of antibody binding sites per cell of a positive population, a cut-off point between the fluorescence intensity of positive and negative cells must be defined. This is not possible for non-disjunct fluorescence intensity distributions. To overcome this Dux *et al.* (1991) have developed a statistical test based on a comparison of the relative number of cells per channel to determine a cut-off point above which the relative number of cells per channel of the test sample significantly exceeds that of the control sample. These workers also included a factor in their calculations for accidental disturbances due to small fluctuations which may cause changes in the shape of distributions and lead to incorrect statistical decisions.

Ideally, quantitation of fluorescence should be performed with linear amplification. The photomultiplier tubes (PMTs) and diode detectors in flow cytometers produce output currents that vary linearly with the amount of total light collected from cells. The detector output currents are converted to voltages by pre-amplifiers. The pre-amplifier output voltages therefore are, ideally, proportional to the amount of light collected from cells. In fluorescence detection, the pre-amplifier output voltage should be a linear function of the number of fluorescent molecules per cell. Although many cellular parameters, e.g. DNA content vary over only a small dynamic range (less than a decade), others, such as the number of antigen molecules on the surface, may vary over a range of three or more decades. Log amplification produces an output voltage (or current) proportional to the logarithm of the input voltage (or current) and this facilitates analysis of heterogeneous populations in which the fluorescence values vary over a wide dynamic range.

On a linear scale, peaks with the same coefficient of variation (CV) differ in width according to the peak location; on a logarithmic scale peaks with the same CV are the same widths regardless of the location. When measurements are made on a linear scale, the difference between values in adjacent channels is constant. For an ideal analysis on a log-scale input signals with a constant ratio of amplitudes should produce output signals that differ by a constant amount (i.e. the log of the ratio) and the relationship between input and output peak amplitudes when plotted on semi-log paper should be a straight line, this is rarely the case (Parks *et al.*, 1988). If mixtures of beads with known fluorescence are analysed at a range of settings of PMT gain, the plots of the difference in channel numbers between peaks *vs* peak location provide a precise indicator of deviations from logarithmic behaviour over the log amplifier (Schmid *et al.*, 1988).

For quantitative analysis if the log-amplifier deviates substantially from ideal behaviour over its range, accurate conversion from log-scale back to linear requires that a calibration curve for the amplifier be available. If signals being studied do not vary over a large dynamic range, it is usually easier to do accurate quantitative measurements on a linear scale than to use log-amplification (Gandler and Shapiro, 1990).

Peripheral blood lymphocyte subpopulations: normal ranges

The reference distribution of peripheral blood lymphocyte subsets has been established for normal Caucasian adults (Table 3.1). Age and sex differences exist for some antigens. Age-related trends have been found to be similar for both sexes (range 0–80 years). Natural killer (NK) cells and CD4$^+$ cells increase significantly with age as a percentage of lymphocytes (Lighart *et al.*, 1986; Utsuyama *et al.*, 1992). The CD8$^+$ cell percentage does not change significantly in adulthood. However, because the CD4$^+$ percentage does change, the CD4/CD8 ratio increases with age in adults. Definite differences between sexes have been found for T cells and NK cells (Levi *et al.*, 1988). The lymphocytes and NK cells of normal individuals also exhibit circadian and diurnal rhythms (Levi *et al.*, 1983; Fry *et al.*, 1992); for this reason in sequential studies venesection should be at the same time on each occasion.

Despite changes in lymphocyte subpopulations the sum of %T + %B + %NK approximates 100% throughout life. The total may be greater than 100% when dual CD8$^+$CD4$^+$ or CD2$^+$CD56$^+$ cells are present or when CD16$^+$CD56$^+$ NK cells have been excluded from the flow-cytometric gate (Lagaay *et al.*, 1990). Dual positive CD4$^+$CD8$^+$ lymphocytes are considered to be immature thymocytes (Fujii *et al.*, 1992; Sancho *et al.*, 1992) but increased numbers have also been found in adult T-cell leukaemia (Kamihira *et al.*, 1992), in Hashimoto's disease and thyroiditis (Iwatani *et al.*, 1992), in myaesthenia gravis and thymoma (Ichikawa *et al.*, 1992) and in HTLV-1 positive T-cell lymphomas (Shih *et al.*, 1992). Most studies have been performed on Caucasian individuals but there is evidence for ethnic variation. For example Chinese individuals have relatively more NK cells (Prince *et al.*, 1985) and therefore studies with such populations will require appropriate reference ranges to be determined.

Table 3.1 Reference range for major lymphocyte subsets

Cell type	Population parameters (%)					
	Mean	Median	Range	s.d.	Variation with age	Sex difference
CD3$^+$ T cell	73	73	60–85	6.5	NS	2.5 F > M
CD19$^+$ B cell	14	13	7–23	4.2	NS	NS
CD4$^+$ T cell	44	43	29–59	7.6	1.2% per decade	3.7 M > F
CD8$^+$ T cell	33	33	19–48	7.4	NS	NS
CD16$^+$ CD56$^+$ NK cell	14	13	6–29	6.0	0.9% per decade	1.6 M > F
CD4/CD8 ratio	1.4	1.3	0.6–2.8	0.6	0.07% per decade	0.19 F > M

From Clinical Monograph 1. Becton Dickinson.
NS, not significant; F, female; M, male.

Immunophenotyping results can be expressed as the absolute number of cells of each lymphocyte subgroup per microlitre or as a percentage of the total lymphocyte population. If an aliquot of the patient's blood is analysed by a haematology counter at the same time as it is analysed by flow cytometry, the WBC count and the lymphocyte differential can be determined. The absolute count for the lymphocyte subsets can be calculated by:

WBC count × % total lymphocytes × % subset

However, studies have shown that the median values obtained for WBC varied greatly from site to site and for samples within the adult normal range (College of American Pathologists, 1988). This variation is caused by the intrinsic differences among haemotology instruments produced by different manufacturers. Until the problem of comparability in absolute counts for the WBC is resolved, both percentage and local absolute values should be considered in making interpretations of lymphocyte subset population parameters.

Dual-colour immunofluorescence

One-colour immunofluorescence is widely used to characterize functional cell types within a heterogeneous population. However, since the expression of one surface antigen is rarely unique and specific for a functional subset, this technique may be inappropriate for the discrimination between cell subsets in heterogeneous populations. This limitation may be reduced through the use of multispecific labels. In this context, two-colour immunolabelling has been practised to detect double staining of cells by using the combination of two fluorochromes, among which FITC and phycoerythrin (PE) together allow good sensitivity. Both fluorochromes are excited by the 488 nm line of argon lasers. However, there is some overlap between the spectral emission of the two fluorochromes but electronic compensation may be used to correct for this overlap when necessary.

Assay procedure

1 Cells are prepared using Ficoll-Paque separation; tissue dispersal or whole blood methods may be used.
2 It is preferable to use directly conjugated monoclonal antibodies (MoAb). However, if these are not available the first-stage antisera should have different isotypes and the FITC/PE conjugated second-stage antisera should then be specific for the two isotypes. Alternatively, one of the first-stage antisera may be biotin conjugated and identified by an avidin-linked fluorochrome.
3 Aliquots of cells are incubated with the antisera; appropriate controls include:

Continued on page 76

(a) unlabelled cells for background fluorescence;

(b) dual-stained mouse immunoglobulin FITC and mouse immunoglobulin PE antibody control for non-specific binding;

(c) single-stained test MoAb-FITC with low and high level fluorescence for adjusting the green PMT gains or voltage and to apply any adjustment to compensate for green spectral overlap into the PE PMT;

(d) single-stained test MoAb-PE with low and high fluorescences for adjusting the PE PMT gains and spectral overlap as in (c);

(e) dual-stained MoAb-FITC plus MoAb-PE on control normal cells and test cells.

4 The negative controls and single-stained test sample are analysed prior to analysis of the dual-labelled cells.

5 The use of compensation may result in loss of sensitivity. To check for this the total number of FITC$^+$ or PE$^+$ cells in the dual-labelled sample should be the same as the single-stained samples without compensation.

6 Loss of sensitivity may also be due to quenching and/or steric hindrance (see below).

Dual fluorescence combined with forward and 90° light scatter has been used to provide an unambiguous identification of monocytes within normal blood (Terstappen *et al.*, 1992). In this procedure monocytes within the lymphocyte gate are identified by their expression or CD14PE and CD45FITC. The CD45 antigen is expressed on all normal leucocytes but not on non-haemopoietic cells or mature erythrocytes (Shah *et al.*, 1988). CD14 antibodies stain monocytes very brightly and have low reactivity with cells of other lineages (Griffin *et al.*, 1981). The clear discrimination of monocytes from other cells may be made based on the surface co-expression of CD14 and CD45.

Three-colour immunofluorescence

Recently, antibodies coupled to fluorochromes with emission spectra above 600 nm have become available (Red 613, Gibco; CyChrome, AMS; Quantum Red, Sigma). These are based on energy transfer between two fluorochromes, PE and cyanine-5 and have made three-colour immunofluorescence more amenable than the previous procedures (Lansdorp *et al.*, 1991). It is preferable to use directly conjugated antibodies and appropriate control should be included.

Quenching

High concentrations of PE can completely quench the fluorescein signal in dual fluorescence analysis of lymphocytes when some combinations of antibodies are used. Reduction in fluorescein signal has been shown to correlate with the intensity of PE staining (Chapple *et al.*, 1990). This

may seriously compromise interpretation of dual fluorescence studies.
It can be avoided by: (a) careful analysis of single colour control; (b) the
use of FITC antibody conjugates with the same or greater F:P ratio
than the PE antibody conjugate; (c) if one antigen has a higher density
distribution than the other labelling this with the FITC-conjugated
antibody; (d) enhancing the FITC by indirect labelling.

Steric hindrance

In dual fluorescence studies steric hindrance of antibody binding may
occur due to close proximity of antigens or in the case of a single
antigen due to adjacent epitopes on the antigen. There is no obvious
solution to this problem except to try antibodies to different epitopes
on the antigens.

Analysis of surface and intracellular antigens

Dual immunofluorescence has been used extensively to examine the
expression of surface molecules in relation to: cytoplasmic IgM (Zipf
et al., 1984; Loftin *et al.*, 1985); viral antigens (Jacobberger *et al.*, 1986);
nuclear Ki-67 antigen (Drach *et al.*, 1989); tumour necrosis factor α
(Andersson *et al.*, 1989); and CD3, CD16 and CD22 (Jacob *et al.*, 1991). A
variety of methods have been used to permeabilize cells including:
ethanol (Braylan *et al.*, 1982); lysolecithin (Schroff *et al.*, 1984); paraformaldehyde (Clevenger *et al.*, 1985); and saponin (Andersson *et al.*, 1989;
Jacob *et al.*, 1991). Saponin has also been used for the simultaneous
analysis of DNA content and cell surface molecules (Rigg *et al.*, 1989).
Schmenti and Jacobberger (1992) comprehensively assessed techniques
for the evaluation of DNA content and this is also discussed further in
Chapter 8.

Clinical implications of cell analysis

Diagnostic applications fall into five categories: (a) initial assessment of
immune status and leukaemia diagnosis; (b) assessment of immune
status following immunotherapy; (c) provision of a reliable correlation
between immunological status and clinical course; (d) molecular definition of new disease states; and (e) pathological study of disease tissue.
The molecular definition of new disease states is a rapidly expanding
area; some of the antigens associated with disease have been tabulated
in Chapter 1. The pathological study of disease tissue is examined
in Chapter 8.

Initial assessment of immune status and leukaemia diagnosis

The initial assessment of newly diagnosed leukaemic patients is important for identifying the type of acute leukaemia, that is, myeloid or
lymphoid as this determines the subsequent form of treatment (Chan

et al., 1985). In most cases the classification of acute leukaemia is based on the morphology and cytochemistry of the blast cells (Table 3.2). The blasts are then categorized according to the FAB (French–American–British Co-operative Group) classification (Bennett *et al.*, 1976; Table 3.3). Cytochemical techniques which use short chain esters as substrates are widely employed for identifying cells of the monocyte and myeloid lineage. Although monocytes usually show an intense diffuse reaction there is increasing evidence to suggest that in clinically abnormal states, and this includes the leukaemias, this reaction may be absent (Inns *et al.*, 1986). It is apparent that accurate assessment of lymphocyte, monocyte and myeloid populations in such patients should ideally be based on a combined cytochemical–immunophenotypic approach.

Immunophenotypic analysis of leukaemias and lymphomas relies on the staining patterns of the blast population with panels of antisera. Different primary panels are used for the acute leukaemias and the chronic lymphoid disorders. The primary panel is designed to allow distinction between myeloid and T/B lymphocytic leukaemias. Depending on the reactivity of the blast with the primary panel, additional panels may also be analysed to identify T-cell subsets and monocytic, erythroid or megakaryocytic lineages. Table 3.4 illustrates the panels suggested in the first Workshop on Immunophenotyping of Leukaemias and Lymphomas by the International Committee for Standardisation in Haematology (1988). The analysis of cytoplasmic IgM μ chains, CD3, myeloperoxidase (MPO) and nuclear terminal deoxynucleotidyl trans-

Table 3.2 Differentiation of leukaemic blast cells

	Lymphoblast	Myeloblast
Nucleoli	Usually one	More than two
Cytoplasm	Scanty High nuclear/ cytoplasmic ratio	Abundant Low nuclear/ cytoplasmic ratio
Auer rods	Absent	Present
Sudan black	Negative	Positive
PAS	Strong block positive	Negative or weak background positive
Acid phosphatase	Negative except in T lymphoblasts	Positive
Naphthol AS Acetate Esterase	Negative	Positive-myeloid resistant to fluoride monocytic abolished by fluoride
Chloracetate esterase	Negative	Positive

Table 3.3 French–American–British (FAB) Co-operative Group classification

(a) FAB classification of myeloid leukaemias

Category	Characteristics
M0	Undifferentiated blasts
M1	AML without maturation
M2	AML with 10–20% of cells differentiating
M3	Acute promyelocytic leukaemia
M4	Acute myeloblastic leukaemia
M5	Acute monoblastic leukaemia
M6	Erythroleukaemia
M7	Megakaryoblastic leukaemia

(b) Classification of ALL

Category	Characteristics
L1	Small, monomorphic
L2	Large convoluted and heterogeneous
L3	Burkitt-cell-type with cytoplasmic basophilia and vacuoles.

Table 3.4 Immunophenotypic panels for leukaemia diagnosis

Cell type identified	Acute leukaemias: panel of antisera		Chronic lymphoid disorders: panel of antisera	
	Primary	Secondary	Primary	Secondary
B cell	CD10 CD19 Cyto CD22 SIg heavy and light chains	Cyto μ-chain SIg μ-chain	CD10 CD20 CD5 SIg heavy and light chains	CD11c CD25 CD38 FMC7
T cell	CD2 Cyto CD3 CD7	CD1 CD3 CD4 CD8	CD3	CD4 CD8 CD11b CD16 CD57
Myeloid/ monocytic	CD13 CD33	CD14 CD15 Cyto myeloperoxidase		
Erythroid		Glycophorin A		
Megakaryocyte		CD41		
Non-specific	HLA-DR TdT	CD45 Cytokeratin	HLA-DR	TdT

Cyto, cytoplasmic; SIg, surface immunoglobulin.

ferase (TdT) is usually performed on slide preparations of fixed cells (Campana *et al.*, 1990a; Janossy and Campana, 1991). However, flow cytometric techniques have also been described for TdT (Syrjala *et al.*, 1992), IgM (Loftin *et al.*, 1985) and MPO (Slaper-Cortenbach *et al.*, 1988).

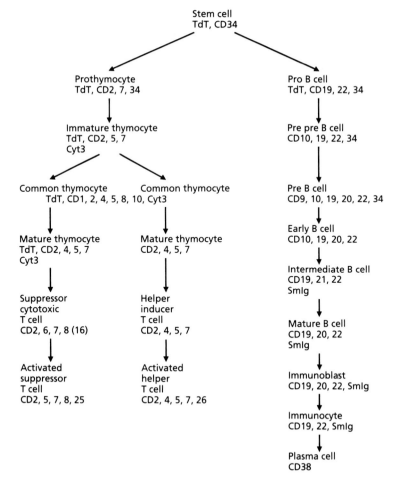

Fig. 3.3 Schematic representation of antigens associated with lymphoid differentiation.

The antigen expression on cells during lymphoid and myeloid differentiation is illustrated in Figs 3.3 and 3.4, respectively.

Phenotypic analysis of the acute lymphoblastic leukaemias

An illustration of the phenotypic analysis of blood from patients with acute lymphoblastic leukaemia (ALL) is given in Table 3.5. It is clear that B-cell ALLs react with CD19 and CD10, while T-cell ALLs react with CD2 and TdT so that different types of lymphoblastic leukaemias may be distinguished.

Detailed immunophenotypic and molecular analysis has shown that ALL subtypes correspond to clonal derivatives of B- and T-cell precursors (Greaves, 1986). Equivalent normal cells proliferate in substantial numbers in fetal tissue, normal or regenerating paediatric bone marrow or thymus. Leukaemic cells, however, are not the perfect replicas of normal cells and their phenotypes may show asynchrony of gene expression.

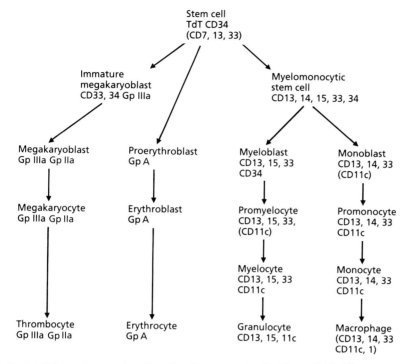

Fig. 3.4 Schematic representation of antigens associated with myeloid differentiation.

Table 3.5 Features of ALL

Feature	Null cell	Common ALL Pre-B	T-ALL	B-ALL
WBC (10⁹/l)	Often <10	Often >50	Often >50	Often <10
Cell type	L1	L1	L1 or L2	L3
Immunophenotype				
CD2	−	−	++	−
CD19	−	++	−	++
CD10	−	++	−	−
CD13	−	−	−	−
CD33	−	−	−	−
Tdt	++	++	++	±
Incidence	9%	70%	20%	1%

Karyotype immunoglobulin and TCR gene rearrangements are always clonal.

These observations accord with the view that leukaemogenesis in ALL involves an uncoupling of growth from differentiation in precursor cells rather than a stringent maturation arrest at a precise development stage.

A proportion of childhood and adult acute leukaemias have 'mixed lineage' (i.e. myeloid plus lymphoid, biphenotypic) phenotypes on individual cells. There has been controversy over whether the pattern of gene expression is due to genetic misprogramming (lineage infidelity) arising as a direct result of leukaemogenic mutations or, alternatively, whether the leukaemic process can immortalize a normal multi-potential progenitor cell, which when proliferating without maturation can express a promiscuous pattern of lineage specific genes (Greaves *et al.*, 1986). Although both possibilities may be at least in part correct, recent evidence indicates that normal multi-potential progenitor cells proliferating continuously in response to interleukin-3 can have a multilineage pattern of gene expression. ALL cells have diverse patterns of immunoglobulin and T-cell receptor gene rearrangements which are clonal and ALL cells are almost always of monoclonal origin (Greaves, 1992).

Phenotypic analysis of the acute myeloblastic leukaemias

The immunophenotypic distinction between different myeloid leukaemias is not so well defined (Table 3.6; Fig. 3.4). Distinction between these leukaemias relies heavily on cytochemistry and cellular morphology. The combined use of CD13, CD33 and anti-MPO, which detects the α-chain as well as the inactive proenzyme, allows recognition of 99% of acute myeloid leukaemia (AML) cases (Catovsky and Matutes, 1992). A major contribution of CD13 and CD33 is in the diagnosis of AML MO (Bennett *et al.*, 1991). In some reports these cases have been classified as ALL 'My' on account of lymphoblastic morphology and negative myeloid cytochemistry, despite evidence of the presence of myeloid antigens. This minimally differentiated form of AML which represents 3% of cases should be classified according to the following features: L2 morphology, negative MPO and Sudan Black B cytochemistry, negative expression of lymphoid antigens (TdT and CD7 may be positive), positive expression of CD13 and/or CD33 and other myeloid antigens, such as CD11b, CD15 and anti-MPO may also be positive. M5 may be defined by CD14 positivity and the M6 and M7

Table 3.6 Features of AML

Feature	Immature		AML	APML	AMML	Monoblastic	Erythroblastic	Megakaryoblastic
Morphology	M0	M1	M2	M3	M4	M5	M6	M7
WBC (10⁹/l)	33% less than normal				33% normal		33% above normal	
Immunophenotype								
CD2	−	−	−	−	−	−	−	−
CD19	−	±	−	−	−	−	−	−
CD10	−	−	−	−	−	±	−	−
CD13	+	+	+	++	++	++	±	±
CD33	+	±	+	++	++	++	±	±
CD14	−	−	−	−	±	+	−	−
CD34	++	++	+	±	±	±	±	±
CD68	−	−	−	−	−	−	++	−
CD41	−	−	−	−	−	−	−	+
Incidence	3%		70%	7%	1−2%	1−2%	1−2%	<1%

APML, acute promyelocytic leukaemia; AMML, acute myeloblastic leukaemia.

lineages are defined by anti-glycophorin-A and CD41, CD42, CD61, respectively.

Analysis of biphenotypic acute leukaemia

The greater use of monoclonal antibodies has brought to light the existence of leukaemias in which expression of lymphoid and myeloid antigens are co-expressed on the same cells; these are termed biphenotypic and are distinct from transforming leukaemias where mixtures of lymphoid and myeloid cells may be present (Catovsky *et al.*, 1991). There is considerable confusion in the literature about the definition of biphenotypic acute leukaemia. One reason for this is that antigens are not always critically assessed for true specificity since non-specific binding of antibodies to Fc receptors may occur. However, atypical antigen expression has been found in cases classified as AML and ALL, with perhaps a higher frequency in adults and in cases of AML.

In cases of leukaemia with biphenotypic expression, the majority express only one, or occasionally two, inappropriate antigens such as TdT, CD2 and CD7. The lineage specificity of these antigens is not clear (Figs 3.3, 3.4). However, there is a distinct group, representing approximately 10% of all cases, and twice as frequent within cases classified as AML by conventional criteria, that appear to express several inappropriate antigens. In a recent study (Hanson *et al.*, 1992) 52 of 746 cases (7%) fulfilled criteria for acute biphenotypic leukaemia and consisted of four major subgroups: $CD2^+$ AML (11 cases); $CD19^+$ AML (8); CD13 and/or $CD33^+$ ALL (24); and $CD11b^+$ ALL and others (9).

A scoring system has been proposed (Catovsky and Matutes, 1992) to distinguish true biphenotypic acute leukaemias which express many antigens (including lineage specific), from cases with minimal phenotypic deviation. The proposal is summarized in Table 3.7. A score of greater than 2 for each lineage is required to qualify the cells as biphenotypic. Most true biphenotypic cases score between 2.5 and 5. CD2 is the most frequently expressed T cell antigen in AML and this expression of CD2 has been supported by the detection of messenger RNA (Ball *et al.*, 1991).

Table 3.7 Scoring system for biphenotypic acute leukaemia

Scoring points	B cell	Lineage T cell	Myeloid
2	cCD22	cCD3	MPO*
1	CD10	CD2	CD13
	CD19	CD5	CD33
0.5	Tdt	Tdt	CD11b/c
		CD7	CD14/15

c, cytoplasmic.
* Demonstration of MPO by any method. To qualify as biphenotypic the score of two separate lineages should be more than 2.

Preliminary data suggest that there is a higher incidence of rearrangement of lymphocyte functional genes, such as the IgH and TCR genes, in cases defined as biphenotypic. Also there is a higher incidence of chromosome translocations, including cases with t(9;22). In the study mentioned above (Hanson *et al.*, 1992) chromosomal analysis was carried out in 42 of 52 acute biphenotypic leukaemic cases; a clonal abnormality was found on 31 of 42 cases. By restricting the criteria for the diagnosis of biphenotypic cases it may be possible to identify a distinct group of acute leukaemias which probably represent stem cell malignancies with multilineage gene expression and distinct clinical and biological features.

Phenotypic analysis of the lymphoproliferative disorders

Lymphoid malignances may be divided into two groups: (a) the leukaemias and lymphomas derived from precursor cells of T and B lymphocytes which are more common in childhood and are represented morphologically by lymphoblasts, i.e. the lymphoblastic leukaemias; (b) chronic lymphoid leukaemias, non-Hodgkin's lymphoma (NHL) and leukaemia/lymphoma syndromes resulting from immunologically competent B- and T-lymphoid cells, which are more common in adults (Fig. 3.5). This latter group is classified according to the FAB group proposals (Bennett *et al.*, 1989). Of these disorders the B-cell diseases are the most common and include chronic lymphocytic leukaemia (CLL), B-cell prolymphocytic leukaemia (B-PLL) and hairy cell leukaemia (HCL) (Catovsky and Foa, 1990). The treatment modalities used for the B-cell leukaemias are often quite different and it is important to make the correct diagnosis. B-PLL, for example does not respond to the chemotherapy used in CLL such as chlorambucil and prednisolone; HCL shows a specific response to interferon-α, deoxycoformycin and chlorodeoxyadenosine, agents which are less active in CLL and B-PLL (Catovsky, 1992). The clinical and phenotypic characteristics of this group are summarized in Table 3.8.

Blood and bone marrow features resembling B-leukaemia may develop from tissue-based NHL. Involvement of the blood is seen in most cases of splenic lymphoma with circulating villous lymphocytes (SLVL) (Mulligan and Catovsky, 1992), in a minority of follicular lymphomas and mantle zone (intermediate or centrocytic) (Pombo de Oliveira *et al.*, 1989) and occasionally in large cell NHL (Bain *et al.*, 1991). Chromosomal abnormalities which are typical of some of these NHLs, are also found in cases in the leukaemic phase (Table 3.9). It may prove useful to sort such cells for subsequent polymerase chain reaction (PCR) analysis (see below).

The importance of these disorders is twofold. First they present problems of differential diagnosis with the other leukaemias, particularly with CLL. Also, cases of large cell NHL often mimic morphologically acute leukaemias of the monoblastic type M5. Second, these diseases have a variable prognosis and often require a different treatment

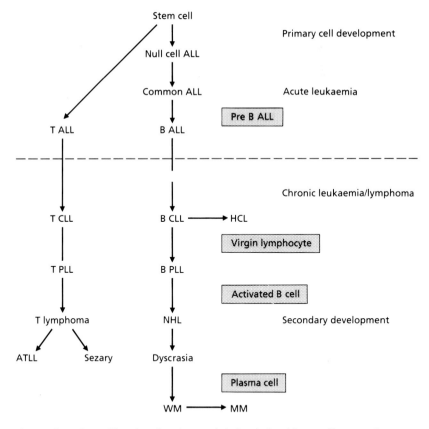

Fig. 3.5 Lymphoproliferative disorders and their relationship to cell maturation.

Table 3.8 Features of mature B-cell leukaemias

Feature	CLL	B-PLL	HCL
WBC (10^9/l)	10–50 (some >50)	>50 (often <100)	<10 (rare >10)
Monocytopenia	−	−	++
Cell type	Lymphocyte	Prolymphocyte	Hairy cell
Immunophenotype*			
CD5	++	±	−
CD23	++	±	−
SmIg	±	++	++
FMC7	±	−	++
B-ly-7	−	−	++

* All cases positive with pan-B MoAb, e.g. CD19, 20, 37 and HLA-DR. FMC7 and B-ly-7 are MoAb with specificity for HCL.

approach. For example SLVL benefits from splenectomy, while chemo-therapy is of little value.

There are two types of leukaemias of mature T cells: T-prolymphocytic leukaemia (Matutes *et al.*, 1991) and large granular lymphocytic (LGL; Mulligan and Catovsky, 1992). The main features of these two disorders are given in Table 3.10 together with features of two common syndromes of mature T-cells, T-cell leukaemia/lymphoma and Sézary's syndrome. The prognosis of most types of mature T cells is poor with survivals less than a year.

Phenotypic analysis of the myeloproliferative disorders

Classification of the myeloproliferative disorders is difficult because there is a spectrum of disease without clearly defined parameters and because one disorder is capable of transforming into another. The most prevalent disorder is chronic granulocytic leukaemia (CGL) also known as chronic myeloid leukaemia (CML). The Philadelphia chromosome (PH') is an acquired translocation between chromosomes 22 and 9 and is highly characteristic of CGL, being present in 96% of cases.

It is clear that AML is a disorder of stem cell common to granulocytopoiesis, erythropoiesis and probably thrombocytopoiesis. Most descendants from the diseased stem cell fail to differentiate and remain as blast cells. In CML the progeny of the leukaemic stem cells have differentiated to some extent and may give rise to functionally useful cells. The mechanism by which useful haemopoiesis is apparently suppressed in the presence of leukaemic cells has remained enigmatic so far (Killmann, 1991). However, of those patients with this disorder 80% transform to acute leukaemia, usually myeloid (Colvin and Newland, 1988).

Cytogenetics of acute leukaemia

An important development for the classification of acute leukaemias has been the recognition of non-random chromosome abnormalities

Table 3.9 Features of B-cell NHL in leukaemic phase

Feature	Follicular lymphoma	Mantle zone	SLVL	Large cell
WBC (10^9/l)	20–200	25–250	10–30	5–100
Cell type	Small	Medium	Villous	Blast-like
Immunophenotype*				
CD5	±	++	–	±
CD23	±	±	–	–
CD10	++	±	±	+
SmIg	++	++	++	++
FMC7	++	++	++	+
'M' band	–	–	++	–
Karyotype	t(14;18)	t(11;14)	t(11;14) in 20%	t(14;18) in 20%

* All cases positive with pan-B MoAb, e.g. CD19, 20, 37, HLA-DR.

associated with certain forms of leukaemia defined by morphology and cytochemistry, such as FAB types L3, M2, M3, and M5, or by immuno-phenotype such as early B, pre-B and B-ALL. This led to the MIC proposals for a classification based on morphology (M), immunology (I) and cytogenetics (C) (First and Second MIC Cooperative Study Groups, 1986, 1988). Although all three parameters contribute to the classification of leukaemias, some types of acute leukaemias can only be defined by their karyotype (Table 3.11). However, although many leukaemias may be defined without their karyotype there is evidence to suggest that some translocations are associated with poor prognosis. Pre-B ALL cases with t(1;19) have a worse prognosis. Similarly, ALLs with t(4;11) and t(9;22) are associated with very poor prognosis in both adults and children (Pui *et al.*, 1991; Fletcher *et al.*, 1991). Such patients are eligible for more radical treatment programmes such as bone marrow transplan-tation, thus their identification is imperative. The relatively rare t(8;16), a form of AML associated with erythrophagocytosis and coagulation features suggestive of fibrinolysis, is also associated with a low remission rate and few long-term survivors (Catovsky and Matutes, 1992).

The importance of chromosomal translocations is not just in disease classification but also in their key role of identifying genes located at breakpoint regions which have a role in the pathogenesis of some leukaemias. M3 and t(15;17) is probably the best example of a well-characterized disease where the cloning and identification of the retinoic acid receptor-α gene has a bearing on the differentiation and therapeutic effect obtained by All-trans retinoic acid in patients with M3 (Lo Coco *et al.*, 1991).

In addition to translocations other structural abnormalities can occur in leukaemic blasts, these include partial deletions and inversions. At the Eleventh Human Gene Mapping Workshop at least 80 different recurrent chromosomal abnormalities were recorded in acute leukaemias

Table 3.10 Features of mature T-cell lymphomas and syndromes

Feature	T-PLL	LGL Leukaemia	ATLL	Sézary's syndrome
WBC (10⁹/l)	>100	>5	>20	>10
Neutropenia	−	++	−	−
Cell type	Prolymphocytic	Large granular	Pleomorphic flower-like	Ceribri form
Immunophenotype*				
CD7	++	+	±	+
CD4	++	±	++	++
CD8	+	++	−	−
CD25	±	−	++	±
CD56,57,11b.16	−	++	−	−
Karyotype	inv(14;18q)	Variable; always clonal		

* Always positive with pan-T MoAb, e.g. CD3 and CD5 and negative with CD1a and anti-TdT.

Table 3.11 Chromosome translocations which define distinct types of acute leukaemia

Translocation	Leukaemia
t(1;19)	Pre-B ALL
t(4;11)	Null-ALL
t(9;22)	Ph$^+$ ALL
t(6;9)	AML with basophilia
t(8;16)	M5 with erythrophagocytosis

In these cases the karyotype is essential to define the leukaemia. In other known associations such as t(8;14) and L3, t(8;21) and M2, t(15;7) and M3 and t(9;11) and M5 the leukaemia is well defined by other criteria.

(Mitelman *et al.*, 1992) and it is evident that this number will increase in coming years (Berger, 1992; Table 3.12). In the early 1980s many of the translocations occurring in malignant cells were claimed to involve genes previously characterized as retroviral oncogenes. It appears now that most of the recently cloned genes involved in chromosomal re-arrangement of acute leukaemia have their DNA characteristic motifs of transcription factors (helix-loop, zinc finger, leucine zipper, homeobox, hormone receptors) that are normally implicated in cell differentiation and proliferation (Hunter, 1991; Cleary, 1991; Table 3.13). Analysis of the proteins encoded by these genes offers a new approach to under-standing the consequences of the alterations, which result in abnormal differentiation and proliferation of the leukaemic cells. Many of these chromosome abnormalities may be detected by PCR. The use of PCR for diagnosis, follow-up and detection of minimal residual disease is highly desirable (see below). Flow cytometry may be used to sort malignant cells for use in PCR and for analysis of mRNA in cells by primed *in situ* hybridization (see Chapter 10).

Flow-sorted chromosomes for use in fluorescent *in situ* hybridization studies has also been developed (Young, 1992). The presence of certain characteristic chromosomal translocations can be detected using break-point specific probes (cosmids or yeast artefactual chromosome, YACs) which either span or lie adjacent to such breakpoints. The same approach can be used to detect both gene deletions and amplifications when seen as homogeneously staining regions (HSRs).

Whole chromosome probe mixtures (or paints) can be used where the precise molecular nature of the event is uncertain. Chromosomal *in situ* hybridization (or painting) has been performed using *Alu* elements and random primer-mediated PCR products from small quan-tities (250–500) of flow-sorted normal and abnormal chromosomes. The *Alu* PCR method allows the amplification of human DNA of unknown sequence from a complex mixture of human DNA (Nelson and Caskey, 1989). The method makes use of the ubiquitous *Alu* repeat sequence found in human DNA. Approximately 900 000 copies of this 300 b.p. sequence are distributed throughout the human genome. Although there is considerable variation between copies of the *Alu* repeat, a

Table 3.12 Structural chromosome abnormalities in acute leukaemias

Rearrangement		Disease	Rearrangement		Disease
t(1;3)	(p36;q21)	AML, MDS	del(9)	(p13−22)	ALL
t(1;7)	(p11;q11)	AML, MDS, PV	del(9)	(q22)	AML
t(1;11)	(p32;q23)	ALL	t(9;11)	(p21−22;q23)	AML, M5, ALL
t(1;11)	(q21;q23)	AML, M4−M5	t(9;12)	(p11;p12)	ALL
t(1;14)	(p32−34;q11)	T-ALL	dic(9;12)	(p11−13;p11−12)	ALL
t(1;17)	(p36;q21)	AML	t(9;22)	(q34;q11)	AML, ALL, CML
t(1;19)	(q23;p13)	Pre B-ALL	t(10;11)	(p12−14;q13−21)	AML, M5
t(1;22)	(p13;q1)	AML, M7	t(10;14)	(q24;q11)	T-ALL
del(2)	(p23)	AML	i(11q)		AML
del(2)	(p21)	AML	del(11)	(p11−12p14−15)	AML
t(2;8)	(p12;q24)	ALL-L3	del(11)	(q14−23)	ALL
ins(3;3)	(q26;q21;q26)	AML, MDS	del(11)	(q23)	AML, M5
inv(3)	(q21;q26)	AML, MDS	t(11;11)	(q23;q25)	AML, M5
t(3;3)	(q21;q31)	AML	t(11;14)	(p15;q11)	T-ALL
t(3;5)	(q25;q34−35)	AML	t(11;14)	(p13;q11)	T-ALL
t(3;21)	(p14;q22)	AML	t(11;17)	(q23;q21)	AML
t(4;11)	(q21;q23)	ALL, AML, mixed AL	t(11;17)	(q23;q25)	AML
del(5)	(q12−31;q31−35)	AML, MDS	t(11;19)	(q23;p13)	AML, ALL, mixed AL
t(5;14)	(q31;q32)	ALL with eosinophils	t(11;20)	(p15;q11)	AML
			t(X11)	(q24−25;q13)	AML
t(5;16)	(q32;q33)	AML	i(12p)		AML
t(5;16)	(q33;q22)	AML	del(12)	(p11;p13)	ALL, AML
del(6)	(q13−14;q21−27)	ALL	t(12;14)	(q24;q32)	AML
t(6;9)	(p23;q34)	AML, M2, MDS	t(12;17)	(p12−13;q12)	ALL
t(6;11)	(p27;q23)	AML, M5	i(14q)		AML
i(7q)		AML, MDS	inv(14)	(q11;q32)	T-CLL, T-ALL
del(7)	(p12;p21)	AML	del(14)	(q11−24;q22−32)	ALL
del(7)	(q11)	ALL	t(14;22)	(q32;q11)	ALL
del(7)	(q22)	AML, MDS	t(15;17)	(q22;q12−21)	AML, M3, M3v
del(7)	(q32)	ALL	del(16)	(q22)	AML, M4EO
dic(7;9)	(p11;q11)	ALL	inv(16)	(p13;q22)	AML, M4EO
t(7;9)	(q35;q32)	T-ALL	t(16;16)	(p13;q22)	AML, M4EO
t(7;9)	(q35;q34)	T-ALL	t(16;21)	(p11;q22)	AML
t(7;11)	(p15;p15)	AML	del(17)	(q22)	AML
t(7;11)	(q35;p13)	T-ALL	del(20)	(q11−13)	AML, MDS MPD, PV
t(7;14)	(q35;q11)	T-ALL	i(21q)		AML, MDS
del(8)	(q22)	AML	del(22)	(q11−13)	ALL, AML
t(8;12)	(p21−22;q13)	ALL	del(X)	(q24)	AML
t(8;14)	(q24;q11)	T-ALL	idic(X)	(q13)	AML
t(8;14)	(q24;q32)	ALL, L3			
t(8;16)	(q11;q13)	AML, M5			
t(8;21)	(q22;q13)	AML, M2			
t(8;22)	(q24;q11)	ALL, L3			
t(9p)		ALL			

ALL, acute lymphoblastic leukaemia; AML, acute myeloblastic leukaemia (M2, M3, M3v, M4, M4EO, M5); CML, chronic myeloid leukaemia; MDS, myeloid dysplastic syndrome; MPD, myeloproliferative disorder; PV, polycythemia vera.

del, deletion; dic, dicentric; i, isochromosome; ins, insertion; inv, inversion; t, translocation; p, short arm of chromosome; q, long arm of chromosome.

For nomenclature see Table 3.13.

consensus sequence has been established and there are regions of the repeat that are reasonably well conserved. PCR primers designed to recognize these conserved regions are used to allow inter-*Alu* amplification for the isolation of human DNA from complex sources. PCR products are generated from a range of normal chromosomes using the designed primers and have been shown to be effective in *in situ* hybridization for the identification of the appropriate chromosome. This technique has been used with abnormal chromosomes and used to generate region-specific paints. A consequence of this work is that chromosome paints specific for common aberrant chromosomes can be generated and made widely available for clinical use.

Further considerations

There are a number of problems associated with flow cytometric immunophenotypic analysis of leukaemias. The first relates to the identification of the blast population. If the blood or bone marrow sample from the patient contains predominantly blast cells, these may be identified by atypical light scattering properties. However, if this is not the case, dual or triple fluorescence studies may be necessary (see Chapter 4). Second, as can be seen from Table 3.14 the number of blasts reactive with a given antibody is highly variable. For these reasons immunophenotyping alone (at least at present) is not sufficient to classify all leukaemias.

Immune equilibrium studies

Helper and suppressor T lymphocytes have been used to study immune equilibrium. Although ratios significantly different from the normal range (0.6−2.8) have been found in many diseases, functional studies have all too often not correlated with immune imbalance, perhaps because there is also normal circadian variation as described above and factors such as exercise, which influence cell numbers (Fry *et al.*, 1992). One exception is the imbalance in the acquired immune deficiency syndrome (AIDS). Early in the course of this disorder, affected individuals have reversed ratio due to profoundly decreased $CD4^+$ T-helper cells, and this is highly predictive of clinical disease (Kidd and Vogt, 1989; Taylor *et al.*, 1989; Smith *et al.*, 1991; Katz *et al.*, 1992; Saah *et al.*, 1992).

A decreased expression of the membrane inhibitor of complement-mediated cytolysis (CD59) on T lymphocytes from human immunodeficiency virus (HIV)-infected patients has also been shown (Weiss *et al.*, 1992). However, the decreased expression does not correlate with the clinical stage of the disease. Decreased CD59 expression may result in increased susceptibility of T lymphocytes from HIV-infected patients to complement mediated lysis.

Table 3.13 Chromosomal abnormalities and genes involved in acute leukaemia

ALL B lineage	Cytogenetics		Genes
Pre-B	t(1;19)	(q23;p13)	PBX1, E2A, homeobox transcription factor
L3	t(8;13)	(q24;q32)	*myc*, IGH oncogene with HLH motif
L3	t(8;22)	(q34;q11)	MVC, IGL
L3	t(2;8)	(p12;q24)	IGK, *myc*
	t(9;22)	(q34;q11)	abl, bcr
	t(5;14)	(q31;q32)	il3, *igh*
ALL T cell	t(1;14)	(p32;q11)	TAL1, TCRD, HLH motif
	t(7;9)	(q35;q32)	TCRB
	t(7;9)	(q35;q34)	TCRB, TANI, homologue of notch
	t(7;10)	(q35;q24)	TCRB, HOX11 homeobox
	t(7;19)	(q35;p13)	TCRB, LYL1 HLH motif
	t(8;14)	(q24;q11)	*myc*, TCRA
	t(10;14)	(q24;q11)	HOX11, TCRD homeobox
	t(11;14)	(p15;q11)	Rhom1, TCRD LIM domain
	t(11;14)	(p13;q11)	Rhom2, TCRD LIM domain
AML	t(6;9)	(p23;q34)	DEK, CAN
	t(8;21)	(q22;q22)	AML1
	t(9;22)	(q34;q11)	abl, bcr
	t(15;17)	(q22;q12−21)	PRL, RARa

IGH, immunoglobulin heavy chain; IGK, immunoglobulin K chain; IGL, immunoglobulin I chain; RARa, retinoic acid receptor-α; Rhom1, Rhom2, Rhombotin 1 and 2; TCRA, TCRB, TCRD T-cell receptor a, b and d chains; *myc, abl, bcr* proto-oncogenes.

Nomenclature
A translocation is indicated by the letter *t* followed by parentheses which include the chromosomes and bands involved, e.g. t(2;5) (q21;q23). This specifies that breakage and reunion have occurred at bands 2q21 and 5q31 in the long arms of chromosomes 2 and 5, respectively. The segments distal to these bands have been exchanged between the two chromosomes. The derivative chromosome with the lowest number (i.e. chromosome 2) is designated first.

Immune status following immunotherapy

The assessment of immune status following immunotherapy, and correlation between immunological status and clinical course, are important in a variety of situations. After bone marrow transplantation the patient is severely immune deficient. It is therefore necessary to monitor lymphocyte subpopulations to ensure that: (a) a normal haemopoietic system develops (Ericson *et al.*, 1992); (b) the onset of graft-*vs*-host disease is identified so that chemotherapy may be modified (Buckner *et al.*, 1992; Goldman, 1992; Santos, 1992); (c) graft-*vs*-leukaemia in CML is followed (Yiang *et al.*, 1991; Goldman, 1992); and (d) development of residual disease is detected (see Chapter 4 and below).

The recovery of lymphocyte subpopulations after bone marrow transplantation may take up to a year (Fig. 3.6), with the CD8$^+$ T-cell population recovering first. These CD8$^+$ cells are LGLs which exhibit natural killer cell activity (Ault *et al.*, 1985; Jacobs *et al.*, 1992). The CD4$^+$ T lymphocytes may not reach normal levels for at least 6 months after transplantation.

During the past few years peripheral blood stem cells (PBSC) have been used as an alternative to bone marrow for use in autologous transplantation (Gale *et al.*, 1992). Their levels are increased after standard chemotherapy and after high dose chemotherapy such as cyclophosphamide. The myeloid growth factors G-CSF and GM-CSF have also been used to enhance stem cell production. The generation of stem cells may be monitored by determining the per cent CD34$^+$ cells.

Detection of MRD

Leukaemia relapse is still the major cause of failure in today's treatment

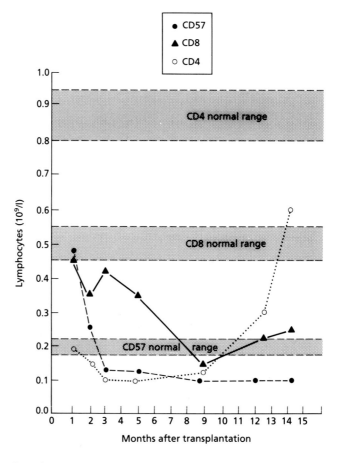

Fig. 3.6 Lymphocyte recovery post bone marrow transplantation.

of acute leukaemia. Relapse rates vary from 60 to 80% after chemotherapy
and from 20 to 50% after allogeneic or autologous bone marrow transplantation respectively. MRD is defined as those relatively few leukaemic
cells which have survived initial remission-induction chemotherapy
(Fig. 3.7). The number of cells in the entire bone marrow compartment
is in the order of 10^{12}. The conventional detection level of MRD of less
than 5% blast cells would require 10^{10} leukaemic cells to be present in
the bone marrow. Thus in the past years, clinical research has focused
on developing methods to decrease the detection level for MRD
(Lowenberg et al., 1990; Hagenbeek, 1992). Detection of MRD in human
leukaemia is currently performed in three ways: (a) immunological
detection of cell surface, cytoplasmic and nuclear antigens; (b) analysis
of abnormal chromosomes; and (c) PCR analysis of DNA and RNA.

Studies with monoclonal antibodies and flow cytometry have been
used to detect MRD. In bone marrow the distribution of MRD is
extremely heterogeneous. Analysis of marrow samples from different
bones yields differences in leukaemic cell frequencies (Martens et al.,
1987). The measured leukaemic frequency in one specific marrow sample
may not reflect the concentration in other compartments. Furthermore,
in humans one bone marrow aspiration contains only 0.0001% of the
entire marrow compartment. Thus quantitation of MRD in a given
patient based on a simple bone marrow aspiration is likely to be
unsuccessful. However, the presence of specific combinations of antigens
on/in normal marrow cells is used to detect small quantities of leukaemic
cells (Table 3.15). Campana et al. (1990b) used these combinations to
detect one leukaemic cell per 10 000 normal cells in marrow samples
which were morphologically in complete remission and the detection of
MRD correlated with the occurrence of subsequent leukaemia relapse.
The majority (75%) of AML blasts are TdT positive (Adriaansen, 1990).

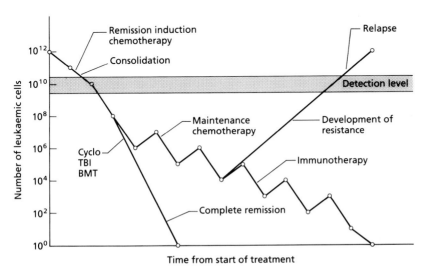

Fig. 3.7 Schematic representation of MRD in acute leukaemia. Cyclo, cyclophosphamide; TBI, total body irradiation; BMT, bone marrow transplantation.

Table 3.14 Antibody reactivity (%) with acute leukaemias
(a) Lymphoblastic leukaemias

Diagnosis	No. of cases		% Reactivity with panel of antibodies					
			CD2	CD19	CD13	CD33	CD10	TdT
Pre-B common ALL	10	Mean	9.2	46.3	8.5	8.5	57.2	—
		Range	0–39	1–47	0.53	0–69	10–77	—
T-ALL	9	Mean	66.2	9.1	4.3	6.1	6.9	85.0
		Range	9–97	0–20	0–7	0–7	0–15	80–90
B-ALL	2	Mean	25.0	40.0	1.0	1.0	3.5	—
		Range	18–31	20–60	1.0	1.0	1–7	—

(b) Myeloblastic leukaemias

Diagnosis	No. of cases		% Reactivity with panel of antibodies						
			CD2	CD19	CD13	CD33	CD10	*R10	CD41
FAB M1	9	Mean	4.4	1.4	23.4	61.7	6.3	—	—
		Range	0–10	1–3	0–70	20–91	0–17	—	—
M2	7	Mean	11.0	5.3	24.3	37.6	2.9	—	—
		Range	1–30	1–16	6–69	7–69	0–11	—	—
M3	1	—	0	0	34.0	6.0	7.0	—	—
M4	6	Mean	7.0	3.5	61.0	79.0	1.0	—	—
		Range	0–16	0–9	6–90	76–90	0–3	—	—
M5	1	—	13.0	16.0	87.0	89.0	20.0	—	—
M6	3	Mean	36.0	5.3	5.9	7.3	1.0	55.3	—
		Range	8–59	2–9	2–8	4–13	0–2	26–88	—
M7	2	Mean	10.0	2.5	32.0	26.0	1.0	—	30.0
		Range	8–12	1–4	24–40	19–33	1.0	—	22–38

* R10 Antibody specific for erythroid glycophorin antibody.

Table 3.15 Detection of MRD in sample morphologically in complete remission

Cell type	Combination
T-ALL	cCD3/TdT
B-lineage ALL	CD13/TdT
	CD33/TdT
Pre-B-ALL	cu/TdT
AML	CD13/TdT
	CD33/TdT
	CD7/TdT

Also the presence of TdT-positive cells in red-cell-free CSF from ALL patients is highly predictive for the development of overt leptomeningeal leukaemia (Hooijkas *et al.*, 1989). TdT-positive cells are not present in normal CSF and TdT detection is more sensitive than conventional cytology.

False-negative results in the immunological detection of MRD may be due to: (a) the presence of less than $10^{-4}-10^{-5}$ leukaemic cells in the sample under study; (b) sampling error due to heterogeneous distribution of cells within the marrow; and (c) phenotypic switch. A limited number of cases have been reported in which a phenotypic switch occurs between analysis at presentation and relapse (Campana *et al.*, 1990b).

Apart from conventional cytogenetic analysis where chromosomal aberrations are derived from metaphases (mitotic cells), flow karyotyping has been developed where chromosomes in suspension are stained with fluorescent dyes. The dyes specifically bind to either C-G or A-T base pairs in the DNA. Upon excitation by dual laser beam flow cytometers every chromosome is individually represented in a flow karyogram (see Chapter 9). In this way numerical aberrations present in 40% of the acute leukaemias and translocations ($10-15\%$ in ALL, $25-30\%$ in AML) can be detected. In addition to conventional karyotyping, flow karyotyping offers the advantage that thousands of chromosomes per second may be analysed in an objective, quantitative way, yielding a detection limit in the order of 10^{-2} as compared with $10^{-1}-10^{-2}$ for conventional cytogenetic analysis. The use of fluorescence *in situ* hybridization with chromosome specific probes has been employed on metaphase spreads (Poddighe *et al.*, 1991) and may be performed on flow-sorted interphase cells (as described above) to detect numerical aberrations and translocations. This procedure will lead to a detection limit of 10^{-3} or lower for MRD.

The PCR may be used to detect MRD by selectively amplifying small defined regions of nucleic acid which are characteristic or unique to the malignant cell. Tumour-specific nucleic acid sequences are found at: (a) breakpoints of chromosomal translocations; (b) junctions of re-arranged receptor genes; and (c) sites of mutations in various oncogenes. These nucleic acid aberrations are used to detect MRD (Van Dongen *et al.*, 1991). PCR has several limitations in detecting MRD due to false-negative and false-positive reactions. False-positives result from: (a) contamination of the reaction by exogenous amplifiable template; and (b) amplification of DNA sequences derived from dead cells or leukaemic cell debris. False-negatives arise from: (a) the presence of multiple, rearranged subclones present at diagnosis (oligoclonality); (b) further recombinations of DNA sequences in a subpopulation of leukaemic cells (clonal evolution); (c) sampling error due to heterogeneous distribution of leukaemic cells in the bone marrow; and (d) the presence of less than $10^{-5}-10^{-6}$ leukaemic cells in the sample. However, the use of PCR enables MRD detection levels of between 10^{-4} and 10^{-6} in the majority of patients.

In conclusion although MRD may be detected by several methods there are a number of questions that remain to be answered. Which fraction of leukaemic cells that are detected are capable of *in vivo* clonogenic expansion? Does detection of MRD predict relapse? Is eradication of all leukaemic cells required to achieve a cure? The answers will come from systematic studies with serial bone marrow sampling in individual patients providing insight into the natural history and kinetics of MRD. This in turn will provide information on the development of leukaemia and lead to the molecular definition of disease states which may be detected by flow cytometry.

References

Adri A, Noorloos A, Beck AM, Mellof CJM (1980) Cryopreservation of cells for immunological typing of non-Hodgkin lymphoma. *Cancer Res.* **40**: 2890–2894.

Adriaansen GJA, van Dongen JJM, Kappers-Klune MC (1990) Terminal deoxynucleotidyl transferase positive subpopulations occur in the majority of ANLL: implications for the detection of minimal disease. *Leukemia* **4**: 404–410.

Andersson U, Gunther A, Dohlsten M, Moller G (1989) Characterisation of individual tumor necrosis factor alpha and beta producing cells after polyclonal T cell activation. *J. Immunol. Methods* **123**: 233–240.

Ashmore LM, Shopp GM, Edwards BS (1989) Lymphocyte subset analysis by flow cytometry. Comparison of three different staining techniques and effects of storage. *J. Immunol. Methods* **118**: 209–215.

Ault KA, Antin JH, Ginsberg SH *et al.* (1985) The phenotype of recovering lymphoid cell populations following bone marrow transplantation. *J. Exp. Med.* **161**: 1483–1502.

Bain B, Matutes E, Robinson D *et al.* (1991) Leukaemia as a manifestation of large cell lymphoma. *Br. J. Haematol.* **77**: 301–310.

Ball ED, Davis RB, Griffin JD, Mayer RJ, Davey FR, Bloomfield CD (1991) Prognostic value of lymphocyte surface markers in acute leukemia. *Blood* **77**: 2242–2250.

Behnken LJ, Rogge H, Emmerich W, Musil J, Lohr G (1984) Measurement of lymphocyte subsets in EDTA blood by flow cytometry: studies on stability and reference range. *Blut* **49**: 286 (Abstr. 204).   ·

Bennett JM, Catovsky D, Daniel MT *et al.* (1976) Proposals for the classification of the acute lymphoblastic leukaemias. French–American–British (FAB) Co-operative group. *Br. J. Haematol.* **33**: 451–458.

Bennett JM, Catovsky D, Daniel MT *et al.* (1989) Proposals for the classification of chronic (mature) B and T cell leukaemias. *J. Clin. Pathol.* **42**: 567–584.

Bennett JM, Catovsky D, Daniel MT *et al.* (1991) Proposal for the recognition of minimally differentiated acute myeloid leukaemia (AML-MO). *Br. J. Haematol.* **78**: 325–329.

Berger R (1992) Cytogenetics of acute leukemia. *Leukemia* **6** (Suppl. 2): 7–11.

Boyum A (1968) Separation of leukocytes from blood and bone marrow. *Scand. J. Clin. Lab. Invest.* **21** (Suppl.): 97.

Braylan RC, Benson NA, Nourse V, Kruth HS (1982) Correlation analysis of cellular DNA membrane antigens and light scatter of human lymphoid cells. *Cytometry* **2**: 337–343.

Brown G, Greaves MF (1974) Enumeration of absolute numbers of T and B lymphocytes in human blood. *Scand. J. Immunol.* **3**: 161–172.

Brunsting A, Mullaney PF (1974) Differential light scattering from spherical mammalian cells. *Biophys. J.* **14**: 439–453.

Buckner C, Doney K, Sanders F, Petersen F, Apellbaum F (1992) Marrow transplantation for patients with acute lymphoblastic leukemia. *Leukemia* **6** (Suppl. 2): 191–193.

Campana D, Coustan-Smith E, Janossy G (1990a) Immunophenotyping in haematological diagnosis. *Bailliére's Clin. Haematol.* **3**: 906–909.

Campana D, Coustan-Smith E, Janossy G (1990b) The immunological detection of minimal residual disease. *Blood* **76**: 163–171.

Carter PH, Resto-Ruiz S, Washington GC *et al.* (1992) Flow cytometric analysis of whole blood, three anticoagulants and five cell preparations. *Cytometry* **13**: 68–74.

Catovsky D (1992) Lymphoproliferative disorders. *Br. J. Haematol.* **82**: 46–49.

Catovsky D, Foa R (1990) *The Lymphoid Leukaemias.* Butterworth, London.

Catovsky D, Matutes E (1992) The classification of acute leukemia. *Leukemia* **6** (Suppl. 2): 1–6.

Catovsky D, Matutes E, Bucchrei MT *et al.* (1991) A classification of acute leukaemia for the 1990's. *Ann. Haematol.* **62**: 16–21.

Chan LC, Pegram SM, Greaves MF (1985) Contribution of immunophenotyping to the classification and differential diagnosis of leukaemia. *Lancet* **i**: 475–479.

Chapple MR, Johnson GD, Davidson RS (1990) Fluorescence quenching, a practical problem in flow cytometry. *J. Microscopy* **159**: 245–253.

Cleary ML (1991) Oncogenic conversion of transcription factors by chromosomal translocations. *Cell* **66**: 619–622.

Clevenger CV, Bauer KD, Epstein AL (1985) A method for simultaneous nuclear immunofluorescence and DNA quantification using monoclonal antibodies and flow cytometry. *Cytometry* **6**: 280–286.

Cline MJ, Lehrer RI (1968) Phagocytosis by human monocytes. *Blood* **32**: 423–430.

College of American Pathologists (1988) *Comprehensive Hematology Limited Coagulation Module Survey.* CAP Surveys Set H1-A.

Colvin BT, Newland AC (1988) *Haematology.* Pocket consultant. Blackwell Scientific Publications, Oxford, pp. 213–214.

Drach J, Gattringer C, Glassi H, Schwarting R, Stein H, Huber H (1989) Simultaneous flow cytometric analysis of surface markers and nuclear Ki-67 antigen in leukaemia and lymphoma. *Cytometry* **10**: 743–749.

Dux R, Kindler A, Lennartz K, Rajewsky MF (1991) Calibration of fluorescent intensities to quantify antibody binding surface determinants of cell subpopulations by flow cytometry. *Cytometry* **12**: 422–428.

Ericson SG, Colby E, Welch L, Ball ED (1992) Engraftment of leukocyte subsets following autologous bone marrow transplantation in acute myeloid leukaemia using antimyeloid (CD14 and CD15) monoclonal antibody-purged bone marrow. *Bone Marrow Transplant.* **9**: 129–137.

Fletcher JA, Lynch EA, Kimbell VM, Donnelly M, Tantravahi R, Sallan SE (1991) Translocation (9;22) is associated with extremely poor prognosis in intensively treated children with acute leukemia. *Blood* **77**: 435–439.

Fletcher MA, Baron GC, Ashman MR, Fischl MA, Klimas NG (1987) Use of whole blood methods in assessment of immune parameters in immunodeficiency states. *Diagn. Clin. Immunol.* **5**: 69–73.

Fry RW, Morton AR, Crawford GP, Keast D (1992) Cell numbers and *in vitro* responses of leukocytes and lymphocyte subpopulations following maximal exercise and interval training sessions of different intensities. *Eur. J. Appl. Physiol.* **64**: 218–227.

Fujii Y, Okamura M, Inada K, Nakahara K, Matsuda H (1992) CD45 isoform expression during T cell development in the thymus. *Eur. J. Immunol.* **22**: 1843–1850.

Gale RP, Heron P, Juttner C (1992) Blood stem cell transplants come of age. *Bone Marrow Transplant.* **9**: 151–155.

Gandler W, Shapiro H (1990) Logarithmic amplifiers. *Cytometry* **11**: 447–450.

Goldman JM (1992) Bone marrow transplantation for chronic myeloid leukemia. *Leukemia* **6** (Suppl. 1): 22–23.

Greaves MF (1986) Differentiation-linked leukaemogenesis in lymphocytes. *Science* **234**: 697–704.

Greaves MF (1992) Acute lymphoblastic leukaemia. *Br. J. Haematol.* **82**: 1–2.

Greaves MF, Chan LC, Furley AJW, Watt SM, Molgaard HV (1986) Lineage promiscuity in haemopoietic differentiation and leukaemia. *Blood* **67**: 1–11.

Griffin JD, Ritz J, Nadler LM, Schlossman SF (1981) Expression of myeloid differentiation antigens on normal and malignant myeloid cells. *J. Clin. Invest.* **68**: 932–941.

Hagenbeek A (1992) Minimal residual disease in leukemia: state of the art 1991. *Leukemia* **6** (Suppl. 1): 12–17.

Hamblin A, Taylor M, Bernhagen J *et al.* (1991) A new method preparing leukocytes for flow cytometry which prevents upregulation of leukocyte integrin expression. *J. Immunol. Methods* **146**: 219–235.

Hanson CA, Abaza M, Sheldon S, Ross CW, Schnitzer B, Stoolman LM (1993) Acute biphenotypic leukaemia; immunophenotypic and cytogenetic analysis. *Br. J. Haematol.* (in press).

Hooijkas H, Hahlen K, Adriaansen HJ, Dekker I, van Dongen JJM (1989) Terminal deoxynucleotidyl transferase (TdT)-positive cells in cerebrospinal fluid and development of overt CNS leukaemia; A 5-year follow-up study in 113 children with TdT-positive leukaemia or non-Hodgkin's disease. *Blood* **74**: 416–422.

Hunter T (1991) Cooperation between oncogenes. *Cell* **64**: 249–270.

Ichikawa Y, Shimizu H, Yoshida M, Arimori S (1992) Two-color flow cytometric analysis of thymic lymphocytes from patients with myesthenia gravis and/or thymoma. *Clin. Immunol. Immunopathol.* **62**: 91–96.

Inns H, Mackerill D, Limbert HJ, Scotts CS (1986) Normal monocyte subpopulations defined by monoclonal antibodies and alpha-napthyl acetate esterase cytochemistry. *Med. Lab. Sci.* **43**: 280–283.

Iwatani Y, Amino N, Hidaka Y *et al.* (1992) Decreases in alpha beta T cell receptor negative T cells and CD8 cells, an increase in CD4$^+$CD8$^+$ cells in active Hashimoto's disease and subacute thyroiditis. *Clin. Exp. Immunol.* **87**: 444–449.

Jacob MC, Favre M, Bensa JC (1991) Membrane permeabilisation with saponin and multiparametric analysis by flow cytometry. *Cytometry* **12**: 550–558.

Jacobberger JW, Fogleman D, Lehman JM (1986) Analysis of intracellular antigens by flow cytometry. *Cytometry* **7**: 356–364.

Jacobs R, Stoll M, Stratmann G, Leo R, Link H, Schmidt RE (1992) CD16, CD56$^+$ natural killer cells after bone marrow transplantation. *Blood* **79**: 3239–3244.

Janossy G, Campana D (1991) In: Catovsky D, ed. *The Leukaemic Cell*, 2nd edn. Churchill Livingstone, Edinburgh, pp. 168–196.

Kamihira S, Sohda H, Atogami S *et al.* (1992) Phenotypic diversity and prognosis of adult T-cell leukaemia. *Leuk. Res.* **16**: 435–441.

Katz MH, Bindman AB, Keane D, Chan AK (1992) CD4 lymphocyte count as an indicator of delay in seeking human immunodeficiency virus-related treatment. *Arch. Intern. Med.* **152**: 1501–1504.

Kidd PG, Vogt RFJ (1989) Report of the workshop on the evaluation of T cell subsets during HIV infection and AIDS. *Clin. Immunol. Immunopathol.* **52**: 3–9.

Killmann SA (1991) Acute leukaemia development, remission/relapse pattern, relationship between normal and leukaemic haemopoiesis, and the 'sleeper-to-feeder' stem cell hypothesis. *Baillières Clin. Haematol.* **4**: 577–598.

Lagaay AM, Bosman CB, Van der Keur M (1990) Gating of so-called 'lymphocytic' cell population for the natural killer cells (CD16$^+$) by flow cytometry causes loss of CD16 positive cells. *J. Immunol. Methods* **133**: 235–244.

Lansdorp PM, Smith C, Safford M, Terstappen LWMM, Thomas TE (1991) Single laser three colour immunofluorescence staining procedures based on energy transfer between phycoerythrin and cyanine 5. *Cytometry* **12**: 723–730.

Levi F, Canon C, Blum JP, Reinberg A, Mathe G (1983) Large amplitude circadian rhythm in helper:suppressor ratio of peripheral blood lymphocytes. *Lancet* **ii**: 462–463.

Levi FA, Canon C, Touitou Y *et al.* (1988) Circadian rhythms in circulating T lymphocyte subsets and plasma testosterone, total and free cortisol in five healthy men. *Clin. Exp. Immunol.* **71**: 329–335.

Lighart GJ, Van Vlokhoven PC, Schuit HRE, Hijmans W (1986) The expanded null cell compartment in ageing: increase in the number of natural killer cells and changes in T cell and NK cell subsets in human blood. *Immunology* **59**: 353–360.

Lo Coco F, Avvisati G, Diverio D, Biondi A, Frontani M, Mandelli F (1991) Rearrangements of the RAR-alpha gene in acute promyelocytic leukaemia: correlations with morphology and immunophenotype. *Br. J. Haematol.* **78**: 494–499.

Loftin KC, Reuben JM, Hersh EM, Sujansky D (1985) Cytoplasmic IgM in leukaemic B cells by flow cytometry. *Leuk. Res.* **9**: 1379–1387.

Loken MR, Shah VO, Datilo KL, Civin CI (1987) Flow cytometric analysis of human bone marrow. *Blood* **70**: 1316–1324.

Lowenberg B, Hagenbeek A (1990) Detection of minimal residual leukaemia by polymerase chain reactions. Proceedings of the Third International Symposium on Minimal Residual Disease in Acute Leukaemia, Rotterdam. *Bone Marrow Transplantation* **6** (Suppl. 1): 1–8.

Martens ACM, Schulz FW, Hagenbeek A (1987) Nonhomogeneous distribution of leukaemia in the bone marrow during minimal residual disease. *Blood* **70**: 1073–1078.

Matutes E, Brito-Babapulle V, Swansbury J *et al.* (1991) Clinical and laboratory features of 78 cases of T-prolymphocytic leukaemia. *Blood* **78**: 3269–3274.

McMann LE, Walterson ML, Hogg LM (1988) Light scattering and cell volume in osmotically stressed and frozen-thawed cells. *Cytometry* **9**: 33–38.

MIC (First) Cooperative Study Group (1986) *Cancer Genet. Cytogenet.* **23**: 189–197.

MIC (Second) Cooperative Study Group (1988) *Cancer Genet. Cytogenet.* **30**: 1–15.

Mitelman F, Kaneko Y, Trent J (1992) Report of the committee on chromosome changes in neoplasia. Human Gene Mapping 11. *Genes. Chromosom. Cancer* **5**: 57–66.

Mullaney PF, Dean PN (1970) The small angle light scattering of biological cells. *Biophys. J.* **10**: 764–772.

Mulligan SP, Catovsky D (1992) Splenic lymphoma with villous lymphocytes. *Leuk. Lymphoma* **6**: 97–105.

Nelson DL, Caskey T (1989) *Alu* PCR: The use of repeat sequence primers for amplification of human DNA from complex sources. In Erlich HA, ed. *PCR Technology. Principles and Applications for DNA Amplification.* Macmillan Stockton Press, pp. 112–118.

Paoli P, Reitano M, Battistin S, Castiglia C, Santini G (1984) Enumeration of human lymphocyte subsets by monoclonal antibodies and flow cytometry: a comparative study using whole blood or mononuclear cells separated by density gradient centrifugation. *J. Immunol. Methods* **72**: 349–353.

Parks DH, Bigos M, Moore WA (1988) Logarithmic amplifier transfer function evaluation and procedures for logamp optimization and data correction. *Cytometry* **9** (Suppl. 2): 27.

Poddighe J, Moesker O, Smeets D, Awwad BH, Ramaekers FCS (1991) Metaphase cytogenetics of haematological cancer: comparison of classical karyotyping and *in situ* hybridisation using a panel of eleven chromosome specific DNA probes. *Cancer Res.* **51**: 1959–1967.

Pombo de Oliveira MS, Jaffe ES, Catovsky D (1989) Leukaemic phase of mantle zone (intermediate) lymphoma: its characterisation in 115 cases. *J. Clin. Pathol.* **42**: 962–972.

Prince HK, Hirji K, Waldbeser S, Paeger-Marshall S, Kleinman S, Lanier L (1985) Influence of racial background on the distribution of T cell subsets and Leu 11 positive lymphocytes in healthy blood donors. *Diag. Immunol.* **3**: 33–39.

Pui CH, Frankel LS, Carroll AJ, Borowitz MJ (1991) Clinical characteristics and treatment outcome of childhood acute lymphoblastic leukaemia with t(4;11) (q21;q23): A collaborative study of 40 cases. *Blood* **77**: 440–447.

Rigg KM, Shenton BK, Murray IA, Givan AL, Taylor RMR, Lennard TWJ (1989) A flow cytometric technique for simultaneous analysis of human monoclonal cell surface antigens and DNA. *J. Immunol. Methods* **123**: 177–184.

Ritson A, Bulmer JN (1987) Extraction of leukocytes from human decidua: A comparison of dispersal techniques. *J. Immunol Methods* **104**: 231–236.

Roe R, Robins RA, Laxton RR, Baldwin RW (1985) Kinetics of divalent monoclonal antibody binding to tumour cell surface antigens using flow cytometry: standardisation and mathematical analysis. *Mol. Immunol.* **22**: 11–21.

Rudberg C, Grimelius L, Johansson H (1986) Alteration in density, morphology and parathyroid hormone release of dispersed parathyroid cells from patients with hyperparathyroidism. *Acta Pathol. Microbiol. Scand.* **A**: 94–253.

Saah AJ, Munoz A, Fuo V *et al.* (1992) Predictors of the risk of developing acquired immunodeficiency syndrome within 24 months among gay men seropositive for immunodeficiency virus type I: a report from the multicentre AIDS cohort study. *Am. J. Epidemiol.* **15**: 1147–1155.

Sancho J, Silverman LB, Castigli E *et al.* (1992) Developmental regulation of transmembrane signalling via the T cell antigen receptor/CD3 complex in human T lymphocytes. *J. Immunol.* **148**: 1315–1321.

Santos GW (1992) Allogeneic and autologous bone marrow transplantation in AML. *Leukemia* **6** (Suppl. 1): 102–104.

Schmenti KJ, Jacobberger JW (1992) Fixation of mammalian cells for flow cytometric evaluation of DNA content and nuclear immunofluorescence. *Cytometry* **13**: 48–59.

Schmid I, Schmid P, Giorgi JV (1988) Conversion of logarithmic channel numbers into relative linear fluorescence intensity. *Cytometry* **9**: 533–538.

Schroff RW, Bucana C, Klein RA, Farrell MM, Morgan AC (1984) Detection of intracytoplasmic antigens by flow cytometry. *J. Immunol. Methods* **70**: 167–177.

Shah VO, Civin CI, Loken MR (1988) Flow cytometric analysis of human bone marrow: IV. differential quantitative expression of T200 common leukocyte antigen during normal haematopoiesis. *J. Immunol.* **140**: 1861–1867.

Shih LY, Kuo TT, Dunn P, Liaw SJ (1992) HTLV-1 positive and HTLV-1 negative peripheral T-cell lymphoma in Taiwan Chinese. *Int. J. Cancer* **21**: 186–191.

Slaper-Cortenbach ICM, Admiraal LG, Kerr JM, van Leeuwen EF, von dem Borne AEGKr, Tetteroo AT (1988) Flow cytometric detection of terminal deoxynucleotidyl transferase and other intracellular antigens in combination with membrane antigens in acute lymphatic leukaemia. *Blood* **72**: 1639–1644.

Slease RB, Wister R, Scher I (1979) Surface immunoglobulin density on human peripheral mononuclear cells. *Blood* **54**: 72–75.

Smith GM, Forbes MA, Cooper J *et al.* (1991) Prognostic indicators for the development of AIDS in HIV antibody positive haemophiliac patients: results of a three-year longitudinal study. *Clin. Lab. Haematol.* **13**: 115–125.

Syrjala MT, Tirikainen M, Jannson SE, Krusius T (1992) Flow cytometric analysis of TdT. *Proceedings of the 24th Congress of the International Society of Haematology.* Blackwell Scientific Publications, Oxford, p. 77. (Abstr. 304).

Taylor J, Fahey J, Detels R, Giorgi J (1989) CD4 percentage, CD4 number and CD4 : CD8 ratio in HIV infection — which to choose and how to use. *J. AIDS* **2**: 114–124.

Terstappen LWMM, Hollander Z, Meiners H, Loken MR (1990) Quantitative comparison of myeloid antigens on five lineages of mature peripheral blood cells. *J. Leuk. Biol.* **48**: 138–148.

Thompson JM, Gralow JR, Levy R, Miller RA (1985) The optimal application of forward and ninety-degree light scatter in flow cytometry for the gating of mononuclear cells. *Cytometry* **6**: 401–406.

Utsuyama M, Hirokawa K, Kurashima C *et al.* (1992) Differential age-change in the numbers of CD4$^+$CD45RA$^+$ and CD4$^+$CD29$^+$ T cell subsets in human peripheral blood. *Mech. Ageing Dev.* **63**: 57–68.

Van Dongen JJM, Wolvers-Tettero ILM (1991) Analysis of immunoglobulin and T-cell receptor genes. *Clin. Chim. Acta* **198**: 1–174.

Weiblen BJ, Debell K, Valeri CR (1983) 'Acquired immune deficiency' of blood stored overnight. *N. Engl. J. Med.* **309**: 793.

Weiss L, Okada N, Haeffner CN *et al.* (1992) Decreased expression of the membrane inhibitor of complement-mediated cytolysis (CD59) on T-lymphocytes of HIV-infected patients. *AIDS* **6**: 379–385.

Yiang YZ, Macdonald D, Cullis JO, Barrett AJ (1991) Is graft versus leukaemia separable from graft versus host disease. *Bone Marrow Transplant* **7** (Suppl. 2): 26.

Young BD (1992) Advances in molecular cytogenetics: Analysis of the leukaemic cell. *Br. J. Haematol.* **82**: 62–63.

Zipf TF, Bryant LD, Koskowich GN, MacGregor SE, Chin L, Johnson H (1984) Enumeration of cytoplasmic μ immunoglobulin positive acute lymphoblastic leukaemia cells by flow cytometry: Comparison with fluorescence microscopy. *Cytometry* **5**: 610–613.

Chapter 4
Cell Differentiation and Maturation in Normal Bone Marrow and Acute Leukaemia

L. W. M. M. TERSTAPPEN

Introduction

Examinations of bone marrow aspirates or biopsies are performed to identify dysfunction in one or more haematopoietic cell lineages, to identify haematopoietic malignancies or to assess bone marrow involvement of other malignancies. Flawless bone marrow examination requires an extensive knowledge of the composition of normal bone marrow against which abnormalities can be recognized. Microscopic examinations of Romanowsky or cytochemically stained bone marrow slides are currently used to examine bone marrow aspirates or biopsies. This technique, however, is subjective and any cell which appears in a frequency below 5% may be overlooked. The introduction of flow cytometry to examine bone marrow has significant advantages over the microscope-based technique in that it is quantitative and has the ability to discriminate between various cell types with objective criteria (Terstappen and Loken, 1988; Terstappen and Levin, 1993).

Multidimensional flow cytometric analysis has proven to be a unique tool for the *in vivo* characterization of haematopoietic cell differentiation and mäturational pathways (Robinson *et al.*, 1981; Sieff *et al.*, 1982; Langlois *et al.*, 1985; Ryan *et al.*, 1986; Loken *et al.*, 1987a,b; Lansdorp *et al.*, 1990; Le Bien *et al.*, 1990; Terstappen *et al.*, 1990b,d, 1991a, 1992a,b). By simultaneous analysis of multiple independent parameters on individual cells passing through a laser beam, a multidimensional space is created in which cells with dissimilar properties emerge in different locations. Static flow cytometric images of haematopoiesis are used to reconstruct *in vivo* maturational pathways by detection of the gradual, co-ordinated changes in the expression of lineage-specific or lineage-associated cell surface and cytoplasmic antigens. In addition, gradual changes in cell morphology are assessed by forward light scatter, related to cell size (Brunsting and Mullaney, 1972) and orthogonal light scatter, related to cell granularity (Salzman *et al.*, 1975; de Grooth *et al.*, 1987). Identification of distinct or gradual changing cell populations in a multidimensional data space can be achieved with the Paint-A-Gate[Plus] software developed for this purpose and reviewed in detail elsewhere (Terstappen *et al.*, 1990c). The differentiation pathway of multipotent haematopoietic stem cells and the maturational pathways of neutrophils, erythroid, B-lymphoid and T-lymphoid cells have been characterized in normal bone marrow and have shown that the differentiation and maturational pathways of all cell lineages are nearly identical in normal individuals (Loken *et al.*, 1987a,b; Terstappen *et al.*, 1990d, 1991a, 1992b).

Comparison of normal differentiation pathways with those observed in acute leukaemias shows that the leukaemic pathways do not match the normal cell differentiation and maturation pathways (Foon and Todd, 1986; Greaves *et al.*, 1986; Roberts *et al.*, 1986; Hurwitz *et al.*, 1988; Janossy *et al.*, 1988, 1989; Ludwig *et al.*, 1988; Terstappen and Loken, 1990; Terstappen *et al.*, 1991c). The 'infidelity' of antigen expressions in leukaemia does not therefore permit a projection of an acute leukaemia on the normal differentiation pathway. For example, the presence of myeloid-specific antigens in acute leukaemia does not imply the presence of a myeloid leukaemia. Likewise, the presence of early or late antigens does not imply the presence of relatively undifferentiated or differentiated leukaemias, respectively.

In general, four patterns of antigen infidelity can be observed: (a) aberrant expression of lineage-specific antigens; (b) asynchronous expression of lineage-associated antigens; (c) overexpression of cell surface antigens; and (d) absence of cell surface antigen expression (Terstappen *et al.*, 1991c). Aberrant expression of lineage-specific antigens refers to the expression of antigens which are lineage-specific in normal bone marrow, but expressed in another lineage in acute leukaemia. Asynchronous expression of lineage-associated antigens refers to the expression of antigens present during maturation of the same lineage, but not co-expressed during the normal maturation process. Overexpression of cell surface antigens refers to a higher cell surface density as compared with normal bone marrow. Absence of expression of cell surface antigens refers to the lack of expression of a cell surface antigen, which should be present at a particular cell differentiation stage.

The large diversity of the antigenic and light scattering profiles of leukaemic cells of patients diagnosed with acute leukaemia further emphasizes the heterogeneity of the disease and can explain the large variation in the clinical course. This diversity is due to the genetic disposition of the leukaemic cells and the influence of external factors on the microenvironment and suggests that leukaemic 'stem cells' can give rise to a large variety of leukaemia cell progeny.

The current value of antigen profiles in acute leukaemias is the ability to assign lineage and define subgroups with different prognostic outcomes. The future clinical value of detailed assessments of the antigen profiles of leukaemic cells is its potential to monitor the effect of therapy on the leukaemic cell population(s) (Wörmann *et al.*, 1991). The high incidence of infidelity of antigen expressions provides a sensitive method for the detection of residual leukaemic cells in patients that are in clinical complete remission.

This review summarizes:

1   The light scatter profiles in normal bone marrow and acute leukaemias.
2   The myeloid maturation pathway in normal bone marrow and acute leukaemias.
3   The B-lymphocyte maturation pathway in normal bone marrow and acute leukaemias.
4   The T-lymphocyte maturation pathway in normal bone marrow, thymus and acute leukaemias.
5   The progenitor cell differentiation pathway in normal bone marrow and acute leukaemias.

Light scatter profiles in normal bone marrow and in acute leukaemia

In flow cytometry, forward light scatter is related to cell size, and orthogonal light scatter is a measure of cell granularity. In the correlative display of both light scatter parameters peripheral blood neutrophils, eosinophils, basophils, monocytes, granular lymphocytes and non-granular lymphocytes each are located in typical positions (Terstappen *et al.*, 1986, 1990a,c; de Grooth *et al.*, 1987). In normal bone marrow aspirates the positions of each of these cell populations are identical to those in peripheral blood. However, the positions are less distinct in bone marrow because of the presence of precursor cells of each of the cell lineages, with distinct light scattering properties. Figure 4.1a shows a typical example of forward and orthogonal light scatter of normal human bone marrow cells. The positions of the end maturational stages of neutrophils (N), monocytes (M), lymphocytes (L) and erythrocytes (E) are indicated. The arrows in the figure start at the position of the progenitor cells and follow the pathways ending at positions of erythro-cytes, B lymphocytes, monocytes and neutrophils.

In contrast with normal bone marrow, the majority of cells in acute leukaemia are located in one specific light scatter region. The position of the predominant cell cluster in the light scatter display varies con-siderably between acute leukaemias as is illustrated for five patients in Fig. 4.1b–f. Analysis of the light scatter patterns between patients shows three prominent light scatter patterns (Terstappen *et al.*, 1991b). The first pattern is characterized by an accumulation of cells with low forward and low orthogonal light scatter (Fig. 4.1b and c). This light scatter profile is typical for acute lymphoid leukaemia and the majority of patients classified as FAB; M0, M1 and M6 (Terstappen *et al.*, 1991b). The second light scatter pattern is characterized by an accumulation of cells with intermediate to high forward light scatter and low to high orthogonal light scatter (Fig. 4.1e). Only acute myeloid leukaemias (AML) display this light scatter profile; the light scatter pattern illustrated in Fig. 4.1e is typical for acute promyelocytic leukaemia (M3). The third

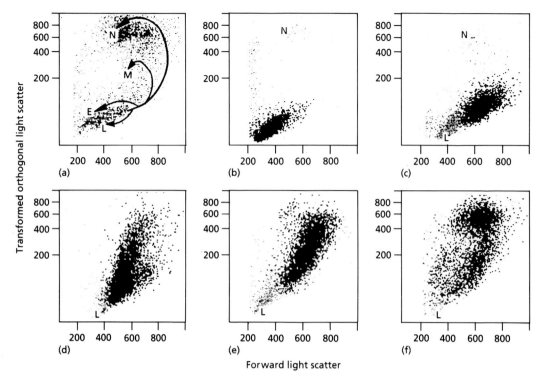

Fig. 4.1 Light scatter profiles. Correlative displays of forward and transformed orthogonal light scatter of bone marrow aspirates illustrated with the Paint-A-Gate^{Plus} software (BDIS) of: (a) normal donor; (b) B-ALL; (c) AML (FAB M1); (d) AML (FAB M2); (e) AML (FAB M3); and (f) AML (FAB M4). The position of the neutrophils (N), monocytes (M), lymphocytes (L) and erythrocytes (E) are indicated in this figure. In (a) the non-lineage committed CD34^{++}, CD38^{-} cells are coloured in black. The arrows indicate the pathway followed during maturation of neutrophils, monocytes, B lymphocytes and erythrocytes in normal bone marrow. In (b) to (f) the leukaemic cells are depicted black and all other cells are depicted grey.

light scatter pattern is characterized by an accumulation of cells with low forward and low orthogonal light scatter but branching towards higher regions (Fig. 4.1d and f). This light scatter pattern also is only observed in myeloid leukaemias. The branching of cells towards regions with higher light scatter indicates the maturation of the leukaemic cells, i.e. increase in granularity.

Although the light scattering profiles are indicative for the type of acute leukaemia, the information present in light scatter measurements on cell morphology of the leukaemic cells is often neglected and is often restricted to a discriminatory function for studying expression of cell surface antigens.

Myeloid maturation pathway in normal bone marrow and in acute leukaemia

The CD33 antigen is one of the earliest antigens to appear on the cell surface of progenitor cells which differentiate into the myeloid lineage

(Peiper *et al.*, 1988; Andrews *et al.*, 1989). Cells co-expressing CD33 and CD34 can give rise to burst-forming unit−erythroid and colony-forming unit−granulocyte macrophage (Andrews *et al.*, 1989). Commitment to the erythroid lineage is accompanied by a loss of CD33 and the expression of the transferrin receptor (CD71) (Loken *et al.*, 1987a). Differentiation of the myeloid cells into the monocyte and neutrophil lineages can be assessed by the differential expression of cell surface antigens as is schematically represented in Fig. 4.2. Expression of CD33 increases during commitment into the monocyte lineage whereas for neutrophils the density remains unchanged. Plate 4.1a and b (facing p. 116) illustrates the expression of CD33 and CD7 in a normal bone marrow. Neutrophils are depicted yellow and characterized by an intermediate CD33 staining and large orthogonal light scatter. Monocytes are depicted green and characterized by a high CD33 staining, large forward light scatter and intermediate orthogonal light scatter. Cells differentiated into the myeloid lineage, but not yet committed to the granulocytic, monocytic or erythroid lineages, are depicted blue and are characterized by an intermediate CD33 staining, large forward light scatter and low orthogonal light scatter. The few cells depicted violet are committed to the monocytic lineage (high CD33 density), but have not yet reached the position in the light scatter display typical for monocytes. The light scatter parameters are of the utmost importance to identify myeloid maturational pathways as is illustrated in Plate 4.1a. T lymphocytes and natural killer (NK) cells identified by CD7 expression and a lack of CD33 are depicted red in Plate 4.1a and b. Distinction of early neutrophils (myeloblasts, promyelocytes) from cells differentiated into the monocyte lineage can be achieved by the differential expression of CD15. Increasing densities of the CD11b occur during both neutrophil and monocyte

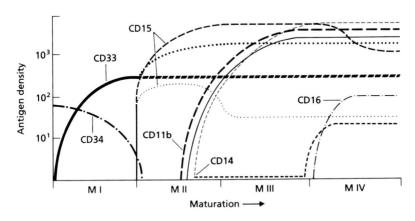

Fig. 4.2 Schematic representation of the sequential expression of cell surface antigens during myeloid cell maturation. The myeloid cells are divided into four stages and indicated with MI, MII, MIII and MIV, respectively. Expression of CD33 concurrently with a loss of CD34 indicates early myeloid commitment. Commitment to the monocyte lineage is indicated with dotted lines and neutrophil commitment with dashed lines. The expression of CD11b, CD14, CD15, CD16 and CD33 is indicated during monocyte and neutrophil maturation.

maturation. Expression of both CD14 and CD16 occurs late during neutrophil maturation (bands, segmented neutrophils). The CD10 antigen present on early B and T lymphocytes appears on the neutrophils concurrently with the CD14 and CD16 antigens. To this date no cell surface antigens are found which specifically identify only the monocyte or neutrophil maturational pathways. Assessment of maturation of these lineages can therefore only be achieved by combining various cell surface antigens with light scattering properties (Andreesen *et al.*, 1986; Falkenburg *et al.*, 1986; Socinski *et al.*, 1988; Terstappen and Loken, 1990; Terstappen *et al.*, 1990d).

In the majority of AMLs cell differentiation and cell maturation pathways can be identified. Assignment of these pathways to either erythroid, monocytic, eosinophilic, basophilic or neutrophilic lineages is often difficult, if not impossible, due to the large variation in the mixture of cells from the various lineages and the frequent diversities of the maturational pathways of each of the cell types from those observed in normal bone marrow. Examples of such deviations are the expression of CD14 in densities normal for monocytes in a light scatter region typical for neutrophils, expression of CD16 in a light scatter region typical for monocytes, lack of expression of CD15 in a light scatter region typical for promyelocytes and expression of CD34 in light scatter regions typical for monocytes and neutrophils. Whether or not a detailed description of the maturational and differentiation pathways in acute leukaemias is clinically useful is still open for discussion. Prognostic significance of specific antigenic profiles (Thiel *et al.*, 1980; Borowitz *et al.*, 1989; Geller *et al.*, 1990; Terstappen *et al.*, 1992c) and the large variation in the sensitivity to chemotherapy of cell subpopulations within individual patients (Wörmann *et al.*, 1993) suggest that treatment protocols can be targeted to specific antigenic profiles.

Expression of T- or B-lineage-specific antigens on myeloid leukaemic cells is frequently observed in AML. Plate 4.1 illustrates the correlated expression of CD33 and CD7 in normal bone marrow and two AML patients. The leukaemic cells in the patient illustrated in Plate 4.1c and d are depicted blue, express the CD33 antigen, aberrantly express the CD7 antigen and display large forward light scatter and intermediate orthogonal light scatter, typical for myeloid leukaemias. Normal T lymphocytes and NK cells are depicted red in the figure. The leukaemic cells in the patient illustrated in Plate 4.1e and f are depicted blue and show two features of infidelity: aberrant expression of CD7 and absence of CD33. The assignment of this leukaemia to the myeloid lineage is obvious from its light scatter characteristics, the expression of the myeloid antigens CD13 and CD15 and the lack of other T-lineage-specific antigens (data not shown). In this patient monocytes and neutrophils are present and depicted green and yellow respectively. Whether or not these are of leukaemic origin is not known. Cell surface antigens frequently found aberrantly expressed in AML are CD2, CD5, CD7, CD19 and CD56 (Roberts *et al.*, 1986; Ludwig *et al.*, 1988; Master *et al.*, 1991; Terstappen *et al.*, 1991c). Antigens found to be frequently co-expressed asynchronously are CD34 with CD15 or CD11b. The antigen which is most frequently overexpressed is CD34. Antigens frequently absent are CD33 and CD13 or CD11b and CD15 on cells with large orthogonal light scattering.

The importance of describing mismatches between normal cell differentiation and that observed in myeloid leukaemia is that the abnormal antigenic and light scatter profiles can be used to detect residual leukaemic cells after treatment of the patients. The sensitivity of this approach will vary for each patient, since it depends on the extent to which the leukaemic cells differ from the normal pathway. For instance, the sensitivity will be larger in the patient illustrated in Plate 4.1e and f than that of the patient illustrated in Plate 4.1c and d. Normal monocytes (see Plate 4.1b) are close to the aberrantly expressing CD7 cells (Plate 4.1d), whereas the distance between normal myeloid cells and leukaemic cells is considerably larger for the aberrantly expressing CD7, and CD33 lacking cells (Plate 4.1f). The first prospective study employing lineage infidelity to detect residual disease in AML patients showed that all patients who reached a clinical complete remission and had detectable residual leukaemic cells by flow cytometry indeed relapsed (Wörmann *et al.*, 1991). Remarkably, the frequency of residual leukaemic cells was larger than expected in this study and was about 1% in most cases.

B-lymphocyte maturation pathway in normal bone marrow and in acute leukaemia

The CD19 antigen is the earliest antigen to appear on the cell surface of progenitor cells, which differentiates into the B-lymphoid lineage and remains present throughout B lymphocyte maturation up to the final

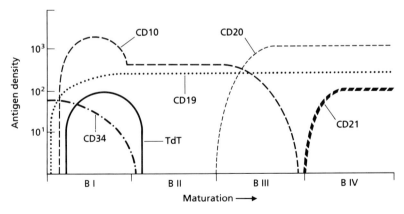

Fig. 4.3 Schematic representation of the sequential expression of cell surface antigens during B-lymphocyte maturation. The B lymphocytes are divided into four stages and indicated with BI, BII, BIII and BIV, respectively (Loken *et al.*, 1987a). Expression of CD10 and CD19 concurrently with a loss of CD34 indicates early B-lymphoid commitment. Terminal deoxynucleotidyl transferase is only present in the CD34 expressing B lymphocytes. The CD20 and CD21 appear only late during B-lymphocyte maturation.

maturation into the plasma cells, at which stage the CD19 antigen is lost (Ryan *et al.*, 1986; Loken *et al.*, 1987b; Le Bien *et al.*, 1990; Terstappen *et al.*, 1990b). The CD10 antigen appears on the cell surface concurrently with the CD19 antigen. CD10 in contrast with CD19 is not B-lineage specific and appears in a similar fashion on T-cell precursors and is expressed late in neutrophil development. The sequential expression of cell surface antigens and intranuclear terminal deoxnucleotidyl transferase expression during B-lymphocyte maturation is schematically represented in Fig. 4.3. Plate 4.2a and b (between pp. 116 and 117) illustrates the expression of the CD10 and CD19 antigens in normal bone marrow. The CD19$^+$, CD10$^-$ late B lymphocytes are depicted green and the early CD19$^+$, CD10$^+$ B lymphocytes are depicted red. The few red-coloured cells which express CD10 the brightest represent the earliest B lymphocytes which co-express CD34 (Loken *et al.*, 1987b).

B-lymphoid leukaemias are often subclassified according to the maturational stages of normal B lymphocytes (Foon and Todd, 1986). In view of the lineage infidelity frequently observed in acute B-lymphoid leukaemias (B-ALL) (Roberts *et al.*, 1986; Hurwitz *et al.*, 1988, Janossy and Campana, 1988; Ludwig *et al.*, 1988, Janossy *et al.*, 1989), this approach to subclassifying B-lymphoid leukaemias is questionable. In Plate 4.2 the correlated expression of CD10 and CD19 of two patients with B-ALL is compared with that of normal bone marrow. In both cases the cells show a low orthogonal light scatter and a large range of forward light scatter typical of lymphoid leukaemias and undifferentiated myeloid leukaemias. However, the position of the leukaemic cells does not match that of the normal bone marrow illustrated in Plate 4.2a and b. In the case illustrated in Plate 4.2c and d there is at least a 10-fold increase in CD10 expression as compared with normal bone marrow and a normal CD19 expression, whereas in the case illustrated in Plate 4.2e and f there is a 10-fold increase in CD19 expression with a normal expression of CD10.

Antigens frequently expressed aberrantly in B-ALL are CD7, CD33 and CD13 (Roberts *et al.*, 1986; Hurwitz *et al.*, 1988; Janossy and Campana, 1988; Ludwig *et al.*, 1988; Janossy *et al.*, 1989). Antigens frequently overexpressed or absent in B-ALL are CD10 and CD19. Asynchronously expressed antigens are CD34 with CD20 and CD22 (Hurwitz *et al.*, 1988; Janossy and Campana, 1988). Although the CD22 antigen is expressed in the cytoplasm of CD34$^+$ B lymphocytes it is not expressed on the cell surface of these B lymphocytes in adult bone marrow (Janossy and Campana, 1988). Co-expression of cell surface CD22 and CD34 is, however, normal in fetal bone marrow.

T-lymphocyte maturation pathway in normal bone marrow/thymus and in acute leukaemia

In normal adult bone marrow the majority, if not all, of the T lymphocytes are mature T cells expressing the T-cell receptor (CD3) on the cell surface (Terstappen *et al.*, 1992b). In contrast with adult bone marrow,

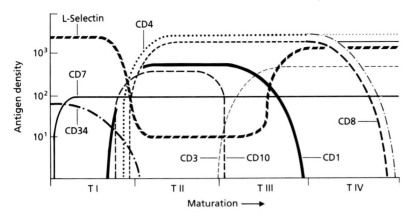

Fig. 4.4 Schematic representation of the sequential expression of cell surface antigens during T-lymphocyte maturation. The T lymphocytes are divided into four stages and indicated with TI, TII, TIII and TIV, respectively. Expression of CD7 and high density of L-selectin concurrently with a loss of CD34 indicates early T-lymphoid commitment and can be found in fetal bone marrow and thymus. Expression of CD1 is restricted to thymus and appears concurrently with CD10 and a decrease in L-selectin, CD1 is down-regulated during T-cell maturation concurrently with CD3 and up-regulation of L-selectin. The majority of thymocytes co-express CD4 and CD8. Expression of CD4 without CD8 (.....) and expression of CD8 without CD4 (– – – –) occurs late in T cell maturation when L-selectin and CD3 reach their highest expression levels.

T-cell precursors can be readily identified in fetal bone marrow and are characterized by co-expression of CD34 with the T-cell-associated antigens CD7, CD2 and CD5 (Terstappen *et al.*, 1992b). The CD7 antigen is the earliest antigen to appear on the cell surface of progenitor cells which differentiate into the T-lymphoid lineage. These T-cell precursors are believed to seed the thymus whose environment then promotes T-cell maturation (Terstappen *et al.*, 1992b). The sequential expression of cell surface antigens during T-lymphocyte maturation is schematically represented in Fig. 4.4. T I cells are found in fetal bone marrow and thymus and T II and T III cells are only found in thymus. Mature T IV cells are found at both sites. The CD10 antigen appears on the cell surface of T-cell precursors in a similar fashion to B cell precursors. During T-cell maturation the CD10 is lost before cell surface expression of the T-cell receptor complex and during B-cell maturation CD10 is lost before cell surface immunoglobulin expression. The majority of the T cells in the thymus co-express both CD4 and CD8. The expression of L-selectin is reciprocal to CD1 expression during T-cell maturation in the thymus. L-selectin (previously known as LAM1, LECAM1 or Leu8) is known for its role in homing of T lymphocytes to peripheral lymph nodes (Picker *et al.*, 1990). Its presence on early T lymphocytes suggests it plays a role in the homing of these early lymphocytes to the thymus (Terstappen *et al.*, 1992). The expression of the CD1 and CD5 antigens in normal adult bone marrow is illustrated in Plate 4.3a and b (between pp. 116 and 117). The CD5$^+$, CD1$^-$ T lymphocytes are depicted red and no T lymphocytes expressing the CD1 antigen are present. CD1 is expressed only during T-cell maturation in the thymus and cannot be found on T cells in adult or fetal bone marrow. The correlated expression of CD1 and CD5 in the thymus is illustrated in Plate 4.3c and d. The plate illustrates an up-regulation of the CD5 antigen concurrently with a down-regulation of CD1. T II lymphocytes (CD1$^+$, CD5$^+$) are depicted green, T III lymphocytes (CD1$^+ \rightarrow$ dim, CD5$^+ \rightarrow ^{++}$) are depicted yellow and the mature T IV lymphocytes (CD5^{++}, CD1$^-$) are depicted red.

T-cell leukaemias are relatively infrequent and consequently lineage infidelity is less well documented (Janossy and Campana, 1988; Janossy *et al.*, 1989; Master *et al.*, 1991). However, for T-cell leukaemias one can distinguish an infidelity which does not exist in B-ALL or AML, i.e. aberrant 'location' of a cell subset with an antigenic profile not found in normal bone marrow. An example of this is shown in Plate 4.3e and f. In the bone marrow of this patient with acute T-lymphocytic leukaemia (T-ALL) the leukaemic cells are depicted violet and a subset of the leukaemic cells is found which expressed the CD1 antigen (coloured blue), a phenomenon normally only observed in thymus. Likewise, leukaemic T cells can be found in T-ALL which express the CD34 antigen as illustrated in Plate 4.4g and h (between pp. 116 and 117).

Progenitor cell differentiation pathway in normal bone marrow and in acute leukaemia

Normal human bone marrow cells expressing the CD34 antigen represent a heterogeneous progenitor cell population of which most of the cells are committed to either erythroid, lymphoid or monomyeloid cell lineages (Andrews *et al.*, 1989, 1990; Lansdorp *et al.*, 1990; Verfaillie *et al.*, 1990; Terstappen *et al.*, 1991a). Lineage commitment of the CD34$^+$ bone marrow cells has been demonstrated by cell morphology, presence of lineage-specific or associated antigens and formation of colonies with lymphoid, erythroid or myeloid features. Enrichment for pluripotent non-committed progenitor cells in the CD34$^+$ cell fraction has been successfully performed by elimination of CD34$^+$ cells expressing lineage-associated antigens (Civin *et al.*, 1987; Andrews *et al.*, 1989, 1990; Terstappen *et al.*, 1991a), lacking HLA-DR (Verfaillie *et al.*, 1990), lacking CD38 (Terstappen *et al.*, 1991a) or expressing Thy1 (Baum *et al.*, 1992).

In this review we examine the correlated expression of the CD34 and CD38 antigens to assess early cell differentiation in normal bone marrow and acute leukaemia. Four cell differentiation stages are identified: (a) PI CD34^{++}, CD38$^-$ cells which can give rise to each of the cell lineages, have the potential to form blast colonies, and have a large self-renewal capacity; (b) PII CD34^{++}, CD38$^+ \rightarrow ^{++}$ cells with a limited ability to form blast colonies and a limited self-renewal capacity; (c) PIII CD34$^{++} \rightarrow ^+$ CD38^{+++} cells, which are all lineage committed and form colonies according to their lineage commitment; (d) PIV CD34$^+ \rightarrow ^-$, CD38^{+++} cells, which are all lineage committed and have only a limited ability to form colonies. Figure 4.5 summarizes the sequential expression

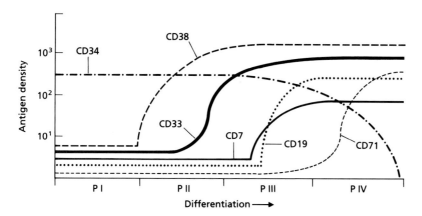

Fig. 4.5 Schematic representation of the sequential expression of cell surface antigens during early haematopoietic cell differentiation. The progenitor cells are divided into four stages and indicated with PI, PII, PIII and PIV, respectively. Expression of CD38 indicates lineage commitment, CD33 myeloid commitment, CD7 T-cell commitment, CD19 B cell commitment and CD71 erythroid commitment.

of lineage-specific or associated cell surface antigens on progenitor cells. Expression of CD33 indicates myeloid commitment, CD7 T-cell commitment, CD19 B-cell commitment and CD71 erythroid commitment. Plate 4.4a and b illustrates the early cell differentiation pathway in an erythrocyte lysed bone marrow of a typical normal donor. In the plate, the expression of CD34 is correlated with CD38, forward and orthogonal light scatter. CD34$^+$ cells are indicated with a colour whereas CD34$^-$cells are depicted grey. PI cells are depicted black, PII cells red, PIII cells blue and PIV cells green. The position of neutrophils, monocytes, erythrocytes, lymphocytes, early B lymphoid cells and plasma cells is indicated in Plate 4.4a and b. The frequency of CD34$^+$ cells in normal bone marrow is remarkably consistent between donors (mean 1%, s.d. 0.3, $n = 10$), as well as the frequency of cells in the CD34 progenitor stages, the PI cells being the most infrequent (1% of CD34 cells, s.d. 0.5, $n = 10$).

In acute leukaemias the early differentiation pathway defined by the correlated expression of CD34 and CD38 is well conserved in that cell differentiation along this pathway can be observed in a large number of patients (Terstappen *et al.*, 1992c). Deviations from the early differentiation pathway include overexpression of the CD34 antigen, asynchrony between light scattering and CD34 and CD38 expression, i.e. intermediate to large orthogonal light scattering on CD34$^+$ cells, and, in most cases, an abnormally high frequency of cells in PI, PII and PIII. Plate 4.4a–h compares the correlated expression of CD34 and CD38 between normal bone marrow and an AML, B-ALL and T-ALL patient, respectively. In all three patients a cell differentiation pathway similar to that of normal bone marrow can be identified and indicated with identical colours: PI, black; PII, red; PIII, blue, and PIV green. The leukaemic cells not expressing the CD34 antigen are depicted yellow. In the AML patient illustrated in Plate 4c and d (CD33$^+$, CD13$^+$) it is obvious that the majority of CD34$^+$ cells belong to the leukaemic cell population. Presence of cells in PI in AML patients has been shown to be a poor prognostic sign in that these patients are less likely to achieve complete remission in addition to having a shorter event-free survival when complete remission is achieved (Terstappen *et al.*, 1992c). In the patient diagnosed with acute B-ALL (CD10$^+$, CD19$^+$) a similar distribution of CD34$^+$ cells is observed as in normal bone marrow except for a lower orthogonal light scatter of the PIV cells, which suggests that these cells belong to the leukaemic cell population. Whether the cells present in PI, PII and PIII in fact represent early precursors of the leukaemic clone is of interest but yet unknown. The early differentiation pathway could also be identified in the T-ALL patient (CD7$^+$, CD5$^+$). In this case, the predominance of CD34$^+$ cells was located in PIII and PIV in a frequency far exceeding that of normal bone marrow. In normal adult bone marrow the frequency of CD34$^+$ T-cell precursors is less than 0.1% of CD34 cells, but can be readily identified in fetal bone marrow and thymus. Detection of CD34$^+$ T-cell precursors in adult bone marrow therefore could be used for the detection of residual leukaemic cells after treatment of these patients.

Summary

Multidimensional flow cytometry permits the identification of cells differentiated into either the myeloid, B-lymphoid or T-lymphoid lineage and the successive maturation of these cells in normal bone marrow. Between normal donors the maturational pathways defined by gradual changes in light scattering properties and by the sequential acquisition and loss of lineage-specific and lineage-associated cell surface antigens is well preserved.

Comparison of the differentiation pathways in bone marrow of normal donors with those of acute leukaemias revealed a deviation from the normal differentiation pathway in the majority of acute leukaemias. This implies that the projection of leukaemias to the normal maturational pathway is an oversimplification and models using this approach to classify leukaemias are incorrect. One can, however, use the antigenic profiles of leukaemias to define subgroups with different prognostic outcomes. The most promising value of an assessment of the antigenic profiles in acute leukaemias is its potential use for residual disease detection.

References

Andreesen R, Brugger W, Scheibenbogen C *et al.* (1990) Surface phenotype analysis of human monocyte to macrophage maturation. *J. Leuk. Biol.* **47**: 490–497.

Andrews RG, Singer JW, Bernstein ID (1989) Precursors of colony-forming cells in humans can be distinguished from colony-forming cells by expression of the CD33 and CD34 antigens and light scattering properties. *J. Exp. Med.* **169**: 1721–1731.

Andrews RG, Singer JW, Bernstein ID (1990) Human hematopoietic precursors in long-term culture: single CD34$^+$ cells that lack detectable T cell, B cell, and myeloid cell antigens produce multiple colony-forming cells when cultured with marrow stromal cells. *J. Exp. Med.* **172**: 355–358.

Baum CM, Weissman IL, Tsukamoto AS, Buckle AM, Peault B (1992) Isolation of a candidate human stem-cell population. *Proc. Natl Acad. Sci. USA* **89**: 2804–2808.

Borowitz MJ, Gockerman JP, Moore JO *et al.* (1989) Clinicopathologic features of CD34 (My10) — positive acute nonlymphocytic leukemia. *Am. J. Clin. Pathol.* **91**: 265–270.

Brunsting A, Mullaney PF (1972) Light scattering from coated spheres: model for biological cells. *Appl. Opt.* **11**: 675–680.

Civin I, Banquerigo ML, Strauss LC, Loken MR (1987) Antigenic analysis of hematopoiesis. IV. Characterization of MY10-positive progenitor cells in normal human bone marrow. *Exp. Hematol.* **15**: 10–17.

de Grooth BG, Terstappen LWMM, Puppels GJ, Greve J (1987) Light-scattering polarization measurements as a new parameter in flow cytometry. *Cytometry* **8**: 539–544.

Falkenburg JH, Koning F, Duinkerken N, Fibbe WE, Voogt PJ, Jansen J (1986) Expression of CD11, CDw15, and transferrin receptor antigens on human hematopoietic progenitor cells. *Exp. Hematol.* **14**: 90–96.

Foon KA, Todd RF (1986) Immunologic classification of leukemia and lymphoma. *Blood* **68**: 1–31.

Geller RB, Zahurak M, Hurwitz CA *et al.* (1990) Prognostic importance of immunophenotyping in adults with acute myelocytic leukaemia: the significance of the stem cell glycoprotein CD34 (My10). *Br. J. Haematol.* **76**: 340–347.

Greaves MF, Chan LC, Furley AJW, Watt SM, Molgaard HV (1986) Lineage promiscuity in hematopoietic differentiation and leukemia. *Blood* **67**: 1–11.

Hurwitz CA, Loken MR, Graham ML *et al.* (1988) Asynchronous antigen expression in B lineage acute lymphoblastic leukemia. *Blood* **72**: 299–307.

Janossy G, Campana D (1988) The pathophysiological basis of immunodiagnosis in acute lymphoblastic leukemia. *Cancer Rev.* **8**: 91–122.

Janossy G, Coustan-Smith E, Campana D (1989) The reliability of cytoplasmic CD3 and CD22 antigen expression in the immunodiagnosis of acute leukemia: a study of 500 cases. *Leukemia* **3**: 170–181.

Langlois RG, Bigbee WL, Hensen RH (1985) Flow cytometric characterization of normal and variant cells with monoclonal antibodies specific for glycophorin A. *J. Immunol.* **134**: 4009–4017.

Lansdorp PM, Sutherland HJ, Eaves CJ (1990) Selective expression of CD45 isoforms on functional subpopulations of CD34 positive hemopoietic cells from human bone marrow. *J. Exp. Med.* **172**: 363–366.

Le Bien TW, Wörmann B, Villablanca JD *et al.* (1990) Multiparameter flow cytometric analysis of human fetal bone marrow B cells. *Leukemia* **4**: 354–360.

Loken MR, Shah VO, Datilio KL, Civin CI (1987a) Flow cytometric analysis of human bone marrow: I. Normal erythroid development. *Blood* **69**: 255–263.

Loken MR, Shah VO, Datilio KL, Civin CI (1987b) Flow cytometric analysis of human bone marrow: II. Normal B lymphoid development. *Blood* **70**: 1316–1324.

Ludwig WD, Bartram CR, Ritter J *et al.* (1988) Ambiguous phenotypes and genotypes in 16 children with acute leukemia as characterized by multiparameter analysis. *Blood* **71**: 1518–1528.

Master PS, Jones RA, Scott CL (1991) Patterns of membrane antigen expression by AML blast: quantitation and histogram analysis. *Leuk. Lymphoma* **5**: 317–325.

Peiper SC, Ashmun RA, Look AT (1988) Molecular cloning, expression, and chromosomal localization of a human gene encoding the CD33 myeloid differentiation antigen. *Blood* **72**: 314–321.

Picker LJ, Terstappen LWMM, Rott LS, Streeter PR, Stein H, Butcher EC (1990) Differential expression of homing-associated adhesion molecules by T-cell subsets in man. *J. Immunol.* **145**: 3247–3255.

Roberts GT, El Badawi SB, Sackey K, Spence D, Sheth KV, Aur RJ (1986) Lineage ambiguity in acute leukemia. *Cancer* **58**: 1473–1478.

Robinson FJ, Sieff C, Deilia D, Edwards PAW, Greaves M (1981) Expression of cell surface HLA-DR, HLA-ABC and glycophorin during eythroid differentiation. *Nature* **289**: 68−71.

Ryan D, Kossover S, Mitchel S, Frantz C, Hennessy L, Cohen H (1986) Subpopulations of common acute lymphoblastic leukemia antigen-positive lymphoid cells in normal bone marrow identified by hematopoietic differentiation antigens. *Blood* **68**: 417−425.

Salzman GC, Growell JM, Martin JC (1975) Cell classification by laser light scattering: Identification and separation of unstained leukocytes. *Acta Cytol.* **19**: 374−377.

Sieff C, Bicknell D, Caine G, Robinson J, Lam G, Greaves MF (1982) Changes in cell surface antigen expression during hemopoietic differentiation. *Blood* **60**: 703−713.

Socinski M, Cannistra SA, Sullivan R *et al.* (1988) Granulocyte-macrophage colony-stimulating factor induces the expression of the CD11b surface adhesion molecule on human granulocytes *in vivo*. *Blood* **72**: 691−697.

Terstappen LWMM, Levin J (1992) Bone marrow differential counts obtained by multidimensional flow cytometry. *Blood Cells* **18**: 311−330.

Terstappen LWMM, Loken MR (1988) 5-dimensional flow cytometry as a new approach for blood and bone marrow differentials. *Cytometry* **9**: 548−556.

Terstappen LWMM, Loken MR (1990) Myeloid cell differentiation in normal bone marrow and acute myeloid leukemia assessed by multi-dimensional flow cytometry. *Anal. Cell. Pathol.* **2**: 229−240.

Terstappen LWMM, de Grooth BG, ten Napel CHH, van Berkel W, Greve J (1986) Discrimination of human cytotoxic lymphocytes from regulatory and B lymphocytes by orthogonal light scattering. *J. Immunol. Methods* **95**: 211−216.

Terstappen LWMM, Hollander Z, Meiners H, Loken MR (1990a) Quantitative comparison of myeloid antigens on five lineages of mature peripheral blood cells. *J. Leukocyte Biol.* **48**: 138−148.

Terstappen LWMM, Johnsen S, Segers-Nolten I, Loken MR (1990b) Identification and characterization of normal human plasma cells by high resolution flow cytometry. *Blood* **76**: 1739−1747.

Terstappen LWMM, Mickaels R, Dost R, Loken MR (1990c) Increased light scattering resolution facilitates multidimensional flow cytometric analysis. *Cytometry* **11**: 506−512.

Terstappen LWMM, Safford M, Loken MR (1990d) Flow cytometric analysis of human bone marrow III. Neutrophil development. *Leukemia* **4**: 657−663.

Terstappen LWMM, Huang S, Safford M, Lansdorp PM, Loken MR (1991a) Sequential generations of hematopoietic colonies derived from single non lineage committed progenitor cells. *Blood* **77**: 1218−1227.

Terstappen LWMM, Könemann S, Safford M *et al.* (1991b) Flow cytometric characterization of acute myeloid leukemias. I. Significance of light scattering properties. *Leukemia* **5**: 315−321.

Terstappen LWMM, Safford M, Könemann S *et al.* (1991c) Flow cytometric characterization of acute myeloid leukemia II. Phenotypic heterogeneity at presentation. *Leukemia* **5**: 757−767.

Terstappen LWMM, Buescher S, Nguyen M, Reading C (1992a) Differentiation and maturation of growth factor expanded early human hematopoeitic progenitors assessed by multidimensional flow cytometry. *Leukemia* **6**: 1001−1011.

Terstappen LWMM, Huang S, Picker LJ (1992b) Flow cytometric assessment of human T-cell differentiation in thymus and bone marrow. *Blood* **79**: 666−667.

Terstappen LWMM, Safford M, Unterhalt M *et al.* (1992c) Flow cytometric characterization of acute myeloid leukemias. IV. Comparison of the differentiation pathway of normal hematopoietic progenitor cells. *Leukemia,* **6**: 993−1001.

Thiel E, Rodt H, Huhn B *et al.* (1980) Multimarker classification of acute lymphoblastic leukemia: evidence for further T subgroups and evaluation of their clinical significance. *Blood* **56**: 759−772.

Verfaillie C, Blakolmer K, McGlave P (1990) Purified primitive human hematopoietic progenitor cells with long-term *in vitro* repopulating capacity adhere selectively to irradiated bone marrow stroma. *J. Exp. Med.* **172**: 509−520.

Wörmann B, Safford M, Könemann S *et al.* (1991) Detection of residual leukemic cells in AML patients in complete remission. *Blood* **78** (Suppl. 1): 1515.

Wörmann B, Könemann S, Safford M *et al*. (1992) Flow cytometric characterization of acute myeloid leukemias. III. Selective elimination of leukemic subpopulations through induction chemotherapy. *Leukemia*, in press.

Chapter 5
Neutrophil Membrane Antigens, Antibodies and Function

P. A. VEYS AND M. G. MACEY

Expression of functional antigens on neutrophils: effects of preparation

At least 29 clusters of differentiation (CDs) have been described for normal human granulocytes and many of the antigens identified by these CDs have been ascribed functions, such as the receptor for the complement component C3bi (Knapp, 1989) and the receptors for the Fc portion of human IgG (Anderson and Looney, 1986). *In vitro* analysis of neutrophil antigen expression is usually assessed on cells isolated from peripheral blood. The most widely used isolation techniques involve: (a) Ficoll-Paque density-gradient centrifugation (Boyum, 1968) and hypotonic lysis of contaminating erythrocytes (Gordon *et al.*, 1989); (b) dextran sedimentation (Skoog and Beck, 1956) followed by Ficoll-Paque density-gradient centrifugation and lysis; or (c) single step Ficoll-Paque separation followed if necessary by lysis. Isolated neutrophils are then usually held at 4°C until analysed (Fearon and Collins, 1983).

Concern that isolation procedures may influence the expression of cell surface antigens, particularly the effect of temperature on CR3, CD11b expression, have been reported (Porteau *et al.*, 1986; Forsyth and Levinsky, 1990). Several studies have shown that if neutrophils which have been kept at 4°C are then warmed to 37°C then the expression of CD18, 11a, 11b and 11c antigens is increased (e.g. Fearon and Collins,

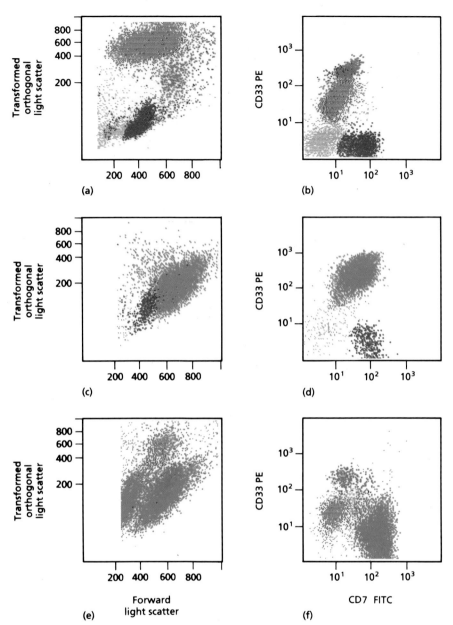

Plate 4.1 Correlative displays of CD7 fluorescein isothiocyanate, CD33 phycoerythrin, forward light scatter and orthogonal light scatter in normal bone marrow and two AML patients. Bone marrow cells were lysed with NH₄Cl and stained with CD7 fluorescein isothiocyanate and CD33 phycoerythrin. Data were acquired on a FACScan and analysed with the Paint-A-Gate^{Plus} software (BDIS). (a) and (b) illustrate the bone marrow cells of a normal donor. T lymphocytes and NK cells expressing CD7 and lacking CD33 are depicted red. Neutrophils expressing CD33 and lacking CD7 are coloured yellow. Monocytes brightly expressing CD33 and lacking CD7 are coloured green. Note the larger autofluorescence of the myeloid cells as compared with the grey-coloured erythroid cells and B lymphocytes. Immature myeloid cells are located in a light scatter region with low orthogonal light scatter and large forward light scatter and coloured blue when dimly expressing CD33 and violet when brightly expressing CD33. (c) and (d) illustrate the bone marrow cells of an AML which aberrantly expresses CD7. The CD33⁺, CD7⁺ leukaemic cells are coloured blue. Residual normal T lymphocytes and NK cells are coloured red. (e) and (f) illustrate the bone marrow cells of an AML which aberrantly expresses CD7 and lack CD33. The CD33⁻, CD7⁺ leukaemic cells are coloured blue. Residual 'normal' neutrophils and monocytes are yellow and green, respectively.

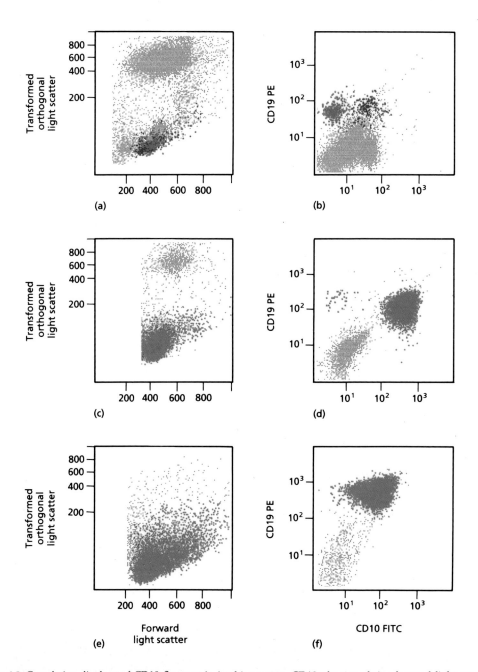

Plate 4.2 Correlative displays of CD10 fluorescein isothiocyanate, CD19 phycoerythrin, forward light scatter and orthogonal light scatter in normal bone marrow and two B-ALL patients. Bone marrow cells were lysed with NH$_4$Cl and stained with CD10 fluorescein isothiocyanate and CD19 phycoerythrin. Data were acquired on a FACScan and analysed with the Paint-A-Gate^{Plus} software (BDIS). (a) and (b) illustrate the bone marrow cells of a normal donor. The CD19$^+$, CD10$^-$ late B lymphocytes (stage B IV, Fig. 4.3) are coloured green and the CD19$^+$, CD10$^+$ early B lymphocytes (stage B I→B III, Fig. 4.3) are coloured red, all other cells are depicted grey. The red-coloured cells with the largest expression of CD10 represent the earliest B lymphocytes (stage B I, Fig. 4.3). (c) and (d) illustrate the bone marrow cells of a B-ALL which overexpresses CD10. The CD19$^+$, CD10$^+$ leukaemic cells are coloured blue. A few potential residual normal B lymphocytes are coloured green (CD19$^+$, CD10$^-$). (e) and (f) illustrate the bone marrow cells of a B-ALL which overexpresses CD19. The CD19$^+$, CD10$^+$ leukaemic cells are coloured blue.

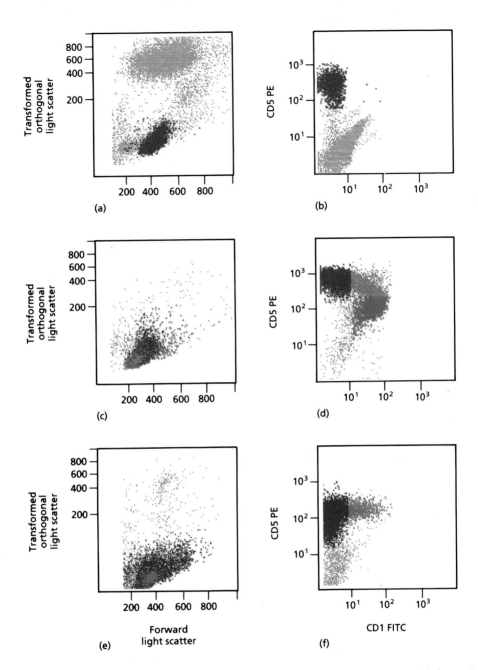

Plate 4.3 Correlative displays of CD1 fluorescein isothiocyanate, CD5 phycoerythrin, forward light scatter and orthogonal light scatter in normal bone marrow, normal thymus and a T-ALL patient. Bone marrow cells were lysed with NH_4Cl and a thymocyte suspension was obtained by density separation, all were stained with CD1 fluorescein isothiocyanate and CD5 phycoerythrin. Data were acquired on a FACScan and analysed with the Paint-A-Gate[Plus] software (BDIS). (a) and (b) illustrate the bone marrow cells of a normal donor. The $CD5^{++}$, $CD1^-$ T lymphocytes (stage TIV, Fig. 4.4) are coloured red and all other cells are depicted grey. No CD1-expressing T cells were detected. (c) and (d) illustrate thymocytes obtained from a normal paediatric patient. The $CD5^{++}$, $CD1^-$, TIV T lymphocytes are coloured red, the $CD5^{++}$, $CD1^+$, TIII T lymphocytes are coloured yellow and the $CD5^+$, $CD1^+$ $TI \rightarrow II$ T lymphocytes are coloured green. (e) and (f) illustrate the bone marrow cells of a T-ALL of which the fraction of leukaemic cells which express CD1 is coloured blue. This expression is aberrant in that in normal donors no CD1-expressing T lymphocytes are found in the bone marrow. All other leukaemic T cells are coloured violet.

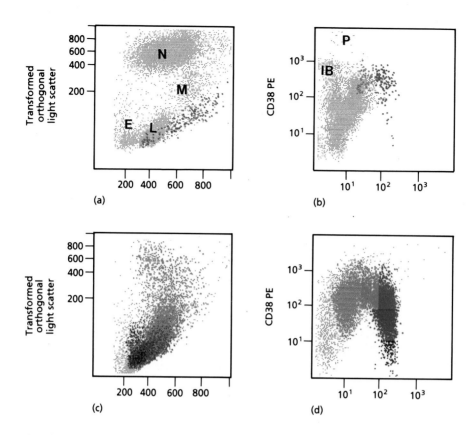

Plate 4.4 Correlative displays of CD34 fluorescein isothiocyanate, CD38 phycoerythrin, forward light scatter and orthogonal light scatter in normal bone marrow, AML, B-ALL and T-ALL. Bone marrow cells were lysed with NH_4Cl and stained with CD34 fluorescein isothiocyanate and CD38 phycoerythrin. Data were acquired on a FACScan and analysed with the Paint-A-Gate[Plus] software (BDIS). (a) and (b) illustrate the bone marrow cells of a normal donor. The position of neutrophils (N), monocytes (M), lymphocytes (L), erythroid cells (E), plasma cells (P) and immature B cells (IB) is indicated in (a) and (b). The $CD34^+$ cells were separated into four differentiation stages and each depicted with a colour. $CD34^-$ cells were coloured grey. Early non-lineage committed progenitors, PI ($CD34^{++}$, $CD38^-$) cells were depicted black, PII ($CD34^{++} \rightarrow {}^+$, $CD38^+ \rightarrow {}^{++}$) cells red, PIII ($CD34^+$, $CD38^{++} \rightarrow {}^{+++}$) cells blue and PIV late lineage committed progenitors ($CD34^+ \rightarrow {}^{dim}$, $CD38^{+++}$) green. Bone marrow cells of AML, B-ALL and T-ALL patients were prepared and illustrated in a similar way to that of the normal donor and shown in (c) and (d), (e) and (f) and (g) and (h), respectively. Similar differentiation pathways can be observed in the acute leukaemias as compared with normal bone marrow, except for a different distribution of the cells along the pathway. The cells depicted yellow are $CD34^-$ cells, which most likely belong to the leukaemic cell population(s).

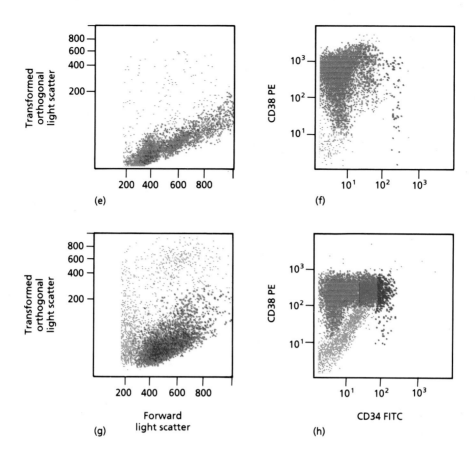

(e)

(f)

(g)

Forward
light scatter

(h)

CD34 FITC

Plate 4.4 (continued)

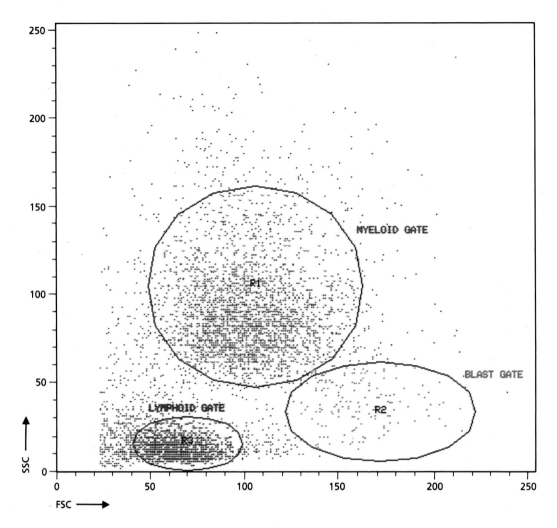

Plate 5.1 Scattergram of a low density mononuclear cell bone marrow population.

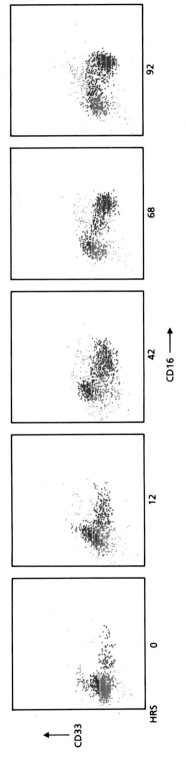

Plate 5.2 Immunological maturation of myeloid cells. Maturation is associated with a loss of CD33 and a gain in CD16 expression.

117

CHAPTER 5
Neutrophil
Membrane
Antigens and
Antibodies

1983; Forsyth and Levinsky, 1990). These changes in expression were shown to be due to activation of the neutrophil.

Even in the absence of temperature changes, the type of preparation procedure itself is also important. Recently flow cytometry has allowed the development of techniques in which whole blood may be used for the analysis of antigen expression on neutrophils without prior cell separation by density gradient centrifugation or dextran sedimentation (Barker, 1988; Hamblin *et al.*, 1991). A recent study (Macey *et al.*, 1992) compared the results obtained using unfixed whole blood anticoagulated with EDTA, dextran-sedimented cells in heparinized blood and formaldehyde-fixed cells on neutrophil expression of five functional antigens (CD11b the C3bi receptor CR3; CD13, aminopeptidase; CD14, the LPS:LPS binding protein receptor; CD16, FcRIII and CDw32, FcRII). In addition the effect of dual antibody labelling was considered. In this study it was shown that the expression of some CD antigens on neutrophils may be influenced by the method of preparation (Fig. 5.1). It was also shown that some antibodies to the Fc receptors on neutrophils may stimulate the cell sufficiently at room temperature to enhance expression of other cell surface molecules such as CR3 (CD11b) (Fig. 5.2). This result is important because it implies that with some combinations of antibodies, dual fluorescence analysis may give misleading results. Clearly, individual antibodies should be examined for this type of interaction where dual fluorescence analyses are undertaken at room temperature. The effect of antibody binding to monocytes has been studied previously (Macintyre *et al.*, 1989). Murine antibodies to CD13, CD14 and class II major histocompatibility complex (MHC) were found to mobilize calcium in normal monocytes. This activation was thought to be due to the formation of antigen–antibody–Fc receptor complexes in which the Fab portion of the antibody bound to the antigen and the Fc portion bound to Fc receptors on the cell. Mab 3G8 (anti-FcRIII) appears to activate neutrophils via this mechanism (Fig. 5.2) as upregulation of CD11b by 3G8 is blocked by a Mab directed against FcRII, and is not seen with the Fab fragment of 3G8. Activation of the respiratory

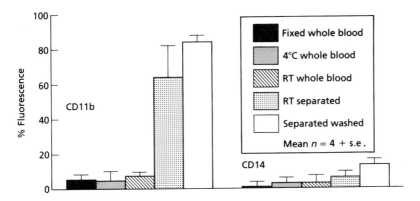

Fig. 5.1 The expression of CD11b and CD14 (% fluorescence) on neutrophils prepared under different conditions.

118

CHAPTER 5
Neutrophil
Membrane
Antigens and
Antibodies

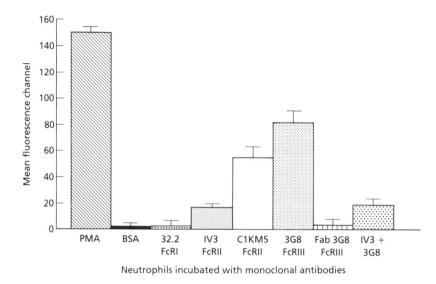

Fig. 5.2 The expression of CD11b on neutrophils which had been prepared by dextran sedimentation and incubated with monoclonal antibodies to FcRI, FcRII and FcRIII.

burst in macrophages has also been shown to be mediated by Fc receptor stimulation (Brozna *et al.*, 1988). Interestingly, Wright *et al.* (1990, 1991) have recently shown that stimulation and upregulation of CD14 also results in increased expression and function of CR3.

In general, neutrophils which are fixed prior to washing and incubation with antibody prevent cell activation. The method described is that of Hamblin *et al.* (1991).

Formaldehyde rapid fix whole blood technique

1 Freshly drawn blood (1 ml) from healthy donors without anticoagulant is mixed with an equal volume of 0.4% formaldehyde in Hank's balanced salt solution (HBSS) without phenol red (Sigma) at 37°C for 4 min.
2 Erythrocytes are then lysed by the addition of 40 ml 0.01 mol/l Hepes (Gibco) buffered ammonium chloride (0.155 mol/l).
3 After incubation at 37°C for 10 min the cells are washed twice in HBSS by centrifugation at 300 g and resuspended to 1 ml of HBSS.
4 Aliquots (50 µl) of cells are then incubated with antisera at room temperature (RT) for 20 min then transferred to 1% formaldehyde before analysis by flow cytometry.

However, in some situations the rapid fix method may alter antigen expression (see below) and it may be preferable to label the cells prior to fixation and lysis of the red blood cells (RBCs).

119

CHAPTER 5
Neutrophil
Membrane
Antigens and
Antibodies

Whole blood technique

1 Aliquots (50 μl) of freshly drawn blood anticoagulated with liquid EDTA (0.25% final concentration Becton Dickinson), sodium citrate (0.105 mol/l Becton Dickinson) or preservative heparin (10 U/ml Monoparin, CP Pharmaceuticals) are incubated with fluorescein-conjugated antisera or isotype control sera either at 4°C or at RT for 20 min.

2 Erythrocytes are lysed and the white cells stabilized and fixed by using either the Coulter Q-Prep system or Becton Dickinson FACS-Lyse.

Further considerations

There are a number of factors which should be considered with regard to these methodologies: (a) the variation in phlebotomy and time of venesection; (b) the anticoagulant used; (c) the length of time prior to fixation; (d) the effect of fixation prior to labelling; (e) the length of fixation; (f) the effect of divalent cations on antibody binding.

Phlebotomy variation and time of venesection

Neutrophils exhibit diurnal variations (Uhlinger *et al.*, 1991) and are affected by exercise (Fry *et al.*, 1992); venesection should therefore be performed at the same time each day if comparative studies are to be undertaken. Also, neutrophils within the bloodstream may become activated by prolonged venocclusion. This is illustrated in Fig. 5.3. Venesection was performed under conditions of no occlusion and occlusion for 1 or 4 min. The blood was immediately processed by the rapid fix method and labelled with phycoerythrin-conjugated CD11b and fluorescein-conjugated CD18 in the presence or absence of divalent cations. The amount of fluorescence associated with the neutrophils in each preparation was determined on a flow cytometer under standard conditions. The cell populations in whole blood were identified on a dual parameter histogram of 90° light scatter and forward angle light (FAL) scatter, which allows clear distinction of granulocytes from monocytes and lymphocytes. The log green and red fluorescence was measured on single parameter histograms. The per cent fluorescence (above background staining with negative control sera) and the mean fluorescence intensity (MFI) were recorded on the granulocyte population for each sample. The MFI for CD11b was up to 50% higher on neutrophils from venesections with 4 min occlusion compared with cells from venesections with no or brief occlusion.

Anticoagulant and the effect of divalent cations

Variation in antigen expression and antibody binding may be influenced

120

CHAPTER 5

Neutrophil
Membrane
Antigens and
Antibodies

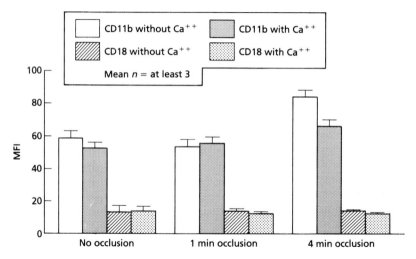

Fig. 5.3 The effect of venocclusion on the neutrophil expression of CD11b and CD18. The cells were processed by the rapid fix whole blood method and labelled either with or without divalent cations.

by the anticoagulant used. In the case of ion chelating agents such as EDTA and acid citrate (AC) this may be due to changes in antigen configuration due to the loss of Ca^{2+} and Mg^{2+} ions (Dransfield, 1991). To illustrate this, blood was either non-anticoagulated or taken into anticoagulants (AC, EDTA and heparin) then immediately processed by the rapid fix method and labelled with CD11b and CD18 in the presence or absence of divalent cations and analysed as above. The binding of CD11b was lower in blood anticoagulated with EDTA while that of CD18 was higher (Fig. 5.4). In these experiments the presence and absence of divalent cations during the labelling procedures was examined. In general the MFI for CD11b was found to be higher in the presence of Ca^{2+} and Mg^{2+} while that of CD18 was higher in the absence of these cations.

Length of time prior to fixation

To examine the stability of neutrophils in anticoagulated blood, blood was taken into EDTA, AC or heparin and held on ice or at 37°C for up to 1 hour. At times 0, 5, 10, 30 and 60 min, aliquots were removed and processed by the rapid fix procedure prior to labelling with CD11b and CD18 in the presence or absence of divalent cations. In general, antigen expression was stable at 4°C but varied with time at 37°C (Fig. 5.5).

The effect of fixation prior to labelling

Some fixative procedures may alter the antigen expression. This has been observed with the Q-prep system in which formic acid is used to

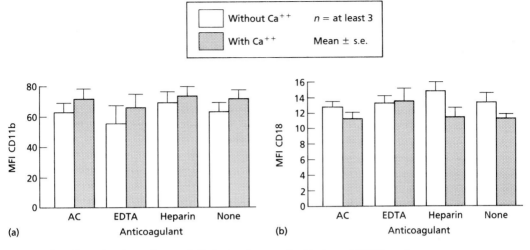

Fig. 5.4 The effect of anticoagulant and divalent cations on the binding of CD11b and CD18 antibodies to neutrophils prepared by the rapid fix whole blood method.

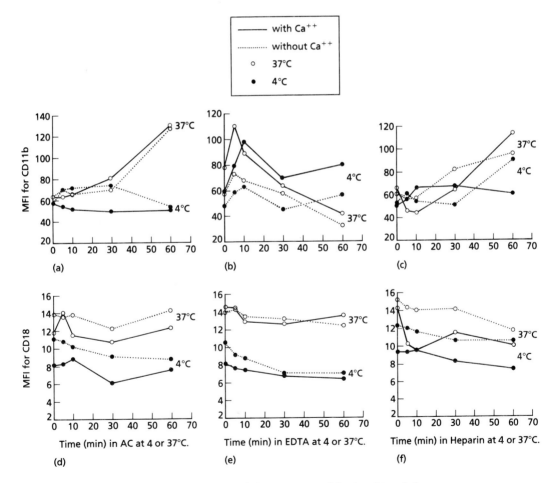

Fig. 5.5 Illustration of the CD11b and CD18 variation on neutrophils stored in whole blood at 4° or 37°C with anticoagulants AC, EDTA and heparin.

122

CHAPTER 5

Neutrophil
Membrane
Antigens and
Antibodies

lyse the RBCs and the leucocytes are fixed with paraformaldehyde (0.1% final concentration). Anticoagulated blood (AC, EDTA, heparin) was processed by the Q-prep system then labelled with CD11b and CD18 and compared with cells labelled prior to Q-prep processing; the results are shown in Fig. 5.6. There was little change in the MFI for CD18, but that of CD11b was markedly reduced on cells that had been labelled prior to Q-prep processing, suggesting that either the antigen/antibody was stripped from the cells, or alternatively, fixation prior to labelling may have activated the cells.

Length of fixation

The concept of fixation is to set molecules such that they do not change. However, many fixatives also act as cellular permeabilizing agents (see Chapter 10). Prolonged periods of fixation may therefore result in subsequent analysis of cell surface and cytoplasmic antigen expression. This is illustrated in Fig. 5.7, where whole blood without anticoagulant was incubated for up to 55 min with 0.4% formaldehyde, the RBCs were then lysed and the leucocytes labelled with CD11b and CD18 in the presence or absence of divalent cations. There was a 50-fold increase in the MFI for CD11b and a 200-fold increase in the MFI for CD18 when divalent cations were present.

In conclusion these findings indicate that the analysis of antigens on neutrophils should be performed under clearly defined and controlled conditions. It is clearly important to prevent cellular activation during isolation and labelling. In this respect the use of whole blood analysis with formaldehyde fixation may be beneficial for analysis of some antigens but it is possible that the antigenicity or expression of others

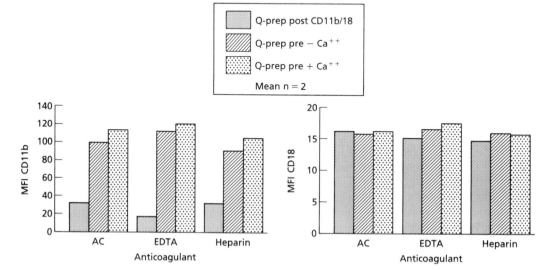

Fig. 5.6 Antigens and/or antibodies may be influenced by fixation prior to labelling as shown here.

123

CHAPTER 5
*Neutrophil
Membrane
Antigens and
Antibodies*

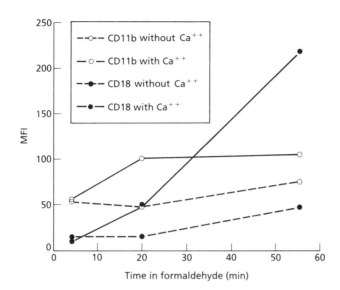

Fig. 5.7 The effect of prolonged neutrophil fixation on the binding of CD11b and CD18 antibodies.

may be altered by this procedure. Recently a method has been described that avoids the use of fixation and lysis in the preparation of leucocytes for analysis by flow cytometry (McCarthy and Macey, 1993). This may prove to be the method of choice.

Clinical studies of neutrophil membrane antigens

The difficulties encountered in the preparation and handling of neutrophil suspensions have largely restricted *in vitro* neutrophil experiments and delayed our understanding of related clinical disorders. Furthermore, changes occurring during *in vitro* handling of neutrophils have all too frequently been attributed to *in vivo* abnormalities where none exist. Flow cytometry provides a ready tool for the analysis of neutrophil populations, which avoids complex purification procedures, and allows a measure of neutrophil activation during experimental manipulation.

As well as leading to upregulation of neutrophil antigens, neutrophil activation may also lead to downregulation or shedding of antigens such as the leucocyte adhesion molecule LAM-1 (Griffin *et al.*, 1990). *In vitro* activation of neutrophil preparations can lead to clinical confusion; this is illustrated by an apparent case of neutrophil CD16 deficiency in an otherwise normal individual (Veys *et al.*, 1991). CD16 which is the Fc receptor III for human IgG is also shed from the neutrophil surface following activation (Huizinga *et al.*, 1988). Following Ficoll-Paque density centrifugation or dextran sedimentation, this subject's neutrophil population appeared to lack CD16 expression; however, following whole blood analysis, CD16 was clearly expressed on all neutrophils; hence activation had led to shedding of neutrophil CD16 *in vitro* and an erroneous result (Fig. 5.8). CD16 deficiency in normal healthy indivi-

124

CHAPTER 5
*Neutrophil
Membrane
Antigens and
Antibodies*

duals can, however, occur; it is a rare phenomenon which has led to CD16 alloimmunization and isoimmune neutropenia (Fromont *et al.*, 1992).

Receptor expression during myeloid maturation

The expression of membrane receptors on developing myeloid cells in the bone marrow is illustrated in Fig. 5.9. Myelopoiesis may be followed both morphologically and immunologically by flow cytometry. Plate 5.1 reveals the scattergram of a low density mononuclear cell bone marrow population; early myeloid precursor cells granulocyte-macrophage colony-stimulating factor (GM-CSF) and myeloblasts are found in the blast gate, metamyelocytes, stab cells and segmented neutrophils in the myeloid gate; promyelocytes and myelocytes are variably split between these two gates (Civin and Loken, 1987). Immunological maturation within these gates can be followed by dual fluorescence immunofluorocytometry, for instance, by the gradual loss of membrane CD33 and gain of CD16 expression which occurs with maturation towards a segmented neutrophil (Plate 5.2).

Monocytic cells also occur within the blast gate and cultured monocytic cells which express $CD16^{+/++}CD33^{++}$ (unpainted cells in Plate 5.2) can be phenotypically distinguished from developing myeloid cells $CD16^{+/++}CD33^{+}$. Dual fluorescence flow cytometry has also shown that the acquisition of membrane CD16 late in myeloid development occurs simultaneously with that of decay accelerating factor (DAF), a complement regulatory protein (Fig. 5.10), probably as a result of attachment of both preformed proteins to the membrane via a common phosphatidyl-inositol glycan (PIG) anchor (Veys *et al.*, 1990a). Acquisition

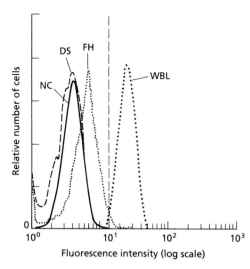

Fig. 5.8 An illustration of the effect of dextran sedimentation (DS), Ficoll-Paque (FH) centrifugation and whole blood lysis (WBL) on the expression of CD16 on neutrophils from a normal healthy individual. NC is the normal isotype control.

125

CHAPTER 5
*Neutrophil
Membrane
Antigens and
Antibodies*

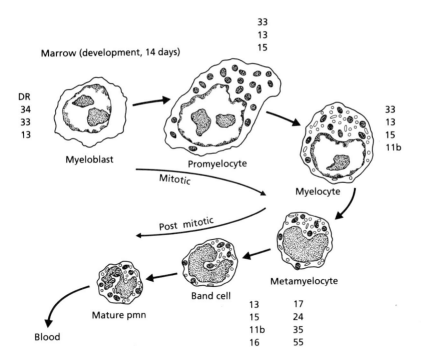

Fig. 5.9 The expression of membrane receptors on developing myeloid cells in bone. marrow. pmn, polymorphonuclear.

of these membrane proteins may differentiate peripheral blood from bone marrow neutrophils (Civin and Loken, 1987).

The final array of mature neutrophil membrane receptors is by no means static, and recent interest has focused on flow cytometric assessment of both up- and down-regulation of neutrophil adhesive receptors to explain rapid movements in body neutrophil pools following infusion of various compounds including GM-CSF and intravenous immunoglobulin (IVIG). GM-CSF has been shown to up-regulate the intercellular adhesion molecule CD11b both *in vivo* and *in vitro* (Arnaout et al., 1986; Devereux et al., 1989). The up-regulation of CD11b induces neutrophil aggregation (Arnaout et al., 1986) and may be responsible for the temporary neutropenia and pulmonary sequestration that occurs after administration of GM-CSF. Further detailed *in vitro* studies have shown that GM-CSF induces a more profound change in surface expression of adhesion molecules, with co-ordinate up-regulation of CD11b and down-regulation of LAM-1 (Fig. 5.11; Griffin et al., 1990). This pattern of response to GM-CSF was the same whichever method of neutrophil preparation was used, although as previously mentioned, the baseline receptor expression differed. IVIG, which also induces a temporary neutropenia following infusion (Majer and Green, 1988; Veys et al., 1988c; Tampi, 1989) has also been shown to up-regulate CD11b (O'Donnell et al., 1988). *In vitro* the up-regulation of CD11b is blocked by monoclonal antibodies to Fc receptors (Fig. 5.12) and as Fc receptors do not bind monomeric IgG (Anderson and Looney, 1986), this implies

126

CHAPTER 5

Neutrophil
Membrane
Antigens and
Antibodies

that the mechanism of neutropenia is through immunoglobulin aggregates in IVIG binding to Fc receptors. This then induces CD11b up-regulation and neutrophil margination/emigration (Veys, 1990b).

The disorders of neutrophil membrane receptors which have been elucidated by flow cytometry can be divided into inherent neutrophil abnormalities and abnormalities induced by *in vivo* stimulation of normal neutrophils. An example of the latter already alluded to is the up-regulation of the adhesive receptor CD11b which helped unravel the mechanism of GM-CSF and IVIG-induced neutropenia. The neutrophil CD11/CD18 receptor is up-regulated several-fold in response to chemotactic factors and this is clinically relevant in neutropenia occurring during dialysis, induced by the generation of C5a (Mazzucchelli *et al.*, 1992) and may be involved in the pathogenesis of rheumatoid arthritis (Macey *et al.*, 1993a).

Inherent abnormalities in CD11b also exist and include diminished expression in congenital leucocyte adhesion deficiency (CD11/CD18 deficiency) where due to a biosynthetic defect of the common β-subunit, CR3, lymphocyte function associated antigen-1 (LFA-1) and p150,95 all have diminished expression on the surface membrane (Harlan *et al.*, 1992). This is an autosomal recessive disorder resulting in neutrophilia,

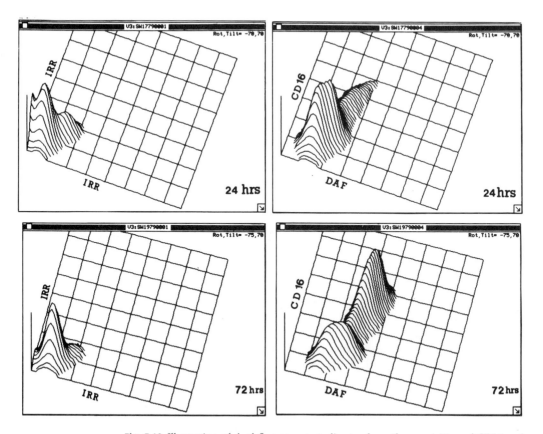

Fig. 5.10 Illustration of dual fluorescent studies to show the acquisition of CD16 and DAF (CD55) late in myeloid development.

defective neutrophil mobilization and recurrent bacterial infection without pus formation (Anderson and Springer, 1987).

127

CHAPTER 5
*Neutrophil
Membrane
Antigens and
Antibodies*

Reduced up-regulation of CR3 from intracellular pools on neonatal
neutrophils exhibit reduced migration *in vitro*, which is believed
to contribute to infectious morbidity and mortality among neonatal
populations (Jones *et al.*, 1990). Other inherent abnormalities include
deficiencies in CD16 DAF (CD55) and other phosphatidyl-inositol
anchored proteins in paroxysmal haemoglobinuria (Selvaraj *et al.*, 1988),
and isolated CD16 deficiency in otherwise normal individuals as mentioned above (Huizinga *et al.*, 1988; Fromont *et al.*, 1992).

Neutrophil antibodies

Neutrophil specific allo-antibodies have been implicated in a number
of clinical disorders including: (a) febrile transfusion reactions (Verheugt
et al., 1977; De Rie *et al.*, 1985); (b) severe pulmonary reactions following
blood transfusion (Thompson *et al.*, 1971; Schiffer *et al.*, 1979); (c)
isoimmune neonatal neutropenia (Lalezari *et al.*, 1986); and (d) failure
of effective granulocyte transfusion (Schiffer *et al.*, 1980; Cairo *et al.*,
1992).

Neutrophil specific auto-antibodies have been identified in auto-

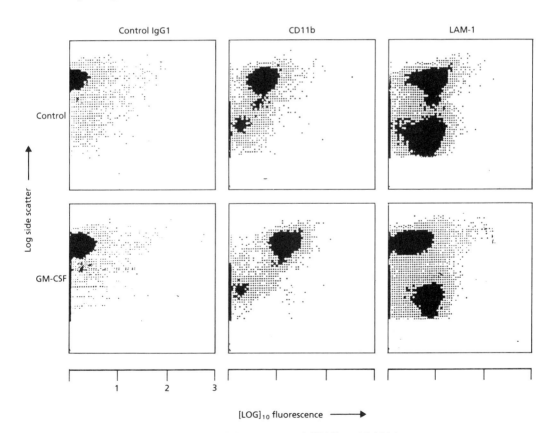

Fig. 5.11 The effect of GM-CSF on neutrophil expression of CD11b and LAM-1.

128

CHAPTER 5
Neutrophil
Membrane
Antigens and
Antibodies

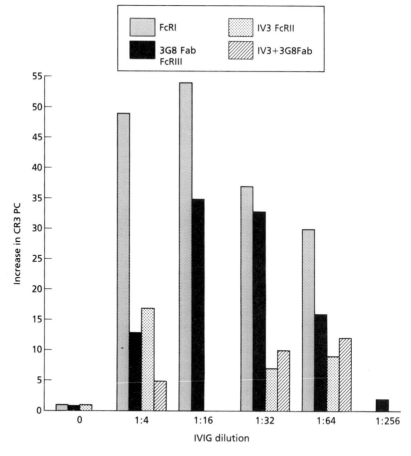

Fig. 5.12 IVIG causes a dose-dependent increase in CR3 (CD11b) expression *in vitro*. This up-regulation may be blocked by prior addition of monoclonal antibodies to receptors FcRII (IV3), partially blocked by antibodies to FcRIII (3G8 Fab) but not blocked by antibodies to FcRI (FcRI). The *y*-axis represents the increase in CR3 (CD11b) peak channel fluorescence.

immune neutropenia in adults (Lalezari *et al.*, 1975, 1986; Verheugt *et al.*, 1978; McCullough *et al.*, 1987; Logue *et al.*, 1991; Beatty and Stroncek, 1992; Bux and Mueller-Eckhardt, 1992) and children (McCullough *et al.*, 1981; Matsubayushi *et al.*, 1991; Lyall *et al.*, 1992). The antigens identified by these granulocyte-specific antibodies were designated the 'N' series (Lalezari and Radel, 1974). McCullough (1983) analysed the clinical significance of this antigen system. The neutrophil-specific NA antigen system has two alleles, NA1 and NA2, which have a phenotypic frequency of 46 and 88% in the Caucasian population (McCullough *et al.*, 1981; von dem Borne *et al.*, 1983; Hartman *et al.*, 1990). Neutrophil FcRIII (CD16) is closely associated with the NA antigen system and has been identified as a 50–80-kDa glycoprotein (GP) on neutrophils that express both NA1 and NA2, a 50–65-kDa GP on neutrophils that express NA1 only and a 65–80-kDa GP on neutrophils that express NA2 only (Logue and Shimm, 1980; Currie *et al.*, 1987).

129

CHAPTER 5
*Neutrophil
Membrane
Antigens and
Antibodies*

Antibodies to FcRIII have been described in numerous cases of auto-immune neutropenia (Stroncek *et al.*, 1991; Rios *et al.*, 1991; Bux *et al.*, 1991a,b,c; Cartron *et al.*, 1992; Fromont *et al.*, 1992). Hartman *et al.* (1990) found that in many cases of autoimmune neutropenia the auto-antibodies were reactive with a 45 kDa antigen that was probably the cytoskeletal, intracellular localized component actin. More recently neutrophil auto-antibodies specific for CD11b/CD18 have been found in patients with autoimmune neutropenia (Hartman and Wright, 1991). This finding suggests that in some patients with autoimmune neutro-penia the presence of antibodies to the functionally important adhesion proteins CD11b/CD18 may interfere with neutrophil function, thereby amplifying the risk of infection associated with neutropenia. Anti-neutrophil antibodies may also be found in drug-induced agranulo-cytosis (Weitzman and Stossel, 1978; Walbroehl and John, 1992). The realization that drug-induced antibodies are involved in the mechanism of an agranulocytosis is important as re-challenge with the offending drug may lead to a dramatic and severe recurrence of neutropenia.

As well as in isolated autoimmune neutropenia, the presence of neutrophil-associated immunoglobulin (NAIg) has been demonstrated in many other diseases where neutropenia may occur, such as the generalized autoimmune diseases, systemic lupus erythematosus (SLE), rheumatoid arthritis and Felty's syndrome (Lasito and Lorusso, 1979; McCullough *et al.*, 1987; Goldschmeding *et al.*, 1988). The presence of different types of antibody as well as immune complexes have both been described in these diseases (Zubler *et al.*, 1976; Lasito and Lorusso, 1979; Starkbaum and Arend, 1979) and they may or may not be associ-ated with neutropenia. Therefore it is unknown whether NAIg in these diseases has an antibody nature or represents immune complexes that have bound to the Fc receptors and complement receptors on the neutrophil membrane. However, either or both may be responsible for inducing neutropenia.

NAIg is also present in chronic infections such as HIV infection (Murphy *et al.*, 1987; Klaassmen *et al.*, 1990). Immune complexes have also been implicated in the pathophysiology of neutropenia in this disease (Bowen *et al.*, 1985). However, recent evidence suggests that NAIg in HIV infections is auto-antibody in nature (Klaassmen *et al.*, 1991b). Neutrophil-associated antibodies have also been implicated in a number of conditions including Hodgkins's disease (Gordon *et al.*, 1991), Crohn's disease (Stevens *et al.*, 1991), primary biliary cirrhosis (Bux *et al.*, 1991a), ulcerative colitis (Shanahan *et al.*, 1992), inflammatory bowel disease (Cambridge *et al.*, 1992) and nutritional copper deficiency (Higuchi *et al.*, 1991).

Detection of anti-neutrophil antibodies

The study of anti-neutrophil antibodies by fluorescence techniques became possible in 1976 with the development of a method to overcome the non-specific binding of IgG from normal serum to neutrophils

130

CHAPTER 5
*Neutrophil
Membrane
Antigens and
Antibodies*

(Verheugt *et al.*, 1977). The method involves the paraformaldehyde fixation of the neutrophil membrane prior to incubation with the test serum. This prevents the binding of normal IgG, but permits the binding of most anti-neutrophil antibodies and some immune complexes (Engelfreit *et al.*, 1984). However, certain specific anti-neutrophil antibodies cannot be detected by immunofluorescence, for example those specific for NB2 antigens; neutrophil agglutination or cytotoxicity assays are required to detect these antigens (Verheugt *et al.*, 1977). In contrast to the study of neutrophil membrane receptors, neutrophil preparation without the use of red cell lysis steps (by Ficoll-Paque or dextran red cell sedimentation) has been found to give better results (Clay and Kline, 1985). Anti-neutrophil antibodies are usually either HLA or neutrophil specific. This distinction requires an additional lympho-

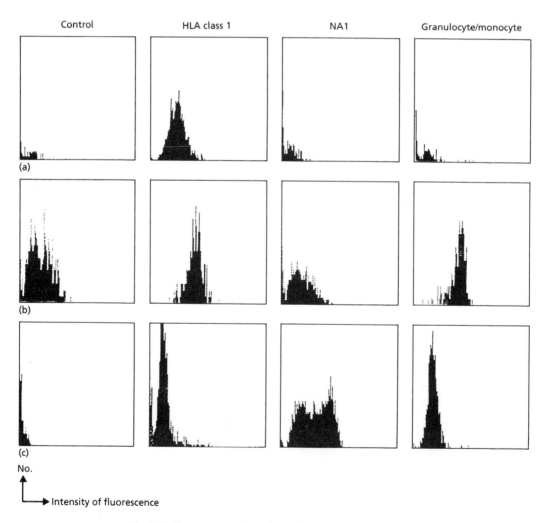

Fig. 5.13 Flow cytometric analysis of lymphocytes, monocytes and neutrophils in a single test allows distinction between HLA, non-specific and neutrophil specific antibodies.

131

CHAPTER 5
*Neutrophil
Membrane
Antigens and
Antibodies*

cytotoxicity test or chloroquine stripping of antigens prior to testing (Minchinton and Waters, 1984).

The differentiation between immune complex and antibody binding may be difficult; a polymorphic pattern of reactivity favours the presence of an antibody as does a positive eluate prepared from the test neutrophils when incubated with control cells. Immune complexes tend to be pan-reactive and can be detected by alternative techniques (Clay and Kline, 1985). Both immune complexes and antibodies may be clinically relevant in the setting of immune neutropenia (Caligaris-Cappio *et al.*, 1979). The detection of IgG bound to the neutrophil membrane *in vivo* is also difficult to interpret as this may reflect anti-neutrophil antibody, immune complex or non-specific IgG binding, as discussed previously, although the absence of neutrophil-associated IgG may help to exclude an immune mechanism. Again elution techniques may provide an answer (Klaassmen *et al.*, 1991a).

Flow cytometric methods for the detection of antineutrophil antibodies have been described and compare favourably with light microscopy (Minchinton *et al.*, 1989). A major concern has been whether flow cytometric methods would be able to exclude from the analysis neutrophils which had been damaged during preparation. These cells fluoresce brightly, but with an abnormal fluorescence pattern which can be discerned by light microscopy (Clay and Kline, 1985). In fact these cells are also excluded by flow cytometry as their light scattering properties are altered (McMann *et al.*, 1988). Flow cytometry enables the use of lymphocytes and monocytes as well as neutrophils as target cells and this permits, in a single test, the distinction between HLA or other antigens and neutrophil-specific antibodies (Veys *et al.*, 1988a; Fig. 5.13); although it is possible that very weak antibodies may be adsorbed onto other cells and missed using this technique (Minchinton *et al.*, 1989). The pattern of fluorescence in the flow cytometric histograms may give some indication as to the presence of antibody or immune complex (Veys *et al.*, 1988a). Flow cytometry also gives slightly superior results with chloroquine-stripped neutrophils (Minchinton *et al.*, 1989). The use of flow cytometry in the investigation of typical cases of autoimmune neutropenia and drug-induced agranulocytosis is illustrated below.

The first patient was a 42-year-old man with a long-standing history of thrombocytopenia eventually requiring splenectomy; autoimmune haemolytic anaemia which responded to steroids; arthralgia, with a positive antinuclear antibody; and a positive four-stranded DNA test. A diagnosis of variant SLE had been made. More recently there was a 1 year history of neutropenia with recurrent mouth ulcers. A bone marrow aspirate and biopsy showed increased myelopoiesis with relative depletion of mature myeloid cells and a clinical diagnosis of autoimmune neutropenia was made. Flow cytometry was used to measure both the neutrophil-associated IgG and the presence of neutrophil antibodies in the patient's serum (for method see below). Both the direct (data not shown) and indirect tests (Fig. 5.14) were strongly positive. Normal

132

CHAPTER 5
Neutrophil
Membrane
Antigens and
Antibodies

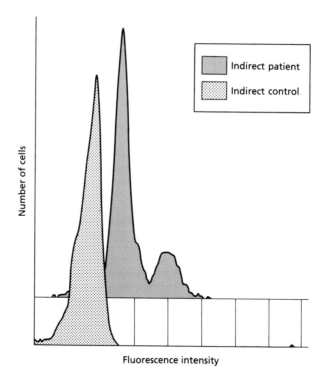

Fig. 5.14 Example of the indirect analysis neutrophil specific IgG in the serum from a neutropenic patient.

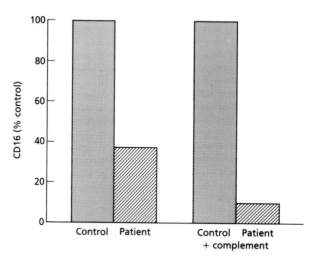

Fig. 5.15 The expression of CD16 on myeloid cells grown in the presence of normal control serum and serum from a neutropenic patient. The patient's serum exhibited myelocytotoxicity with and without complement.

donor bone marrow precursor cells were cultured in a liquid system in the presence of patient serum or normal serum with or without the addition of complement (for method see below). Myeloid growth was assessed at 108 hours by absolute numbers of myeloid cells expressing

133

CHAPTER 5
*Neutrophil
Membrane
Antigens and
Antibodies*

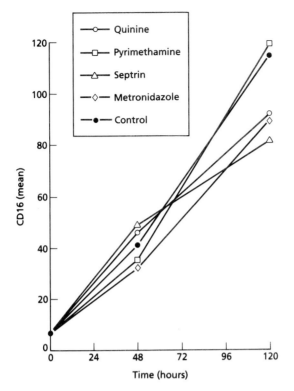

Fig. 5.16 Bone marrow, from a patient with suspected drug-induced neutropenia, was cultured in a liquid system in the presence of four drugs. The cultures were analysed at 108 hours for absolute numbers of cells expressing CD16. The graph shows that none of the drugs caused significant myelotoxicity in the assay.

the late differentiation antigen CD16 (Veys *et al.*, 1992) and Fig. 5.15 shows that the patient serum exhibited a significant myelotoxicity both with and without the addition of complement. Hence the presence of an anti-neutrophil antibody/immune complex had been identified by three independent flow cytometric assays and the diagnosis confirmed.

The second patient was a 34-year-old woman who had just returned from West Africa. She had become unwell with a high swinging fever and was found to have a deep-seated skin abscess and malarial parasites on the blood film. She was treated with a combination of drugs including metronidazole, septrin, pyrimethamine and quinine. There was an initial improvement but 10 days later she became unwell again with a recrudescence of fever and a neutrophil count of zero. A drug agranulocytosis was suspected and a bone marrow aspirate at that time showed markedly reduced myelopoiesis with promyelocytes only present. The marrow was cultured in a liquid system in the presence of metronidazole, septrin, pyrimethamine and quinine at twice steady-state concentrations. Cultures were analysed at 108 hours for absolute numbers of cells expressing CD16. Figure 5.16 shows the results of these cultures. None of the drugs caused significant myelotoxicity in this assay, suggesting that the drugs were not exhibiting direct toxicity on the bone marrow.

134

CHAPTER 5
*Neutrophil
Membrane
Antigens and
Antibodies*

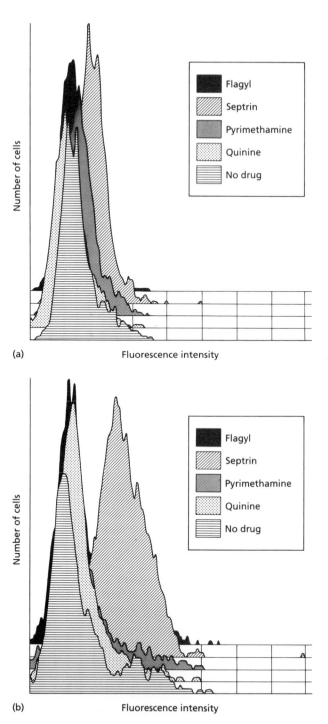

Fig. 5.17 Flow cytometric immunofluorescent identification of a septrin-dependent IgM anti-neutrophil antibody in the serum from a patient with suspected drug-induced neutropenia. (a) Cells incubated with anti-IgG. (b) Cells incubated with anti-IgM.

135

CHAPTER 5
*Neutrophil
Membrane
Antigens and
Antibodies*

On day 3 of each culture, an aliquot of cells was pelleted, fixed with 1% paraformaldehyde and presented as target cells in an indirect immuno-fluorescent test to the patient's serum taken at the time of neutropenia (see below). Further drug was added to this incubation. The target cells were then analysed for neutrophil-associated IgG and IgM by flow cytometry. Figure 5.17, shows the presence of a septrin-dependent IgM anti-neutrophil antibody. A diagnosis of immune neutropenia due to septrin was made, the patient was rechallenged with the non-implicated drugs and she made an uneventful recovery.

Flow cytometry has provided a ready tool for the study of neutrophil disorders. Some of these techniques are now used on a routine basis, while other research applications promise to unravel the further role of neutrophils in both body defence and disease mechanisms.

Assay of NAIg and anti-neutrophil antibodies

A single-step separation of mononuclear cells, neutrophils and erythro-cytes is performed using a discontinuous Histopaque (Sigma) gradient centrifugation assay (English and Anderson, 1974). This method elimin-ates the need for hypotonic lysis of red cells, which may cause damage to the neutrophil membrane (Clay and Kline, 1985). It is also the preferred method for preparation of leucocytes for functional assays because it results in minimal activation of granulocytes (Macey and McCarthy, 1993).

Method

1 Whole blood (10 ml) anticoagulated with Na₂EDTA (5 g/ml, Sigma) is diluted with an equal volume of HBSS without phenol red (Sigma).

2 Histopaque 1119 (3 ml) is added to 15 ml round bottom tubes, then 3 ml Histopaque 1077 is carefully layered onto the Histopaque 1119. Blood (6 ml) is layered on top of the upper gradient.

3 The gradient is centrifuged at 700 g for 30 min at RT after which the mononuclear cells are harvested from the plasma/1077 inter-face and the neutrophils are collected from the 1077/1119 interface. Erythrocytes are pelleted to the bottom of the tube.

4 The granulocytes and mononuclear cells are then washed sep-arately (×2) in HBSS containing 0.2% globulin-free bovine serum albumin (BSA) (Sigma) by centrifugation at 250 g for 5 min at RT.

5 The cells are then fixed with filtered 1% paraformaldehyde (Sigma) in HBSS pH 7.2 for 5 min at RT. Paraformaldehyde should be freshly prepared from a stock 4% solution, which should be made monthly or aliquoted and stored frozen.

6 After fixation the cells are washed (×2) in HBSS-BSA and neutro-phils and mononuclear cells are mixed in equal numbers to give a

Continued on p.136

136

CHAPTER 5

Neutrophil
Membrane
Antigens and
Antibodies

leucocyte suspension of $2-4 \times 10^6$/ml in HBSS-BSA. The average platelet contamination is 5×10^6/ml.

7 Leucocytes (100 μl) are then incubated with 5 μl FITC rabbit F(ab')$_2$ anti-human IgG, IgM and control-serum (DAKO) for 30 min at 4°C. After a final wash in HBSS-BSA the cells are resuspended in the same, ready for analysis.

8 For indirect antibody testing, aliquots (100 μl) of leucocyte suspension are incubated with 100 μl of test serum for 30 min at 37°C, washed twice in HBSS-BSA then labelled as above. Negative controls (serum from non-transfused, blood group AB healthy males) and positive controls (anti-NA1, multispecific anti-HLA or serum from patients with immune complex disorders such as rheumatoid arthritis) should be included in the study.

Flow cytometric analysis

Cell populations are separated by analysis of their light scattering properties. Adequate separation of the cells is confirmed by labelling the cells with monoclonal antibodies, CD2, CD14 and CD16. Lymphocytes are CD2$^+$, CD14$^-$, CD16$^-$; monocytes are CD2$^-$, CD14$^+$, CD16$^-$; and neutrophils are CD2$^-$, CD14$^-$, CD16$^+$.

Short-term liquid bone marrow cultures

This is based on a method described by Nagler *et al.* (1990).

Procedure

1 Bone marrow (10 ml) is collected into 300 U preservative-free heparin (Monoparin) and mixed with 10 ml Iscove's modified Dulbecco's medium (IMDM) (Gibco).

2 The cells are layered over an equal volume of Ficoll-Paque (density 1077) and the gradient centrifuged at 400 g for 30 min at RT.

3 Mononuclear cells at the interface with the medium and Ficoll are collected then washed twice and resuspended in IMDM supplemented with 5% fetal calf serum (FCS) (Gibco).

4 The cells are then incubated for 1 hour at 37°C in 3.5 cm Petri dishes (Nunc) to allow adherence of monocytic cells.

5 The non-adherent cells are collected, washed and resuspended in IMDM-5% FCS and counted.

6 Aliquots (2×10^7 cells/ml) are incubated with: (a) 65 μl My8 antiserum (Coulter); (b) 5 μl anti-glycophorin A (DAKO) at 4°C for 20 min. After which the cells are washed in cold medium, resuspended in 3 ml IMDM-5% FCS and poured into prepared goat anti-mouse coated Petri dishes (see below).

137

CHAPTER 5
Neutrophil
Membrane
Antigens and
Antibodies

7 The cells are incubated for 70 min at 4°C. The dishes are then washed with IMDM to recover non-bound cells which are washed and resuspended in IMDM-15% FCS containing 10 ng G-CSF (Amgen).

Goat anti-mouse Petri dishes

1 To prepare the goat anti-mouse Petri dishes, 0.05 mol/l Tris-buffered saline (TBS) pH 9.5 is filtered onto 100×15 mm Nunc Petri dishes.
2 Goat anti-mouse immunoglobulin (500 µl) is added and the dishes incubated at 23°C for 40 min.
3 After which the TBS is decanted and the dishes are washed four times in phosphate-buffered saline (PBS) prior to addition of IMDM-1% FCS for 15 min at 4°C.

Detection of drug-associated anti-myeloid precursor antibodies

1 Cells are prepared as above, then incubated with a predetermined non-toxic concentration of the suspect drug together with:
    (a) 10% control serum which has had complement inactivated by heating at 56°C for 30 min;
    (b) 10% test serum (heat treated as above).
2 The cells are then cultured in IMDM-15% FCS containing 10 ng G-CSF at 37°C in an atmosphere of 5% CO_2. The expression of CD33 and CD16 is monitored at 132 hours.

Detection of drug-associated complement-dependent anti-myeloid precursor antibodies

1 Cells prepared as above are incubated with a predetermined, non-toxic concentration of the suspect drug.
2 After 12 hours the cells are pelleted and resuspended in IMDM containing:
    (a) 5% control serum (heat treated) plus 5% test serum; and
    (b) 5% test serum (heat treated) plus 5% control serum.
3 The cells are incubated for 1 hour at 37°C, washed twice and resuspended in IMDM-15% FCS with 10 ng G-CSF.
4 The cells are then cultured and haematopoiesis is monitored at 132 hours by determining the percentage of CD33- and CD16-positive cells.

Neutrophil function

The oxidative burst associated with stimulation by Texas Red labelled, opsonized bacteria has been described for dual laser flow cytometry (Bass *et al.*, 1983; Szejda *et al.*, 1984). This was modified for use on a

138

CHAPTER 5
Neutrophil
Membrane
Antigens and
Antibodies

single laser flow cytometer (Macey *et al.*, 1990) and two assays were used to measure the functional ability of the isolated neutrophils. First, the rate of uptake of IgG opsonized bacteria labelled with propidium iodide and second the oxidative burst associated with stimulation by either opsonized bacteria or the phorbol ester, phorbol myristate acetate (PMA). In the latter assay the oxidative burst is measured by quantifying the increase in fluorescence associated with the oxidation of non-fluorescent 2',7'-dichlorofluorescein diacetate (DCFH-DA) to the highly fluorescent 2',7'-dichlorofluorescein (DCF). The substrate DCFH-DA is a stable non-polar molecule that readily diffuses through the cell membrane of the neutrophil. Once inside the cell the acetyl groups are cleaved by enzymes in the cytoplasm to produce a polar molecule (DCFH) which is trapped within the cell. DCFH is non-fluorescent but becomes highly fluorescent when oxidized by hydrogen peroxide (H_2O_2), which is produced during the oxidative burst in neutrophils. The increase in fluorescence associated with the oxidation of DCFH is therefore a direct measure of the oxidative burst.

Assay procedure

Bacterial culture

Staphylococcus aureus strain Wood 45 (Protein A negative; NCTC CPHL; Code NCo7121) are maintained on agar slopes, plated on blood agar, then colonies picked off into peptone water. Cultures are agitated at 37°C overnight. The cells are washed three times in HBSS without phenol red (Gibco) then fixed with 70% ethanol at 4°C for 30 min. The fixed cells are then washed twice in PBS containing 1% gelatine and 1% glucose (Sigma) (PBSg) pH 7.2, then resuspended to a final concentration of 1×10^8 organisms/ml as determined by optical density measurement at 580 nm in an LKB Ultraspec II (Pharmacia).

Opsonization of bacteria

Bacteria 10^8 in PBSg are mixed with 1 ml (30 mg/ml) human IgG (Sandoz) and 1 ml 0.2 mol/l carbonate buffer pH 8.6, then incubated with vigorous agitation at 37°C for 30 min. The bacteria are then washed twice in PBSg and resuspended to a final concentration of 1×10^8/ml.

Propidium iodide labelling of bacteria

Bacteria 10^8 in PBSg are incubated with propidium iodide (Sigma) at a final concentration of 50 μg/ml at 37°C for 30 min then washed twice with PBSg. The labelled bacteria are resuspended in PBSg to a final concentration of 10^8/ml.

139

CHAPTER 5
*Neutrophil
Membrane
Antigens and
Antibodies*

Preparation of PMA

A stock solution of phorbol 12-myristate 13-acetate (Sigma) 1 mg/ml is made in absolute ethanol, aliquoted and stored at −20°. Immediately prior to use the PMA is diluted in PBSg to a final concentration of 100 ng/ml.

Preparation of DCFH-DA

A stock solution (10 mmol/l) of DCFH-DA (Molecular Probes) is made in absolute ethanol and stored in the dark at 4°C. Immediately prior to use the DCFH-DA is diluted in PBSg to a final concentration of 5 μmol/l.

Assay of oxidative product formation

1   Neutrophils in whole blood (1 ml) are preincubated for 15 min with 5 μmol/l DCFH-DA in PBSg with agitation at 37°C.
2   After 15 min incubation 100 μl aliquots of cells are incubated in sterile round-bottom tubes with 100 μl, PBSg (negative control), opsonized bacteria at a bacteria : cell ratio of 500 : 1 (test), non-opsonized bacteria at the same ratio (test control), and PMA at a final concentration of 100 ng/ml (positive control).
3   The tubes are incubated at 37°C with vigorous agitation.
4   Aliquots for each type of stimulation are set up in quadruple, such that samples can be removed at times from 0 to 60 min after commencement of the assay.
5   The reaction is stopped by the addition of 2 ml FACS-Lyse for 10 min. The cells are then washed twice in PBSg, re-suspended in the same and analysed by flow cytometry.

Assay of bacterial uptake

1   Aliquots (100 ml) of blood are incubated in round-bottom tubes with 100 μl of, PBSg (negative control), opsonized propidium iodide labelled bacteria at a cell : bacteria ratio of 1 : 500 (test) and non-opsonized labelled bacteria (test control).
2   Assays are set up in triplicate and samples removed after 10, 20 and 30 min. The reaction is stopped as above, and the samples are analysed by flow cytometry.
3   The rate of increase in red fluorescence per minute is taken to be directly related to the rate of uptake of bacteria.

Flow cytometry

All studies are performed on a flow cytometer equipped with an argon laser (488 nm emission). FAL scatter, 90° light scatter, green (510−550 nm)

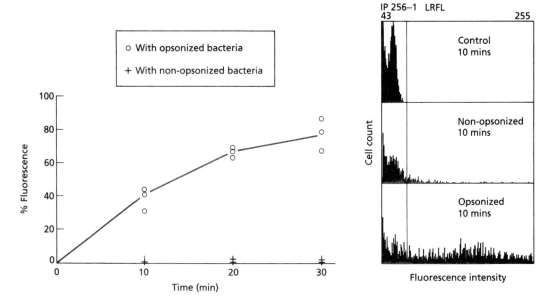

Fig. 5.18 Illustration of the time-dependent increase of red fluorescence associated with neutrophils incubated with propidium iodide labelled, IgG opsonized *Staphylococcus aureus*.

and red (>580 nm) fluorescence are recorded. The assay for neutrophil stimulation is performed in parallel with that for bacterial uptake. Typical results are illustrated in Figs 5.18 and 5.19.

Alternative assays

Recently, a number of assays have been described for measurement of neutrophil function by other techniques. The important point of distinction between internalized and membrane bound particles was addressed by Fattorossi *et al.* (1989). In this assay fluorescein-conjugated heat-killed *Candida albicans* was opsonized by purified antibodies and used as targets for human polymorphonuclear granulocytes (PMNs). The procedure is based on the observation that the targets lose their green fluorescence upon incubation with ethidium bromide (EB) through the resonance energy transfer phenomenon occurring between the two fluorochromes. PMNs are incubated with the opsonized target for 20 min at 4 or 37°C, in the presence of cytochalsin B, an inhibitor of the phagocytic process that does not affect membrane binding of fluorescein. EB is added and the green and red fluorescence associated with PMNs is evaluated. EB does not penetrate intact cell membranes so internalized particles are not affected by EB and remain green, whereas membrane bound particles assume an intense red stain. By dual fluorescence analysis the number of PMNs containing and/or binding fluorescein-labelled targets can be assessed.

The oxidation of hydroethidine (HE) to EB has been used to measure the oxidative metabolic burst in neutrophils stimulated with opsonized

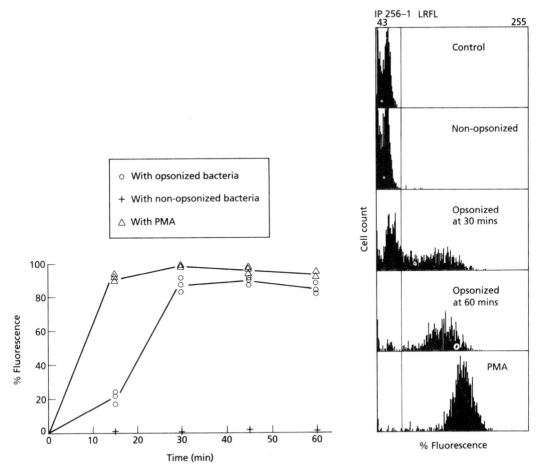

Fig. 5.19 Illustration of the green fluorescence associated with DCFH oxidation in neutrophils stimulated by non-opsonized bacteria, opsonized bacteria and the phorbol ester PMA.

fluorescein-labelled bacteria (Perticarari *et al.*, 1991). Dual fluorescence analysis was used to measure the red EB emission together with the green fluorescence associated with ingested bacteria. In this assay crystal violet is added to quench the fluorescence associated with membrane bound bacteria such that only internalized bacteria are assayed.

The relative involvement, in phagocytosis, of receptors for the Fc portion of IgG and the complement components C3b and C4b has also been studied (Andoh *et al.*, 1991). Fluorescent latex beads coated specifically with IgG or complement components were used in this study. To evaluate bead attachment, the phagocytic assay was performed with 3 μmol/l cytochalasin D treated cells, which inhibited internalization. The per cent cells with ingested beads and the number of ingested beads per 100 cells was assessed. This allowed quantitative analysis of the function of cell surface receptors for IgG and complement components.

The fluorescent dye LDS-751 is specific for nucleated cells and has

142

CHAPTER 5
Neutrophil
Membrane
Antigens and
Antibodies

been used in whole blood assays to eliminate erythrocytes from analysis of granulocyte oxidative metabolic burst (Himmelfarb *et al.*, 1992). The detection of reactive oxygen species is facilitated by oxidation of DCFH-DA (as above). The effect of lipopolysaccharide on phagocytosis and metabolic burst has also been assessed in whole blood (Bohmer *et al.*, 1992).

Neutrophil IgG Fc receptor expression and function

Neutrophils express two receptors for the Fc portion of human IgG, termed FcRII and FcRIII (Anderson and Looney, 1986). These receptors are necessary for the phagocytosis of IgG opsonized particles. The expression of these receptors is therefore a useful measure of potential function.

Assay of Fc receptor expression

Neutrophils in whole blood are processed by the rapid fix procedure, then incubated with 5 µl FITC IV3 (Medarex) or 15 µl FITC Leu11a for 20 min at 4°C. Appropriate negative controls are included in each assay. The cells are washed in cold (4°C) PBS containing 1% BSA then resuspended in the same buffer before flow cytometric analysis. The per cent fluorescence positivity above the negative control is determined and the mean fluorescence channel recorded.

Clinical applications

The combination of a flow cytometric phagocytosis assay with flow cytometric assay of oxidative metabolism has been used to determine the functional abilities of neutrophils from patients with autoimmune neutropenia (AIN; Macey *et al.*, 1990). These patients inherently have low numbers of neutrophils, thus the ability to use flow cytometry, which is a highly sensitive system, is greatly beneficial. In this study the finding of a weak correlation between the neutrophil count and the NAIgG was contradictory to previous reports (Hadley *et al.*, 1987) and was perhaps due to the increased sensitivity of the flow cytometric assay compared with light microscopy.

The data presented showed that neutropenic patients do have a reduced ability to respond to opsonized bacteria compared to normal controls and patients with other autoimmune disorders. Also the data confirmed that the degree of metabolic burst is related to the rate of uptake of bacteria. The rate of bacterial uptake was not found to be related to the amount of IgG on the neutrophil surface or the number of neutrophils circulating in the patient. However, the rate of phagocytosis was found to correlate with the expression of FcR11 and FcRIII. The expression of these receptors was found to be lower than normal, which would be consistent with the presence of increased numbers of immature cells. These findings suggest that the functional ability of neutrophils in AIN patients is influenced by IgG Fc receptor expression (Veys *et al.*, 1988b). Neutrophil function may also be influenced by C3b receptor expression (Fearon and Collins, 1983). Reduced IgG Fc receptor expression has also been found on neutrophils from patients after bone marrow transplantation. These cells also have reduced functional abilities (Macey *et al.*, 1993b).

143

CHAPTER 5
*Neutrophil
Membrane
Antigens and
Antibodies*

References

Anderson CL, Looney RJ (1986) Human leucocyte IgG Fc receptors. *Immunol. Today* **7**: 264−266.

Anderson DC, Springer TA (1987) Leukocyte adhesion deficiency: An inherited defect in the MAC-1, LFA-1 and p150,95 glycoprotein. *Annu. Rev. Med.* **38**: 175.

Andoh A, Fujiyama Y, Kitoh K, Hodohara K, Bamba T, Hosada S (1991) Flow cytometric assay for phagocytosis of human monocytes mediated via Fc-gamma receptors and complement receptor CR1 (CD35). *Cytometry* **12**: 677−686.

Arnaout MA, Wang EA, Clark SC, Sieff CA (1986) Human recombinant granulocyte colony stimulating factor increases cell to cell adhesion promoting glycoproteins on mature granulocytes. *J. Clin. Invest.* **78**: 597−601.

Barker JW (1988) An innovative lymphocyte preparation system for flow cytometry. *Am. Clin. Lab.* **9**: 26−32.

Bass DA, Parce JW, Dechatelet LR, Sjejda P, Seeds MC, Thomas M (1983) Flow cytometric studies of oxidative product formation by neutrophils. A graded response to membrane stimulation. *J. Immunol.* **130**: 1910−1917.

Beatty PA, Stroncek DF (1992) Autoimmune neutropenia in Sheboygan County, Wisconsin. *J. Lab. Clin. Med.* **119**: 718−723.

Bohmer RH, Trinkle LS, Staneck JL (1992) Dose effect of LPS on neutrophils in whole blood flow cytometric assay of phagocytosis and oxidative burst. *Cytometry* **13**: 525−531.

Bowen DL, Lane HC, Fauci AS (1985) Immunopathogenesis of the acquired immuno-deficiency syndrome. *Ann. Intern. Med.* **103**: 704−709.

Boyum A (1968) Isolation of mononuclear cells and granulocytes from human peripheral blood. *Scand. J. Clin. Lab. Invest.* **21** (Suppl. 97): 77.

Brozna J, Hauff N, Phillips W, Johnston R (1988) Activation of the respiratory burst in macrophages. Phosphorylation specifically associated with Fc receptor mediated stimulation. *J. Immunol.* **141**: 1642−1647.

Bux J, Mueller-Eckhardt C (1992) Autoimmune neutropenia. *Semin. Haematol.* **29**: 45−53.

Bux J, Kissel K, Nowak K, Spengel U, Mueller-Eckhardt C (1991a) Autoimmune neutropenia: clinical and laboratory studies in 143 patients. *Ann. Haematol.* **63**: 249−252.

Bux J, Robertz Vaupel GM, Glasmacher A, Dengler HJ, Mueller-Eckhardt C (1991b) Autoimmune neutropenia due to NA1 specific antibodies in primary biliary cirrhosis. *Br. J. Haematol.* **77**: 121−122.

Bux J, Mueller-Eckhardt G, Mueller-Eckhardt C (1991c) Autoimmunisation against the neutrophil-specific NA1 antigen is associated with HLA-DR2. *Human Biol.* **30**: 18−21.

Cairo MS, Worcester CC, Rucker RW *et al.* (1992) Randomised trial of granulocyte transfusion versus intravenous immunoglobulin therapy for neonatal neutropenia and sepsis. *J. Pediatr.* **120**: 281−285.

Caligaris-Cappio F, Gamussi G, Gavosto A (1979) Idiopathic neutropenia with nor-mocellular bone marrow: An immune complex disease. *Br. J. Haematol.* **43**: 595−605.

Cambridge G, Rampton DS, Stevens TR, McCarthy DA, Kamm M, Laeker B (1992) Anti-neutrophil antibodies in inflammatory bowel disease: prevalence and diag-

144

CHAPTER 5
*Neutrophil
Membrane
Antigens and
Antibodies*

nostic role. *Gut* **33**: 668–674.

Cartron J, Celton JL, Gane P *et al.* (1992) Iso-immune neonatal neutropenia due to an anti-Fc receptor III (CD16) antibody. *Eur. J. Pediatr.* **151**: 438–441.

Civin CL, Loken MR (1987) Cell surface antigens on human marrow cells dissection of haematopoietic development using monoclonal antibodies and multiparameter flow cytometry. *Int. J. Cell Cloning* **5**: 267–286.

Clay ME, Kline WE (1985) Detection of granulocyte antigens and antibodies: current perspectives and approaches. In: Garratty G, ed., *Current Concepts in Transfusion Therapy*. Arlington, pp. 183–265.

Currie M, Weinberg JB, Rustugi K, Logue G (1987) Antibodies to granulocyte precursors in selective myeloid hypoplasia and other suspected autoimmune neutropenias. *Blood* **69**: 529–536.

De Rie MA, van des Plas-van Dalen CM, Engelfriet CP, von dem Borne AEGKr (1985) Serology of febrile transfusion-reactions. *Vox Sang.* **49**: 126–134.

Devereux S, Bull HA, Campos-Costa D, Saib R, Linch DC (1989) Granulocyte macrophage colony stimulating factor induced changes in cellular adhesion molecule expression and adherence to endothelium: *in-vitro* and *in-vivo* studies in man. *Br. J. Haematol.* **71**: 323–330.

Dransfield I (1991) Regulation of leukocyte integrin function. In: Hogg N, ed., *Integrins and ICAM-1 in Immune Responses. Chem. Immunol.* Karger, Basel, Vol. 50. pp. 13–33.

Engelfreit CP, Tetteroo JPW, van der Veen JPW, Werner WF, van Plas-van Dalen C, von dem Borne AEGKr (1984) Granulocyte-specific antigens and methods for their detection. In: McCullough J, Sandler RM, eds, *Blood Cell Antigens and Bone Marrow Transplantation, Progress in Clinical and Biological Research*. Advances in Immunobiology: AR Liss, New York, pp. 122–154.

English D, Anderson BR (1974) Single-step separation of red blood cells, granulocytes and mononuclear leukocytes on discontinuous density gradients of Ficoll Hypaque. *J. Immunol. Methods* **5**: 249–252.

Fattorossi F, Nisini R, Pizzola JG, D'Amelio R (1989) New simple flow cytometry technique to discriminate between internalized and membrane-bound particles in phagocytosis. *Cytometry* **10**: 320–325.

Fearon D, Collins L (1983) Increased expression of C3b receptors on polymorphonuclear leukocytes induced by chemotactic factors and by purification procedures. *J. Immunol.* **130**: 370–375.

Forsyth K, Levinsky R (1990) Preparative procedures of cooling and re-warming increase leukocyte integrin expression and function on neutrophils. *J. Immunol. Methods* **128**: 159–163.

Fromont P, Bettaieb A, Skouri H *et al.* (1992) Frequency of the polymorphonuclear neutrophil Fc gamma receptor III deficiency in the French population and its involvement in the development of neonatal alloimmune neutropenia. *Blood* **79**: 2131–2134.

Fry RW, Morton AR, Crawford GP, Keast D (1992) Cell numbers and *in vitro* responses of leukocytes and lymphocytes following maximal exercise and interval training sessions of different intensities. *Eur. J. Appl. Physiol.* **64**: 218–227.

Goldschmeding R, Breedveld FC, Engelfreit CP, von dem Borne AEGKr (1988) Lack of evidence for the presence of neutrophil autoantibodies in the serum of patients with Felty's syndrome. *Br. J. Haematol.* **68**: 37–40.

Gordon BG, Kiwauka J, Kadushin J (1991) Autoimmune neutropenia and Hodgkin's disease: successful treatment with intravenous immunoglobulin. *Am. J. Pediatr. Hematol. Oncol.* **13**: 164–167.

Gordon DL, Rice JL, MacDonald PJ (1989) Regulation of human neutrophil type 3 complement receptor (iC3b receptor) expression during phagocytosis of *Staphylococcus aureus* and *Escherichia coli*. *Immunology* **67**: 460–465.

Griffin JD, Spertini O, Ernst TJ *et al.* (1990) Granulocyte-macrophage colony-stimulating factor and other cytokines regulate surface expression of leukocyte adhesion molecule-1 on human neutrophils and their precursors. *J. Immunol.* **145**: 576–584.

Hadley AG, Byran MA, Chapel HM, Bunch C, Holburn AM (1987) Anti-granulocyte opsonic activity in sera from patients with systemic lupus erythematosus. *Br. J. Haematol.* **65**: 61–65.

145

CHAPTER 5
Neutrophil
Membrane
Antigens and
Antibodies

Hamblin A, Taylor M, Bernhagen J *et al.* (1991) A new method preparing blood leukocytes for flow cytometry which prevents upregulation of leukocyte integrin expression. *J. Immunol. Methods* **146**: 219−235.

Harlan JM, Winn RK, Vedder NB, Doerschuk CM, Rice CL (1992) *In vivo* models of leukocyte adherence to endothelium. In: Harlan JM, Liu, eds, *Adhesion its Role in Inflammatory Disease*. WH Freeman and Company, New York, pp. 117−150.

Hartman KR, Wright DG (1991) Identification of autoantibodies specific for the neutrophil adhesion glycoproteins CD11b/CD18 in patients with autoimmune neutropenia. *Blood* **78**: 1096−1104.

Hartman KR, Mallet MK, Nath J, Wright DG (1990) Antibodies to actin in autoimmune neutropenia. *Blood* **75**: 736−743.

Higuchi S, Higashi A, Nakamura T, Yanabe Y, Matsuda I (1991) Anti-neutrophil antibodies in patients with nutritional copper deficiency. *Eur. J. Pediatr.* **150**: 327−330.

Himmelfarb J, Hakim RM, Holbrook DG, Leeber DA, Ault KA (1992) Detection of granulocyte reactive oxygen species formation in whole blood using flow cytometry. *Cytometry* **13**: 83−89.

Huizinga TW, van der Schoot CE, Jost C *et al.* (1988) The PI-linked receptor for FcR III is released on stimulation of neutrophils. *Nature* **333**: 667−669.

Jones DH, Schmalsteig FC, Dempsey K *et al.* (1990) Subcellular distribution and mobilization of MAC-1 (CD11b/CD18) in neonatal neutrophils. *Blood* **75**: 488−498.

Klaassmen RJL, Mulder JW, Vlekke ABJ *et al.* (1990) Autoantibodies against peripheral blood cells appear early in HIV infection and their prevalence increases with disease progression. *Clin. Exp. Immunol.* **81**: 11−17.

Klaassmen RJL, Goldschmeding R, Vlekke ABJ, Rozendaal R, von dem Borne AEGKr (1991a) Differentiation between neutrophil-bound antibodies and immune complexes. *Br. J. Haematol.* **77**: 398−402.

Klaassmen RJL, Vlekke ABJ, von dem Borne AEGKr (1991b) Neutrophil-bound immunoglobulin in HIV infection is of autoantibody nature. *Br. J. Haematol.* **77**: 403−409.

Knapp W (1989) Leukocyte typing IV. In: Knapp K, Dorken B, Gilks WR, Reibor EP, Schmidt RE, Stein H, von dem Borne AEGKr, eds, *White Cell Differentiation Antigens*. Oxford University Press, pp. 781−946.

Lalezari P, Radel E (1974) Neutrophil specific antigens: Immunologic and clinical significance. *Semin. Hematol.* **11**: 281−290.

Lalezari P, An-Fu J, Yegen L, Santorineou M (1975) Chronic autoimmune neutropenia due to anti-NA2 antibody. *N. Engl. J. Med.* **293**: 744−747.

Lalezari AP, Khorshidi M, Petrosova M (1986) Autoimmune neutropenia of infancy. *J. Pediatr.* **109**: 764−769.

Lasito A, Lorusso L (1979) Polymorphonuclear leukocyte fluorescence and cryoglobulin phagocytosis in systemic lupus erythematosus. *Clin. Exp. Immunol.* **35**: 376−379.

Logue GL, Shimm DS (1980) Autoimmune granulocytopenia. *Annu. Rev. Med.* **31**: 191−200.

Logue GL, Shastri KA, Laughlin M, Shimm DS, Ziolkowski LM, Iglehart JL (1991) Idiopathic neutropenia: antineutrophil antibodies and clinical correlations. *Am. J. Med.* **90**: 211−216.

Lyall EG, Lucas GF, Eden OB (1992) Autoimmune neutropenia of infancy. *J. Clin. Pathol.* **45**: 431−434.

McCarthy DA, Macey MG (1993) A simple flow cytometric procedure for the determination of surface antigens on unfixed leucocytes in whole blood. *J. Immunol. Methods* **163**: 155−160.

McCullough J, Clay ME, Priest JR *et al.* (1981) A comparison of methods for detecting leukocyte antibodies in autoimmune neutropenia. *Transfusion* **21**: 483−488.

McCullough JJ (1983) Granulocyte antigen systems and their clinical significance. *Human Pathol.* **14**: 228−234.

McCullough JJ, Clay ME, Thompson HW (1987a) Autoimmune granulocytopenia. In: Engelfreit CP, von dem Borne AEGKr, eds, *Ballière's Clin. Immunol. Allergy* Vol. 1 no. 2.

McCullough J, Clay M, Kline W (1987b) Granulocyte antigens and antibodies. *Trans-*

146

CHAPTER 5
*Neutrophil
Membrane
Antigens and
Antibodies*

fusion Med. Rev. **1**: 150–160.

Macey MG, McCarthy D (1993) Leukocyte activation during *in vitro* preparation procedures. *Cytometry* (in press).

Macey MG, Sangster J, Veys P, Newland A (1990) Flow cytometric analysis of the functional ability of neutrophils from patients with autoimmune neutropenia. *J. Microscopy* **159**: 277–283.

Macey MG, Jiang XP, Veys P, McCarthy D, Newland AC (1992) Expression of functional antigens on neutrophils. Effects of preparation. *J. Immunol. Methods* **149**: 37–42.

Macey MG, Wilton JMA, Carbon R, Edmonds S, Perry JD, McCarthy D (1993a) Leukocyte activation and function-associated antigens in inflammatory disease. *J. Rheumatol. Agents Actions* **38**: 39–40.

Macey MG, Sangster J, Kelsey S, Newland AC (1993b) *Ex-vivo* studies of neutrophil function in patients post bone marrow transplantation. *Clin. Lab. Haemat.* **15**: 79–85.

Macintyre E, Roberts P, Jones M *et al.* (1989) Activation of human monocytes occurs on cross-linking monocyte antigens to an Fc receptor. *J. Immunol.* **142**: 2377–2383.

McMann LE, Walterson ML, Hogg LM (1988) Light scattering and cell volumes in osmotically stressed and frozen-thawed cells. *Cytometry* **9**: 33–38.

Majer RV, Green PJ (1988) Neutropenia caused by intravenous immunoglobulin. *Br. Med. J.* **296**: 1262.

Matsubayashi T, Arakawa H, Kawase R (1991) Two siblings with autoimmune neutropenia of infancy. *Acta Paediatr.* **33**: 734–736.

Mazzucchelli J, Mazzone A, Pasotti D *et al.* (1992) Role of hemostasis and inflammation of increase of adhesion molecule of phagocytes. ISH 24th Congress BJH. p. 208 (Abstr. 797).

Minchinton RM, Waters AH (1984) Chloroquin stripping of HLA antigens from neutrophils without removal of neutrophil specific antigens. *Br. J. Haematol.* **57**: 703–706.

Minchinton RM, Rockman S, McGrath KM (1989) Evaluation and calibration of a fluorescence-activated cell sorter for the interpretation of the granulocyte immuno-fluorescence test (GIFT) *Clin. Lab. Haematol.* **11**: 349–359.

Murphy MF, Metcalf P, Waters AH *et al.* (1987) Incidence and mechanism of neutropenia and thrombocytopenia in patients with human immunodeficiency virus infection. *Br. J. Haematol.* **66**: 22–24.

Nagler A, Binet C, Mickichan M *et al.* (1990) Impact of marrow cytogenetics and morphology on *in vitro* haematopoiesis in the myelodysplastic syndromes: comparison between recombinant human granulocyte colony stimulating factor and granulocyte-monocyte CSF. *Blood* **76**: 1299–1307.

O'Donnell JL, Bradley J, Ahern MJ, Roberts-Thomson PH (1988) Alteration in circulating neutrophil CR3 density associated with immunoglobulin infusion. *Aust. N.Z. J. Med.* **18**: 95–100.

Perticarari S, Presani G, Mangiarotti MA, Banfi E (1991) Simultaneous flow cytometric method to measure phagocytosis and oxidative products by neutrophils. *Cytometry* **12**: 687–683.

Porteau F, Fischer A, Descamps-Latscha B, Halbwachs L (1986) Defective complement receptors (CR1 and CR3) on erythrocytes and leukocytes of factor I (C3b-inactivator) deficient patients. *Clin. Exp. Immunol.* **66**: 463–471.

Rios E, Heresi G, Arevalo M (1991) Familial alloimmune neutropenia of NA-2 specificity. *Am. J. Pediatr. Hematol. Oncol.* **13**: 296–299.

Schiffer CA (1980) Granulocyte transfusions: an established or still experimental therapeutic procedure. *Vox Sang.* **38**: 56–58.

Schiffer CA, Aisner J, Daly PA, Schimpff SC, Wiernik PH (1979) Alloimmunisation following prophylactic granulocyte transfusion. *Blood* **54**: 766–774.

Selvaraj P, Rosse WF, Silber R, Springer TA (1988) The major Fc receptor in blood has a phosphatidylinositol anchor and is deficient in paroxysmal nocturnal haemoglobinuria. *Nature* **333**: 565–567.

Shanahan F, Duerr RH, Rotter JI *et al.* (1992) Neutrophil autoantibodies in ulcerative colitis: familial aggregation and genetic heterogeneity. *Gastroenterology* **103**: 456–461.

147

CHAPTER 5
*Neutrophil
Membrane
Antigens and
Antibodies*

Skoog WA, Beck WS (1956) Studies on the fibrinogen, dextran and phytohaem-agglutinin methods of isolating leukocytes. *Blood* **11**: 436–454.

Starkbaum G, Arend WP (1979) Neutrophil-binding immunoglobulin in systemic lupus erythematosus. Evidence for the presence of both soluble immune complexes and immunoglobulin G antibodies to neutrophils. *J. Clin. Invest.* **64**: 902–912.

Stevens C, Peppercorn MA, Grand RJ (1991) Crohn's disease associated with auto-immune neutropenia. *J. Clin. Gastroenterol.* **13**: 328–330.

Stroncek DF, Skubitz KM, Plachta LB *et al.* (1991) Alloimmune neonatal neutropenia due to an antibody to the neutrophil Fc-gamma receptor III with maternal deficiency of CD16 antigen. *Blood* **77**: 1572–1580.

Szejda P, Parce JW, Seeds MS, Bass DA (1984) Flow cytometric quantitation of oxidative product formation by polymorphonuclear leukocytes during phago-cytosis. *J. Immunol.* **133**: 3303–3307.

Tampi R (1989) Fall in the neutrophil count during immunoglobulin infusion. *Aust. N.Z. J. Med.* **19**: 515–516.

Thompson JS, Severon CD, Parmley MJ, Marmorstein BL, Simmons A (1971) Pulmonary 'hypersensitivity' reactions induced by transfusion of non-HLA leukoagglutinins. *N. Engl. J. Med.* **284**: 1120–1125.

Uhlinger DJ, Burnham DN, Mullins RE *et al.* (1991) Functional differences in human neutrophils isolated pre- and post-prandial. *FEBS Lett.* **286**: 28–32.

Verheugt FWA, von dem Borne AEGKr, Decary F, Engelfreit CP (1977) The detection of granulocyte alloantibodies with an indirect immunofluorescent test. *Br. J. Haematol.* **36**: 533–544.

Verheugt FWA, von dem Borne AEGKr, van Noord-Bokhorst JC, Engelfreit CP (1978) Autoimmune granulocytopenia: the detection of granulocyte antibodies with an immunofluorescent test. *Br. J. Haematol.* **39**: 339–350.

Veys PA, Macey MG, Newland AC (1988a) Detection of granulocyte antibodies using flow cytometric analysis of leucocyte immunofluorescence. *Vox Sang.* **56**: 42–47.

Veys PA, Macey MG, Newland AC (1988b) Autoimmune neutropenia and the neutro-phil FcR. *Biochem. Soc. Trans.* **16**: 732.

Veys PA, Macey MG, Owens CM, Newland AC (1988c) Neutropenia following intravenous immunoglobulin. *Br. Med. J.* **216**: 1800.

Veys PA, Wilkes S, Ellis G, Hoffbrand AV (1990a) Deficiency in DAF and CD16 on PNH neutrophils. *Br. J. Haematol.* **76**: 318.

Veys PA, Wilkes S, Ellis G (1990b) Fall in the neutrophil count during immunoglobulin infusion. *Aust. N.Z. J. Med.* **20**: 291.

Veys PA, Wilkes S, Hoffbrand AV (1991) Deficiency of neutrophil FcRIII. *Blood* **78**: 852–853.

Veys PA, Wilkes S, Shah S, Noyelle R, Hoffbrand AV (1992) Clinical experience of Clozapine-induced neutropenia in the UK. Laboratory investigation using liquid culture systems and immunofluorocytometry. *Drug Safety* **7** (Suppl. 1): 26–32.

von dem Borne AEGKr, van der Plas van Dalen CM, Engelfreit CP (1983) Immuno-fluorescence antiglobulin test. In: McMillan R, ed., *Immune Cytopenias*. Churchill Livingstone, New York, p. 106.

Walbroehl GS, John PG (1992) Antibiotic associated neutropenia. *Am. Fam. Physician* **45**: 2237–2241.

Weitzman SA, Stossel TP (1978) Drug-induced immunological neutropenia. *Lancet* **i**: 1068–1071.

Wright S, Ramos R, Tobias P, Ulevitch R, Mathison J (1990) CD14, a receptor for complexes of lipopolysaccharide (LPS) and LPS binding protein. *Science* **249**: 1431–1436.

Wright S, Ramos R, Hermanowski-Vosakta A, Rockwell P, Detmers P (1991) Activation of adhesive capacity of CR3 on neutrophils by endotoxin: Dependence on lipo-polysaccharide binding protein and CD14. *J. Exp. Med.* **173**: 1281–1286.

Zubler RH, Nydegger UE, Perrin LH *et al.* (1976) Circulating and intra-articular immune complexes in patients with rheumatoid arthritis. *J. Clin. Invest.* **57**: 1308–1319.

Chapter 6
Platelet-associated Molecules and Immunoglobulins

A. H. GOODALL AND M. G. MACEY

Detection of platelet-associated immunoglobulin (PAIg) and auto-antibodies

In 1956 Harrington *et al.* suggested that idiopathic thrombocytopenic purpura (ITP) was an autoimmune disease. Since then a number of investigators have confirmed that elevated levels of PAIg are found in a significant proportion of these patients (Dixon *et al.*, 1975; Hymes *et al.*, 1979; Mueller-Eckhardt *et al.*, 1980a). Most of these assays are qualitative rather than quantitative and lack reproducibility at the low platelet counts encountered. To overcome this, free antibodies (i.e. un-bound) in the serum of such patients have also been looked for. The use of flow cytometry for the detection of PAIg has many advantages and fulfils many of the criteria required for antibody detection. It can distinguish between the various immunoglobulin classes, it allows the distinction of complement-fixing antibodies and identification of immune complexes is made possible by the use of fluorescein isothio-cyanate (FITC)-conjugated Staphylococcal Protein A, which has been shown to bind to the Fc portion of the antibody but not to immune complexes (Harmon *et al.*, 1980). The technique is simple and both qualitative and quantitative. Lazarchick and Hall (1986) described a semi-quantitative method to measure PAIgG by flow cytometry utilizing the mean fluorescence intensity channel as a measure of increased fluorescence intensity. For non-Gaussian fluorescence histograms the mean fluorescence intensity channel may not provide a reliable quan-titative measure of increased fluorescence intensity. In the method described below the total fluorescence above background is used to quantitate the amount of PAIg. In addition the distinction between antibodies specific for platelets and other cells may be made so that the platelet-specific and HLA antibodies may be identified.

Clinical relevance of PAIg

The detection of antibodies directed against and immune complexes attached to platelets is important in the diagnosis of immune thrombo-cytopenia. With the introduction of high dose intravenous immuno-globulin as a mode of therapy in ITP (Imbach *et al.*, 1981; Newland *et al.*, 1983) with its rapid effect on platelet count there has developed an interest in monitoring PAIg and serum platelet antibodies during treatment; in part to study the potential mechanism of action since it is

Detection of PAIg and PDIg

Sera

Sera from normal healthy volunteers who have not received blood transfusions are used as negative controls. Test sera are from patients with ITP diagnosed by standard criteria.

Antisera

FITC rabbit (F(ab')$_2$ fragments) anti-human IgG and IgM (DAKO) are used to identify the PAIg. FITC mouse anti-glycoprotein Ib or

Continued on page 150

IIIa (GpIb or GpIIIa; DAKO) is used as the positive control. For analysis of indirect PAIg, the optimal antiserum dilution may be determined by a chequer-board titration with various dilutions of antibody containing sera and normal sera. The optimal dilution is that which gives maximal fluorescence with antibody containing sera and minimal fluorescence with normal sera.

Blood collection and analysis

Blood should be analysed as soon after collection as possible. Storage of platelets results in activation, degranulation and expression of increased amounts of internalized IgG on the platelet surface (Fijnheer *et al.*, 1990a; Morris *et al.*, 1991). Blood that has been stored for more than 24 hours should not be analysed as the results will be spurious.

Preparation of a suspension of platelets

1 Blood is collected into liquid K_3EDTA (5 mg/ml blood). Platelet-rich plasma (PRP) is obtained by centrifugation of EDTA blood at $80g$ for 20 min at room temperature.

2 The platelets are obtained by centrifugation of the PRP at $640g$ for 10 min at room temperature then washed three times in filtered (0.22 µm filter) EDTA phosphate-buffered saline (PBS; 0.009 mol/l Na_2EDTA, 0.15 mol/l Na_2HPO_4, 0.15 mol/l KH_2, 0.14 mol/l NaCl pH 6.5).

3 The platelets are resuspended in the same buffer containing 1% bovine serum albumin (BSA) (Sigma; this must be globulin free) to a final concentration of $1-2 \times 10^7$/ml.

4 Contamination by red cells or other white cells should be less than 0.01×10^9/l as determined by the Coulter S Plus IV differential counter.

considered that alterations in PAIg may mirror clinical response. More recently a protein A-immunosorption technique has been developed for the treatment of immune thrombocytopenia (Snyder *et al.*, 1992). This too is a regime in which PAIg and serum platelet-directed immunoglobulin (PDIg) need to be monitored.

Platelets — direct immunofluorescence test

1 A suspension of patients' platelets (0.1 ml) is incubated with FITC-conjugated rabbit anti-human IgG or IgM for 20 min at room temperature.

2 The platelets are then washed twice with EDTA-PBS and resuspended in 1 ml of EDTA-PBS and analysed by flow cytometry.

3 Cells examined by flow cytometry are analysed using log forward angle light scatter and log 90° light scatter; this allows distinction by size and granularity of contaminating red cells and platelet aggregates or fragments. Thus only single intact platelets are gated for analysis of fluorescence.

4 Negative controls consist of platelets incubated with 5 μl FITC rabbit anti-mouse immunoglobulins. Positive controls consist of platelets incubated with 5 μl FITC anti-Gp1b or GpIIIa. Ten thousand platelets are counted for each analysis.

5 Background immunofluorescence is established on the negative control for each patient then all settings are retained unchanged during subsequent analysis.

Platelets — indirect immunofluorescence test

1 A suspension (0.1 ml) of platelets (pooled blood group O) is incubated with 0.1 ml of patients' or control serum for 30 min at room temperature.

2 After incubation the platelets are washed twice with filtered EDTA-PBS and then incubated with 5 μl of FITC-conjugated rabbit anti-human IgG or IgM at room temperature for 30 min.

3 Platelets are washed twice and resuspended for examination as above.

4 Negative controls consist of platelets incubated with serum followed by washing and then incubation with FITC-conjugated rabbit anti-mouse immunoglobulin. Positive controls are set up and flow cytometric analysis is performed as above.

Fluorescent polystyrene microspheres

Calibration standard 5 and 10 μm full bright microspheres (Coulter Electronics or Becton Dickinson) are used to calibrate the flow cytometer.

Platelets are always analysed fresh because paraformaldehyde (PFA)-fixed or liquid nitrogen frozen platelets exhibit high levels of non-specific and/or autofluorescence. The wash buffer used is at pH 6.5 to reduce binding of immune complexes (Myllyla, 1973) and prevent platelet activation (Lagarden *et al.*, 1980).

Whole blood assay for direct detection of PAIg

It is possible to detect immunoglobulin directly on platelets in whole blood. Anticoagulated whole blood (1 ml) is washed three times in 20 ml PBS-EDTA buffer then resuspended in buffer containing 1% BSA. One-hundred-microlitre aliquots are then incubated with antisera as described above, washed twice and resuspended in 2 ml of buffer for analysis. This method is not quicker than the above but does have the advantage that more than one cell type may be analysed for the presence of surface immunoglobulin binding. This is useful for the distinction of HLA, non-specific and specific platelet antibodies (see below).

Analysis of platelet-specific immunoglobulin and HLA or other antibodies

The identification of antibodies to platelet-specific antigens is important for correctly diagnosing neonatal alloimmune thrombocytopenia, post-transfusion purpura and refractoriness due to platelet-specific antibodies. Sera containing platelet-specific antibodies are often contaminated with HLA antibodies reactive with platelets (Taaning *et al.*, 1983). HLA immunization seems to be far more frequent than immunization towards platelet-specific antigens. The importance of HLA immunization in causing alloimmune neonatal thrombocytopenia seems doubtful (Mueller-Eckhardt *et al.*, 1980b) because HLA antibodies give shortened survival of HLA-incompatible platelets. However, post-transfusional purpura is a serious problem and seems to be caused only by platelet-specific antibodies (Mueller-Eckhardt *et al.*, 1982). Thus it is important to identify platelet-specific antibodies in sera containing high titres of platelet-reactive HLA antibodies, particularly in patients whose condition is refractory to platelet transfusions (Murphy and Waters, 1985).

Chloroquine and acid treatment for detection of HLA antibodies

The use of Chloroquine to remove HLA antigens on platelets has been described (Blumberg *et al.*, 1984). Nordhagen and Flaathen (1985) introduced Chloroquine treatment of platelets to discriminate between HLA- and platelet-specific alloantibodies. They showed that in platelet suspension immunofluorescence, the reactivity of HLA antibodies with platelets was practically abrogated, while platelet-specific antibodies (anti-PI^{A1}, anti-Bak^a) retained full reactivity. However, Langenscheidt *et al.* (1989) showed that Chloroquine treatment is not specific for HLA antigens but may also alter GpIIb/IIIa epitopes, so affecting subsequent antibody binding. In addition Chloroquine treatment causes loss of platelet viability and high autofluorescence.

Acid treatment of platelets

1 The acid mixture (pH 3.0) is prepared by mixing equal volumes of 0.263 mol/l citric acid and 0.123 mol/l Na_2HPO_4 and adding 1% BSA.
2 Platelets are prepared by differential centrifugation.
3 Pellets containing 10×10^8 platelets are resuspended in 500 µl of the acid solution or PBS and left for 10 min at 0°C.

4 The acid-treated platelets are immediately neutralized with excess citrate buffer (pH 6.5). The platelets are washed once in PBS then fixed in 1% paraformaldehyde solution at room temperature for 5 min.

5 After washing three times, the platelets are resuspended in PBS to a platelet count of 150×10^6/ml. Fifty microlitres of this platelet suspension is incubated with monospecific HLA alloantisera or 50 µl of patient's serum for 45 min at 37°C.

6 After washing three times, the platelets are incubated with FITC-conjugated rabbit F(ab')$_2$ anti-human immunoglobulin (Dako) for 30 min at room temperature.

7 After a final wash the samples are analysed by flow cytometry.

8 A fluorescence intensity threshold is established at which 99% of the platelets sensitized with pooled serum from 10 healthy subjects, blood type AB, are negative. Pooled sera should be used as a negative control for all investigations.

Recently a method in which platelets are acid treated has been described for distinguishing platelet-specific antibodies from anti-HLA antibodies (Kurata *et al.*, 1990). The viability of acid-treated platelets has been shown to be greater than Chloroquine-treated and also allows platelets to be analysed by flow cytometry (Kurata *et al.*, 1990).

Whole blood method for detection of platelet-specific antibodies

The sera from patients with high levels of PAIg are incubated with Group O blood according to the method of Veys *et al.* (1987).

Assay procedure

1 Aliquots (100 µl) of whole blood anticoagulated with liquid K$_3$EDTA are mixed with 100 µl of a red cell lysing agent (platelet diluting fluid, Mercia).

2 When red cell lysis is complete, usually within 2–3 min, 1 ml of 1% paraformaldehyde (pH 7.2) freshly prepared from a stock 4% solution is added to prevent lysis of the white cells.

3 The white cell preparation is washed in 10 ml of Hank's balanced salt solution (HBSS) without phenol red (Gibco). Phenol red within cells is excited at 488 nm and causes high 560 nm autofluorescence.

4 The washed white cell preparation is incubated with the patient's serum for 30 min at 37°C, then washed twice in HBSS before addition of 5 µl FITC rabbit anti-human IgG or IgM F(ab')$_2$ fragments (DAKO).

5 The negative control consists of cells incubated with FITC rabbit anti-mouse immunoglobulins (F(ab')$_2$ fragments).

6 The cell preparations are then examined by flow cytometry.

Table 6.1 The reactivity of sera containing platelet associated IgG with other cell types

Serum	Platelet	Lymphocyte	Monocyte	Neutrophil
AB-ve (−ve control)	* 23	11	4	7
Anti-Pl[A1] (+ve control)	82	3	1	11
Anti-HLA (HLA control)	3	95	92	97
ChITP (Platelet)	58	3	0	2
ChITP (Platelet + monocyte)	76	13	30	11
TP (Platelet + HLA)	62	74	6	13
TP (Platelet + HLA)	34	76	40	44
ChITP (Platelet)	97	5	16	1
TP (Platelet + HLA)	87	90	64	97
ChITP (Platelet + lymphocyte)	61	20	1	1
ChITP (Platelet)	36	8	4	4
ChITP (Platelet)	45	7	3	3
Post BMT** (Platelet + lymphocyte)	39	35	1	1

* % fluorescence. ** Post bone-marrow transplantation.
ChITP, chronic ITP; TP, thrombocytopenic. Brackets indicate antibody specificity.

Analysis of the cells allows distinction between the lymphocytes, monocytes and neutrophils. The presence of auto-antibodies to any of these cells within a patient's serum would indicate the presence of HLA or other antibodies that are not platelet specific (Table 6.1).

Detection of antigen-specific antibodies

Chronic ITP is a syndrome characterized by thrombocytopenia due to circulating auto-antibody, which is most commonly IgG. Recently, several reports have demonstrated the presence of antibodies specific for platelet glycoproteins Ib, IIb and/or IIIa in the sera from some patients with chronic ITP (van Leeuwen *et al.*, 1982; Varon and Karpatkin, 1983; Beardsley *et al.*, 1984; Woods *et al.*, 1984a,b; Szatkowski *et al.*, 1986; Tomiyama *et al.*, 1987). In most of these reports, investigators employed circulating anti-platelet antibodies because of the difficulty in dealing with platelet-associated antibodies. However recently, the so-called 'capture assays', have been developed. These methods utilize murine monoclonal antibodies (MoAbs) specific for epitopes on the platelet membrane to capture the epitope-carrying molecules from a platelet lysate onto a solid phase. They are then exposed to human antibodies which are detected by a labelled ligand. At present three different modifications have been published: the 'immunobead assay' reported by McMillan *et al.* (1987); the 'capture ELISA' described by Furihata *et al.* (1987); and the monoclonal antibody specific immobilization of platelet antigens (MAIPA) assay developed by Kiefel *et al.* (1987). A modification of the immunobead assay has been developed for use with flow cytometry.

Immunobead method for detection of antigen-specific antibodies

The immunobead assay may be used to measure either platelet-associated auto-antibodies or plasma auto-antibodies.

Immunobead preparation

1 Anti-IgG-coated beads are prepared by incubating polystyrene beads (Polybead, Polysciences) with murine monoclonal anti-human IgG (DAKO) in 0.1 mol/l $NaHCO_2$, pH 8.5 for 60 min at a bead/antibody ratio of 2000:1 by weight (typically 100 mg of beads with 50 μl of anti-IgG dilute in saline).
2 The beads are washed by centrifugation for 10 min at 900 g in 10 ml PBS containing 0.05% Tween-20 pH 7.4 (PBS-Tween).
3 Non-specific binding sites are blocked by incubating the beads with PBS-Tween containing 2% BSA for 60 min.
4 The beads are then washed four times in PBS-Tween and stored at 4°C until used.

Platelet preparation

1 Platelets from EDTA anticoagulated blood are prepared by differential centrifugation, as above, but washed twice in citrate buffer (0.05 mol/l) at 900 g for 10 min.
2 For the preparation of antibody-sensitized platelets, washed normal platelets [10^8 platelets in buffer are incubated with 900 μl of patient or control plasma containing PGE_1 (1 μg/ml) and theophylline (1 μmol/l)] for 20 min at room temperature then washed with 0.05 mol/l citrate buffer containing PGE_1 and theophylline.
3 Patient platelets (10^8) or antibody-sensitized platelets are resuspended in 900 μl citrate buffer containing leupeptin (100 μg/ml) and then solubilized by the addition of 10% Triton X-100.
4 Control samples are handled similarly.

Continued on page 156

Assay

1 The solubilized platelets from each sample are centrifuged at $12000\,g$ for 5 min.
2 Aliquots (900 µl) of the supernatant are then incubated with 100 mg of anti-IgG coated beads for 20 min at room temperature to allow attachment of IgG and any bound antigen.
3 After two washes with PBS-Tween, the presence of specific antibody is demonstrated by incubation with a cocktail of mouse FITC anti-human GpIIb-IIIa or GpIb at room temperature for 20 min.
4 The beads are then washed in PBS-Tween and analysed by flow cytometry.

An alternative method has also been employed which does not require immunobead preparation. In this method platelets are sensitized with control and test sera, washed and incubated with mouse anti-human glycoprotein antisera prior to solubilization. The supernatant from the solubilized platelets is then incubated with commercially available beads coated with antibodies to mouse immunoglobulins (Polysciences). After washing the beads are labelled with FITC rabbit anti-human IgG and IgM (DAKO).

The effect of anticoagulants on direct PAIg

Von dem Borne *et al*. (1986) have suggested that use of EDTA as an anticoagulant may lead to expression of crypt-antigens and so antibodies to these antigens may be detected *in vitro* but are unlikely to occur *in vivo*. The effect of anticoagulant has also been studied by Lucas and Holburn (1987), who found that blood anticoagulated with solid K_3EDTA had PAIgG levels some fivefold greater than in citrated blood and that platelet fragments caused by the solid K_3EDTA were responsible for the elevated levels of PAIgG. In addition PAIgG values of blood anticoagulated with a 5% w/v solution of K_3EDTA were found to be intermittent between values for citrated blood and blood anticoagulated with solid K_3EDTA. We have examined four anticoagulants for use in flow cytometry. Blood from 10 normal individuals was collected into four anticoagulants: solid K_3EDTA, liquid EDTA, sodium citrate and acid citrate dextrose (ACD). The platelets were then prepared and stained as above. Statistical analysis, using the Student's *t*-test, was employed to examine the differences observed between the different preparations. In this study little difference was found between the PAIgG and PAIgM in blood treated with four different anticoagulants. This may be due to the ability to exclude fluorescence due to platelet fragments from the flow cytometric analysis (Table 6.2).

Table 6.2 The effect of different anticoagulants on PAIgG and PAIgM

157

CHAPTER 6
*Platelet-associated
Molecules and
Immunoglobulins*

Specimen	K₃EDTA liquid		K₃EDTA solid		Sodium citrate		ACD*	
	IgG	IgM	IgG	IgM	IgG	IgM	IgG	IgM
1	2.5	3.5	4.6	1.0	0.5	1.7	2.9	2.7
2	5.8	0.0	1.5	2.0	0.8	0.4	1.3	0.7
3	1.2	3.9	1.6	1.9	4.8	0.4	1.5	7.4
4	0.9	1.3	1.0	1.2	1.1	0.4	0.0	0.2
5	0.7	3.2	0.6	1.9	3.0	4.9	0.1	0.5
6	6.0	0.5	4.4	0.7	8.2	0.6	2.6	4.2
7	6.5	0.5	6.6	0.7	8.2	0.6	2.6	4.2
8	1.4	0.4	7.7	0.7	1.7	0.2	1.2	0.4
9	0.4	0.6	5.6	0.7	2.3	0.0	1.2	0.3
10	1.0	1.0	0.8	0.2	0.4	0.7	0.2	0.0
Mean	2.64	1.60	3.44	1.04	2.53	1.07	1.42	1.89
s.d.	2.46	1.51	2.65	0.70	2.41	1.51	0.84	2.48
s.e.	0.78	0.48	0.84	0.22	0.76	0.48	0.27	0.78

* ACD, acid citrate dextrose.

PAIg detection by flow cytometry compared with other methods

Although there are numerous methods for detecting PAIg (Karpatkin and Siskind, 1969; Dixon *et al.*, 1975; Hauch and Rosse, 1977; Hegde *et al.*, 1977, 1981; Mueller-Eckhardt *et al.*, 1978; Cines and Schreiber, 1979; Kelton *et al.*, 1979; von dem Borne *et al.*, 1980) direct fluorescence microscopy of cells in suspension is thought to be the first-line assay in platelet serology (Mueller-Eckhardt *et al.*, 1989). We therefore compared the flow cytometric method described with fluorescence microscopy. Platelets prepared as described were either resuspended in one drop of glycerol mountant (40 ml glycine buffer and 60 ml glycerol, pH 8.6), mounted on a glass slide, covered with a coverslip and examined by fluorescence microscopy or assayed by flow cytometry. Immunofluorescence was read on a Leitz Ortholux microscope with a mercury lamp and a filter set comprising: an exciter filter BP450–490; a beam splitter FT510; and a barrier filter LP520. Good comparison was found between the two techniques (Table 6.3).

The assessment of platelet antibody by flow cytometry and ELISA has also been compared (Lin *et al.*, 1990). IgG and IgM values showed significant correlations between the two methods of measurement.

Nomenclature of platelet-specific antigens

Improvement in the methodology of detection of platelet antigens has led to the discovery of a number of new platelet-specific alloantigen systems. However, many of the new systems, as well as the older ones, are known under different names. In order to avoid confusion a Working Party on Platelet Serology was set up (von dem Borne and Decary, 1990)

Table 6.3 Comparison of flow cytometric and microscopical methods for determining PAIg by immunofluorescence

| Patient | Immunofluorescence | | | |
| | Indirect | | Direct | |
	G	M	G	M
1	+(20)	+(2.9)	−(1.8)	+(13)
2	±(12)	+(12)	−(10)	−(9)
3	±(17)	−(1.8)	−(10)	−(1.8)
4	±(13)	−(1.8)	+(18)	−(1.8)
5	±(21)	+(2.6)	+(21)	+(2.8)
6	±(20)	±(10)	±(15)	+(3)
7	±(16)	±(18)	+(20)	±(5)
8	+(20)	+(20)	+(37)	±(2.3)
9	−(1.0)	±(21)	−(10)	+(30)
10	+(34)	−(6)	++(56)	−(0.6)
11	±(4)	++(55)	+(20)	±(6)
12	±(2.2)	++(60)	−(10)	+(30)
13	++(33)	+(10)	++(50)	+(3.4)
14	++(32)	−(4)	+(37)	−(1.6)
15	++(60)	±(20)	++(51)	−(5)
16	++(30)	+(20)	+(20)	+(10)
17	+(20)	+(16)	+(15)	+(10)
18	+(10)	+(9)	+(16)	±(5)
19	±(5)	±(10)	−(10)	+(30)
20	+(16)	±(10)	+(50)	±(11)

Immunofluorescence determined microscopically: −, negative; ±, weak positive; +, positive; ++, strong positive.
Figures in parentheses are per cent fluorescence as determined by flow cytometry.
Normal range (mean ± s.e.).
Indirect IgG 23.2 ± 1.6, IgM 4.6 ± 0.9, direct IgG 7.9 ± 4, IgM 0.8 ± 0.2.

to formulate a new nomenclature system for such antigen systems.

The nomenclature is as follows:

1 Platelet-specific antigen systems will be called HPA for human platelet antigen(s).

2 The different antigen systems will be numbered chronologically in order of the date of publication.

3 The allelic antigens will be designated alphabetically, in order of their frequency in the population from high to low.

4 The inclusion of new HPA systems will need the approval of the working party.

The HPA systems recognized to date are given in Table 6.4.

Platelet activation antigens

Platelets normally circulate in a resting state and only after stimulation with one of several physiological agonists do they undergo the changes that lead to platelet adhesion and aggregation. These changes can occur *in vivo* or can be effected *in vitro* and can be monitored by changes on the platelet surface, as illustrated in Fig. 6.1.

Table 6.4 Nomenclature of platelet-specific antigens

Antigen system	Glycoprotein (GP) location	Other names	Antigens	Other names	Phenotype frequency % Caucasian	Japanese
HPA-1	GPIIa	Zw^a, P1^A	HPA-1a	Zw^a, P1^{Al}	97.9	99.9
			HPA-1b	Zw^b, P1^{Al}	26.5	3.7
HPA-2	GP1b	Ko, Sib	HPA-2a	Ko^b	99.3	nt
			HPA-2b	Ko^b, Sib^a	14.6	25.4
HPA-3	GPIIb	Bak, Lek	HPA-3a	Bak^a, Lek^a	87.7	78.9
			HPA-3b	Bak^b	64.1	nt
HPA-4	GPIIIa	Pen, Yuk	HPA-4a	Pen^a, Yuk^b	99.9	99.9
			HPA-4b	Pen^b, Yuk^a	0.2	1.7
HPA-5	GPIa	Br, He, Zav	HPA-5a	Br^b, Zav^b	99.2	nt
			HPA-5b	Br^a, Zav^a, He^a	20.6	nt

nt, not tested.

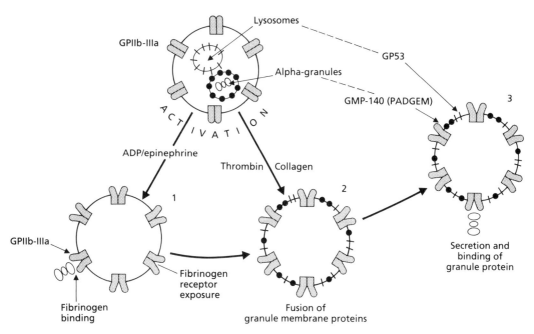

Fig. 6.1 Schematic diagram of changes occurring on the platelet surface following activation.

Stimulation with weak agonists such as adenosine diphosphate (ADP) or epinephrine causes a conformational change in the platelet GPIIb-IIIa complex, exposing the receptor site for fibrinogen, leading to fibrinogen binding and, if platelet–platelet contact is maintained, to aggregation. When platelets aggregate, or when they are stimulated with a strong agonist such as thrombin or vessel wall collagen, degranulation occurs. Degranulation leads to the translocation of granule membranes to the platelet surface, carrying with them specific membrane glycoproteins that appear as neo-antigens on the surface of the activated platelet. Proteins released from the platelet granules can also bind to the platelet surface. These changes, reviewed comprehensively by Abrams and Shattil (1991), can be readily detected by flow cytometry.

Changes in the GPIIb-IIIa complex can be detected in a number of ways, as illustrated in Fig. 6.2. Shattil *et al.* (1985) described a MoAb, PAC-1, that binds to activated GPIIb-IIIa at, or very close to, the fibrinogen receptor, and competes with fibrinogen at this site. Once the fibrinogen receptor is exposed, plasma fibrinogen can bind to the complex and be detected with polyclonal antibodies or MoAbs. Jackson and Jennings (1989) and Warkentin *et al.* (1990) have described the use of commercially available, polyclonal anti-fibrinogen antibodies linked to FITC to detect activated platelets *in vitro*. Warkentin *et al.* (1990) demonstrated that the binding of polyclonal anti-fibrinogen antibody to ADP-stimulated platelets correlated closely with that of PAC-1. Activated GPIIb-IIIa is also a receptor for von Willebrand's factor (vWF) and fibronectin (Phillips *et al.*, 1988), albeit with a lower affinity than for fibrinogen, and the binding of these molecules to activated platelets can also be detected with MoAbs or polyclonal antibodies (Adelman *et al.*, 1987; Ejim *et al.*, 1990; Cox *et al.*, 1991).

When fibrinogen binds to the activated complex, the fibrinogen molecule itself undergoes a conformational change. New structural epitopes on this molecule can be identified with MoAbs that discriminate fibrinogen bound to GPIIb-IIIa from fibrinogen in the plasma (Abrams *et al.*, 1990; Zamarron *et al.*, 1990). These have been termed receptor-induced binding sites (RIBS; Zamarron *et al.*, 1989).

When fibrinogen binds to the GPIIb-IIIa complex, or when the fibrinogen receptor is occupied by a small RGD-containing peptide, the GPIIb-IIIa complex undergoes a further conformational change, exposing new epitopes which have been termed ligand-induced binding sites (LIBS; Frelinger *et al.*, 1988, 1990). These are distinct from the PAC-1 site.

All of these changes represent sensitive markers for small alterations in platelet activation status but are susceptible to *in vitro* handling

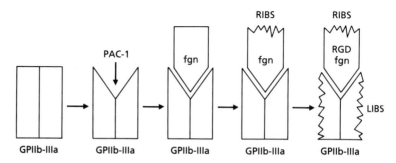

Fig. 6.2 Changes in the platelet membrane GPIIb-IIIa complex following activation (see text for explanation). fgn, fibrinogen; RIBS, receptor-induced binding site; LIBS, ligand-induced binding site; RGD, peptide containing arg-gly-ala sequence of amino acids.

artefacts and to reversal by fixative, and careful preparation of samples
is thus required (Abrams *et al.*, 1990).

161

CHAPTER 6
*Platelet-associated
Molecules and
Immunoglobulins*

More profound platelet activation, associated with degranulation,
can be monitored by the appearance of granule membrane antigens.
The first described and best characterized is the GMP140 (McEver and
Martin, 1984) or PADGEM (Hsu-Lin *et al.*, 1984) antigen, also known
as the CD62 antigen and more recently termed P-selectin (Bevilacqua
et al., 1991). This is found on α-granule membranes (Stenberg *et al.*,
1985; Berman *et al.*, 1986), and has also been described on the membranes
of dense granules (Israels *et al.*, 1992). It is present at less than 1000
molecules on the surface of resting platelets but at more than 10 000
molecules per cell following activation (Stenberg *et al.*, 1985; Berman
et al., 1986). P-selectin is an adhesion molecule, a member of the selectin
family which includes ELAM-1 (E-selectin) and the lymphocyte homing
receptor (L-selectin; Stoolman, 1989; Bevilacqua *et al.*, 1991). It acts as
an attachment site for neutrophils and monocytes (Larsen *et al.*, 1989),
and may help to clear activated platelets from the circulation, into the
reticulo-endothelial system. In addition to P-selectin, Metzelaar *et al.*
(1992) have described a 33 kDa antigen, GMP-33, associated with
α-granule membranes. This can be detected at low levels on resting
platelets but its expression is increased on stimulation.

Platelet lysosomes also have characteristic antigens, reviewed by
Metzelaar and Clevers (1992). The GP53 or CD63 antigen is a 30−60 kDa
glycoprotein found in detectable amounts on the platelet surface only
after activation (Nieuwenhuis *et al.*, 1987; Cox and Goodall, 1991).
Recent data suggest CD63 may be one of a family of molecules, the
function of which is unclear, found in many cells and associated with
tumour cells (Horejsi and Vlcek, 1991; Metzelaar and Clevers, 1992).
CD63 has exact homology with a melanoma-associated antigen known
as ME491 (Metzelaar and Clevers, 1992) and with a 40 kDa glycoprotein
recently described by Azorsa *et al.* (1991). Two homologous integral
membrane proteins of molecular weight 90−120 kDa, known as LAMP1
and LAMP2 are also seen in lysosomal membranes (Chen *et al.*, 1985;
Fukuda *et al.*, 1988) and are expressed on activated platelets (Febbraio
and Silverstein, 1990).

Other granule membrane antigens have been described. A glycoprotein of about 40 kDa has been identified, associated with dense
body membranes, and called granulophysin (Gerrard *et al.*, 1991; Israels
et al., 1992), while Sutherland *et al.* (1991) have described a 150 170 kDa
antigen found on activated platelets and T cells.

The contents of the platelet α-granules such as thrombospondin
(Aiken *et al.*, 1987) and platelet factor 4 (Capitanio *et al.*, 1985) can, once
released from the degranulated platelets, bind to receptors on the platelet
surface. Thrombospondin has been used as a marker of activated platelets
(George *et al.*, 1986); however, it binds to a number of sites which
include the GPIV (or CD36) antigen (Silverstein *et al.*, 1989) and platelet-
associated fibrinogen (Leung and Nachman, 1982), and as such represents a rather variable and heterogeneous marker of platelet activation.

When platelets are activated by certain agonists, such as the calcium ionophore A23187, or by a mixture of thrombin and collagen, or by the C5 component of complement, they undergo a further change which results in two events. Phosphatidyl serine, which is normally found on the inner bilayer of the platelet membrane, becomes exposed on the outer surface of the membrane (Bevers *et al.*, 1983). In addition small microparticles or vesicles bud from the platelet surface. These can be detected in the flow cytometer by their light scatter characteristics (Sims *et al.*, 1988; Abrams *et al.*, 1990; Warkentin *et al.*, 1992; Wenche *et al.*, 1992). These particles are particularly rich in the exposed, negatively charged phosphatidyl serine which can bind the procoagulant proteins Factor VIIIa (Gilbert *et al.*, 1991), Factor Va (Sims *et al.*, 1988) and FIXa (Hoffman *et al.*, 1992).

Thrombin also induces an increased expression of the GPIIb-IIIa complex (George *et al.*, 1986; Michelson and Barnard, 1987) which is translocated from the surface connecting canalicular system (SCCS) and α-granule membranes to the platelet surface (Wencel-Drake *et al.*, 1986; Woods *et al.*, 1986). This is matched by a down-regulation in the expression of GPIb (George *et al.*, 1986; Michelson and Barnard, 1987; Michelson *et al.*, 1991) which is sequestered into the SCCS (Hourdille *et al.*, 1990). In some situations, proteolysis of GPIb by plasmin results in the loss of the glycocalicin portion of the GPIb molecule (Adelman *et al.*, 1985). Recent reports have also demonstrated increases in the expression of CD36 (GPIV) on activated platelets (Kestin *et al.*, 1991).

All of these changes can be detected by flow cytometry, and many have been used to analyse the activation process *in vitro* or to detect activated platelets in various clinical situations, as indicated in Table 6.5.

Detection of activated platelets by flow cytometry

Platelets offer a number of challenges to the flow cytometrist. First, their small size means that they have similar light scatter characteristics to dust particles. This problem can be avoided simply by filtering all buffers used in the preparation of samples through a 0.22 μm filter and by fitting a 0.22 μm filter in the sheath fluid delivery line.

Platelets are also extremely labile and subject to artefactual activation *ex vivo* by separation procedures such as washing and centrifugation which can increase the expression of many, if not all, of the platelet activation antigens. Methods that minimize such artefacts essentially fall into three categories: those which inhibit platelets, those which fix the platelets and those which reduce handling to a minimum. The former two approaches can be applied to the detection of platelet granule membrane antigens as most are recognized with MoAbs raised against fixed platelets, and platelet degranulation, once it has occurred, is not reversed by inhibitors of platelet activation. Fixation and inhibition are, however, inappropriate for analysis of changes in the GPIIb-IIIa complex (ligand binding, PAC-1 binding, detection of LIBS and RIBS

Table 6.5 Activation-induced changes on the platelet surface

163

CHAPTER 6
*Platelet-associated
Molecules and
Immunoglobulins*

Platelet activation antigens	References
Changes in the GPIIb-IIIa complex	
Fibrinogen receptor exposure*	Shattil *et al.* (1985)
Fibrinogen binding*	Jackson and Jennings (1989)
	Abrams *et al.* (1990)
	Warkentin *et al.* (1990)
vWF binding	Adelman *et al.* (1987)
	Cox *et al.* (1991)
Fibronectin binding*	Ejim *et al.* (1990)
RIBS*	Abrams *et al.* (1990)
	Zamarron *et al.* (1990)
LIBS	Frelinger *et al.* (1988, 1990)
Markers of degranulation	
α-granules	
GMP140/PADGEM/CD62/P-selectin*	McEver and Martin (1984)
	Hsu-Lin *et al.* (1984)
Granulophysin	Gerrard *et al.* (1991)
GMP33*	Metzelaar *et al.* (1992)
Bound thrombospondin	George *et al.* (1986)
Lysosomes	
GP53/CD63*	Nieuwenhuis *et al.* (1987)
	Cox and Goodall (1991)
	Azorsa *et al.* (1991)
Lamp 1, Lamp 2	Chen *et al.* (1985)
Dense bodies	
Granulophysin	Gerrard *et al.* (1991)
Changes to cell surface antigen expression	
Increased GPIIb-IIIa*	⎧ George *et al.* (1986)
Decreased GPIb*	⎩ Michelson and Barnard (1987)
Increased GPIV*	Kestin *et al.* (1991)
Changes to the plasma membrane/vesicle formation	
PS flip-flop	Bevers *et al.* (1983)
Microparticle budding*	Sims *et al.* (1988)
	Abrams *et al.* (1990)
Binding of procoagulant proteins	
Factor VIIIa*	Gilbert *et al.* (1991)
Factor Va	Sims *et al.* (1988)
Factor IXa	Hoffman *et al.* (1992)

* Markers used in clinical studies.

epitopes, etc.), which can be affected by fixatives and inhibitors (Abrams *et al.*, 1990).

For analysis of these activation markers, minimum handling of the platelets is advised. This can be effected by the use of whole blood assays (Abrams and Shattil, 1991). These rely on the ability of the flow cytometer to distinguish individual populations of cells in a complex mixture by their light scatter characteristics. This avoids the need for physical separations of the platelets from other blood components, and hence for fixation or the use of inhibitors, which are required to prevent platelet activation during processes such as centrifugation or filtration. The platelet population, discriminated from other cells by their forward angle and 90° light scatter characteristics, can be identified by a fluorescent antibody that binds to all platelets (e.g. anti-GPIb).

Whole blood assays

The term 'whole blood assay' covers a number of different approaches to flow cytometry. To a white cell immunologist a whole blood assay entails a red cell lysis or removal step and various kits and protocols are available from different manufacturers to facilitate such assays. These methods are, however, inappropriate for platelet studies. The separation or lysis of the red cells is accompanied by release of ADP and consequent platelet activation. Separation of the red cells is unnecessary as platelets, unlike lymphocytes, can be differentiated from red cells in the flow cytometer on the basis of their light scatter properties. In this chapter we describe two alternative 'whole blood assay' methods. Detection of PAIg in whole blood is described using a method in which the cells are first washed to remove the majority of the plasma immunoglobulin. However, for the detection of platelet activation antigens, where problems of cross-reactivity of antibodies with plasma proteins are either irrelevant or can be overcome, whole blood assays can be used in which the only post-venepuncture manipulation step is a simple dilution in buffer.

While these methods are particularly suited to the analysis of changes in the GPIIb-IIIa complex, whole blood assays are also applicable to the detection of granule membrane antigens. In addition, the absence of fixatives or inhibitors allows the investigation of platelet responses to agonists *in vitro*, thus allowing the detection of hypo- or hyper-responsive platelets.

Whole blood flow cytometric detection of platelets was first described by Jennings *et al.* (1986) and developed by Shattil's group (Shattil *et al.*, 1987; Abrams *et al.*, 1990). Modifications of this original method have been described by Michelson *et al.* (1991) and by the RFHSM group (Warkentin *et al.*, 1990; Janes *et al.*, 1993).

Detection of changes occurring on the platelet surface following activation *in vivo*

Sample collection

Collection of blood samples for flow cytometric measurement of platelet activation requires essentially the same conditions as other assays of platelet activation status (e.g. plasma β-thromboglobulin (βTG) assay). Blood is collected into citrate, with minimum stasis, using a 21-gauge (or larger) needle or butterfly. It has been suggested that the use of butterfly needles can cause activation of the blood as it passes through the catheter but we do not find this to be the case, provided the first

2 ml are not used for platelet assays and the tourniquet, if used, is removed once free blood flow is established. If anything, the butterfly is more reliable as it minimizes damage during the venepuncture. Blood is collected slowly, to avoid turbulence and the formation of air bubbles. If any one of these criteria is not fulfilled, the samples should not be analysed.

Samples collected into EDTA or heparin are inappropriate for studies in which changes in the GPIIb-IIIa complex are to be monitored, or when agonist stimulation is to be examined. EDTA can alter the GPIIb-IIIa complex and can reverse fibrinogen binding, and both anticoagulants can inhibit agonist stimulation *in vitro*.

Antibodies

Directly conjugated antibodies are, in most cases, the preferred reagent for these studies (Abrams *et al.*, 1990). Biotin-linked antibodies, visualized with a streptavidin fluorochrome complex, can be used, but the incubation time is increased. Indirect immunofluorescence, using an anti-mouse immunoglobulin-fluorochrome conjugate is the least satisfactory, as cross-linking of the bound second layer can lead to agglutination of the platelets and there is an increased risk of Fc receptor-mediated platelet activation (Lindahl *et al.*, 1992). If a second layer antibody is used, a F(ab')₂ or even better, a Fab fragment is recommended. Removal of excess first layer antibody by a washing step is not recommended as this will induce some platelet activation.

All reagents need to be standardized and used at optimum concentrations. Appropriate isotype controls should be used for each antibody in each subject analysed. It is recommended that the subjects' platelets are also labelled with a 'pan-platelet' MoAb to allow confirmation that the particles analysed are platelets. The best such markers are GPIb (Shattil *et al.*, 1987) or GPIIb-IIIa, because of the high number of these molecules per platelets, although expression of both antigens is modulated during platelet activation. Directly conjugated MoAbs to GPIb may, therefore, be the best reagents for this purpose. Other pan-platelet antigens such as GPIV may be used, but are present at lower density per platelet and GPIV is also up-regulated when platelets are stimulated with thrombin (Kestin *et al.*, 1991).

Abrams *et al.* (1990) recommend two-colour analysis, labelling each sample with both a FITC-conjugated pan-platelet marker (e.g. GPIb) and a biotinylated, activation specific antibody; identifying the platelets by size and granularity, then gating on the pan-platelet antibody. This has the advantage of ensuring platelet identity in each sample but

Whole blood analysis
1 Within 10 min of collection, a small aliquot (5 µl) of blood is added to a tube containing 50 µl of Hepes-buffered saline (0.145 mol/l

Continued on page 166

NaCl; 5×10^{-3} mol/l KCl; 1×10^{-3} mol/l MgSO$_4$; 0.01 mol/l Hepes; pH 7.4) and 5 µl of an appropriate dilution of one of a number of antibodies to platelet activation antigens. In some tubes an agonist such as ADP can be added to promote platelet activation *in vitro*.

2 The samples are incubated between 22 and 28°C. In our laboratory, incubation with directly conjugated antibodies is for 20 min.

3 If an indirect antibody system is used, the diluted blood samples are incubated with the first antibody for 15 min, and an appropriate amount of second layer is added for a further 15 min.

4 After incubation at room temperature the platelets are diluted and fixed by the addition of 0.5 ml of 0.2% formyl saline (0.2% formaldehyde on 0.9% NaCl), and analysed in the flow cytometer within 2 hours of fixation.

single colour analysis has the advantages of lower cost, and ease of sample preparation, and avoids the need for colour compensation which can reduce the sensitivity of the fluorescent signal, a particular problem when a bright signal from the pan-platelet marker may spill over into a weak signal from an activation antigen expressed at low level.

Shattil's original method (Shattil *et al.*, 1987), and that described by Michelson *et al.* (1991), rely on a 1 : 10 dilution of blood in buffer prior to aliquoting and adding the antibodies. We favour dilution of the blood directly into the buffer—antibody mixtures as it offers practical advantages when using a number of different antibodies on the same sample. The two methods are equally valid but data cannot be interchanged as platelets prepared by Shattil's method require slightly higher concentrations of exogenous agonist to achieve full agonist response (N. Chronos and A.H. Goodall, unpublished observation).

Mild fixation with 0.2% formaldehyde does not alter fibrinogen binding to unstimulated samples and is effective in preventing changes in fibrinogen binding for up to 2 hours after fixation. In samples diluted with buffered saline, without fixative (Shattil *et al.*, 1987; Abrams *et al.*, 1990), the percentage of positive platelets fell by 40–50% at 2 hours (Janes *et al.*, 1993). Fixation of platelets with 0.2% formyl saline, after stimulation of the blood with 10^{-5} mol/l ADP, produced a small but significant increase in the amount of bound fibrinogen measured, as reported previously by Abrams *et al.* (1990) but the level of bound fibrinogen then remained constant for 2 hours at 22°C or for 24 hours at 4°C.

When blood samples are passed through the flow cytometer the signals from the cells can be separated by means of their forward scatter and side scatter characteristics as shown in Fig. 6.3. Region 1 represents machine noise and dust particles and is present when filtered buffer is run through the flow cytometer. Region 2 comprises the platelets and is distinct from regions 1 and 3, the latter representing red blood cells. The platelets are enclosed in an electronic bit-map and analysed for the expression of the fluorescent antibodies.

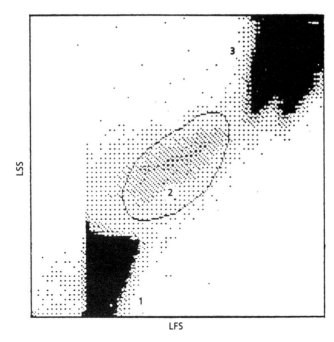

Fig. 6.3 Analysis of platelets in whole blood. Particles are discriminated by means of their forward scatter (x-axis) and side scatter (y-axis) characteristics, both analysed on a logarithmic scale. Region 1, noise/small dust particles; region 2, platelets; region 3, red cells.

Assay variables

The detection of platelet-bound fibrinogen is particularly sensitive to handling artefacts. Thus this parameter has been used to define the optimal conditions for whole blood assay.

The time between phlebotomy and assay is critical. If the blood is left for more than 10 min before dilution and subsequent assay there is a small but significant, spontaneous increase in PAC-1 expression (Abrams *et al.*, 1990), and in platelet-bound fibrinogen (Janes *et al.*, 1993). We also found that blood added to the tubes within the first 2 min after phlebotomy had slightly lower levels of fibrinogen bound to the platelets although the differences were not statistically significant. The blood is therefore added to the tubes between 2 and 10 min of collection; a method that can be readily achieved if the laboratory is close to the site of phlebotomy.

The temperature at which the assays are performed is important (Janes *et al.*, 1993). Platelets become activated at low temperatures but we have found that if the assay is performed outside the temperature range 22–26°C, small but significant rises in the level of fibrinogen bound to resting platelets are seen. The same range of temperatures has been found to be suitable for analysis of granule membrane antigens (S.L. Janes, unpublished observation). Incubation at 37°C causes a small increase in fibrinogen binding to resting platelets but a decreased *in vitro* response to agonists, compared with parallel samples incubated at 22°C (Wilson, unpublished observation).

Attempts to fix the blood, or to inhibit platelet activation after phlebotomy, and prior to assay, altered the level of platelet-bound fibrinogen that was measured (Janes *et al.*, 1993). Blood samples fixed with formaldehyde (0.01−0.1%) or glutaraldehyde (0.05−0.1%), with or without neutralizing glycine, all showed reduced fibrinogen binding as compared with unfixed samples run in parallel. Inhibition of platelet activation by prostacyclin (PGE_1) reversed fibrinogen binding in a dose-dependent manner. Reductions in fibrinogen binding were also caused by an inhibitory cocktail of EDTA, adenosine and theophylline and by indomethacin or lignocaine. EDTA alone, caused an immediate reduction in platelet-bound fibrinogen but thereafter, allowed a spontaneous increase in fibrinogen binding to occur. Sodium azide (0.1% w/v) failed to prevent spontaneous binding of fibrinogen, as did 2−10 units/ ml hirudin.

Detection of changes occurring on the platelet surface following activation *in vitro*

Platelet response to agonists *in vitro* can be determined in the whole blood assay by the addition of 5 µl of appropriate dilutions of agonist to the assay tubes. Shattil *et al.* (1987) and Warkentin *et al.* (1990) have examined the effects of ADP on platelet GPIIb-IIIa changes (PAC-1 and RIBS binding and fibrinogen binding, respectively), while Shattil *et al.* (1989) have used flow cytometry to demonstrate the direct action of supra-physiological concentrations of adrenaline on platelets. Michelson *et al.* (1991) have described a method that enables investigation of the effects of thrombin on platelets in whole blood, and used the method to detail changes in the level of expression of the GPIb-IX and GPIIb-IIIa complexes. In this assay, thrombin-induced clot formation is prevented by the addition of a synthetic peptide, GPRP, which prevents fibrin cross-linking (Laudano and Doolittle, 1980) but allows thrombin activation to proceed. The presence of fibrin monomer does not interfere with platelet fibrinogen binding (Harfenist *et al.*, 1985).

Conditions for single cell analysis

For flow cytometric analysis it is essential that the platelets remain as a suspension of single cells. Platelets in citrated blood, bearing bound fibrinogen, would normally aggregate, if stirred. Micro-aggregates thus formed would fall within the platelet bit-map and give an apparent false increase in fluorescence, while larger platelet aggregates would fall outside the bit-map and be lost to analysis. The conditions used in whole blood flow cytometric assays are designed to avoid aggregation in the samples, despite the presence of activated platelets, with bound fibrinogen. Dilution of the blood reduces cell to cell contact. After an initial mixing step, the samples remain static for the 20 or 30 min incubation with antibody, until further dilution and fixation. Blood samples prepared in this way, and analysed in a whole blood counter, showed no loss of platelets, indicative of aggregation, even when antibody was added ·or in the presence of high concentrations of agonist and when more than 90% of the platelets had bound fibrinogen (Janes *et al.*, 1993).

A number of anti-platelet antibodies, in particular MoAbs to certain epitopes on GPIIb-IIIa and on the CD9 antigen, can activate platelets by an Fc receptor-mediated mechanism (e.g. Rubinstein *et al.*, 1991). This can be avoided by the use of non-activating MoAbs or the use of F(ab')$_2$ or Fab fragments.

If the antibody to the activation antigen on the platelet also recognizes antigen present in the plasma, as for example a polyclonal antibody to fibrinogen, conditions must be used that avoid the formation of immune complexes between antibody and serum antigen, as these complexes could activate the platelets, and they can appear as particles in the flow cytometer and interfere with the analysis (Warkentin *et al.*, 1990). Formation of immune complexes can be avoided by optimization of the concentration of antibody so that a high level of specific binding to activated platelets is seen, in the absence of immune complexes (Warkentin *et al.*, 1990). Addition of the MoAb IV.3, which blocks the binding of IgG to FcγRII *in vivo*, had no effect on the binding of anti-fibrinogen antibody to either resting (Janes *et al.*, 1993) or activated (Warkentin *et al.*, 1990) platelets. Lindahl *et al.* (1992) have used a polyclonal chicken antiserum to human fibrinogen to avoid this potential problem; however, we find the conditions described by Warkentin *et al.* (1990) and Janes *et al.* (1993) do not produce immune complex formation in the samples.

Analysis of PRP

Flow cytometric analysis of platelets in PRP has been carried out in some studies (e.g. Jennings *et al.*, 1986; Lindahl *et al.*, 1992). Preparation of PRP results in a small but significant loss of platelets which may represent the larger, and thus possibly more active cells (Martin, 1990). It can also cause a small increase in platelet-bound fibrinogen. This activation can be prevented by collecting the blood into a cocktail of platelet inhibitors, which can include PGE$_1$, theophylline, adenosine, EDTA or EGTA, apyrase, hirudin, PPACK, etc. Appropriate cocktails will inhibit further degranulation occurring during processing of the blood but all inhibitors will either reverse existing fibrinogen binding (PGE$_1$, EDTA, adenosine, theophylline, indomethacin) or fail to prevent spontaneous fibrinogen binding *in vitro* (EDTA, azide, hirudin) (Janes *et al.*, 1993). The presence of inhibitors also mitigates against the evaluation of platelet responsiveness to agonists *in vitro*. These methods are, however, suitable for analysing platelet granule membrane antigens and the following method, a modification of the whole blood assay described earlier, can be used.

Blood is collected into citrate containing a cocktail of inhibitors (0.13 mol/l EDTA; 0.01 mol/l adenosine; 0.02 mol/l theophylline). The samples are immediately centrifuged for 10 min at room temperature, at 200 g, the PRP removed, and 5 μl aliquots added to 50 μl Hepes-buffered saline containing 5 μl of an appropriate antibody. Samples are incubated for 20 min, fixed with 0.2% formyl saline and analysed, as described earlier.

Analysis of washed platelets

Preparation of washed or gel filtered platelets, in the absence of inhibitors or fixatives, can cause increases in platelet activation antigen expression. However, blood fixed with 0.5–1% glutaraldehyde or PFA can be processed and analysed for expression of granule membrane antigens. Several methods for analysing fixed, washed platelets have appeared in the literature (Adelman *et al.*, 1985; George *et al.*, 1986; Nieuwenhuis *et al.*, 1987; Johnston *et al.*, 1987; Tschöpe *et al.*, 1990); the method described here is essentially that developed by Tschöpe *et al.* (1990).

Method

1 Blood (5 ml) is collected into citrate anticoagulant containing a cocktail of inhibitors. Tschöpe's method recommends soluble aspirin and PGE_1.

2 The blood is mixed immediately with an equal volume of 1% PFA and fixed, at room temperature, for 15 min.

3 PRP is prepared from the sample, by centrifugation for 10 min, at 250 g and the platelets separated by further centrifugation for 5 min at 700 g.

4 The platelet pellet is resuspended in 2 ml PBS containing 3.8% sodium citrate and 10% (v/v) non-immune rabbit serum, to reduce non-specific binding of antibodies to the platelets.

5 Following a further 5 min centrifugation at 700 g the platelet pellet is resuspended in 0.5 ml PBS, counted and adjusted to 2×10^5 platelets/ml.

6 Fifty-microlitre aliquots are dispensed into suitable tubes and 5 μl aliquots of antibody added.

7 The samples are incubated for 20 min at room temperature, diluted with 0.5 ml PBS and analysed in the flow cytometer.

Unstimulated blood samples run in this assay, and compared with paired samples run in parallel in the whole blood assay described earlier, showed identical expression of P-selectin ($3.4 \pm 0.9\%$ and $3.0 \pm 0.6\%$, respectively; $P > 0.5$; $n = 11$). PAC-1, however, bound to $65 \pm 12\%$ of the fixed, washed platelets, illustrating the unsuitability of this method

Table 6.6 Detection of platelet activation in clinical situations by flow cytometry

Condition studied	Assay method	Activation marker	↑ / ↓	Reference
Cardiopulmonary bypass	Fixed, washed platelets	CD62	↑	Metzelaar et al. (1990)
				Corash (1990)
				Rinder et al. (1991a)
		CD63	↑	Nieuwenhuis et al. (1987)
				Metzelaar et al. (1992)
		GMP-33	↑	Metzelaar (1992)
	Whole blood	CD62	↑	Abrams et al. (1990)
		Fibrinogen‡	↑	Abrams et al. (1990)
Haemofiltration	Whole blood	CD63	↑	Janes et al. (1993)
		Fibrinogen§	↑ *	Janes et al. (1993)
Bleeding time wounds	Whole blood	CD63	↑	Abrams et al. (1990)
		Fibrinogen‡	↑	Abrams et al. (1990)
		GPIb	↓	Michelson et al. (1991)
Myeloproliferative disease	Fixed, washed platelets	CD62	↑	Wehmeier et al. (1991)
		CD63	↑	Wehmeier et al. (1991)
Essential thrombocythaemia	Fixed, washed platelets	CD62	↑	Metzelaar et al. (1992)
		CD63	↑	Metzelaar et al. (1992)
		GMP-33	N	Metzelaar et al. (1992)
Diabetes	Fixed, washed platelets	CD62	↑	Tschöpe et al. (1990)
		CD63	↑	Tschöpe et al. (1990)
Deep vein thrombosis	Fixed, washed platelets	CD62	N	Metzelaar et al. (1992)
		GMP-33	N	Metzelaar et al. (1992)
		CD63	N	Metzelaar et al. (1992)
Peripheral vascular disease	Whole blood	CD63	N†	Mookerjee et al. (1992)
Pre-eclampsia of pregnancy	Whole blood	CD63	↑ †	Janes et al. (1991)
		Fibrinogens§	↑	Janes et al. (1991)
Exercise	Whole blood	CD62	N	Kestin et al. (1991)
		GPIb-IX	↓	Kestin et al. (1991)

↑, Increased antibody binding; ↓, Decreased antibody binding; N, No difference in antibody binding from controls; * Decreased expression in response to ADP; † Increased expression in response to ADP; ‡ PAC-1 and RIBS (9F9) binding; § Detected with polyclonal anti-fibrinogen antibody.

of preparation for the analysis of changes in the GPIIb-IIIa complex (N. Chronos and M. de Olivera Domingos, unpublished observation).

Clinical studies of platelet activation

Various laboratories have investigated the presence of activated platelets in clinical situations, using one or more of the various markers (Table 6.6). Most studies have used fixed, washed platelet assays and there is considerable variability between assay methods.

Several groups have examined platelets from patients undergoing cardiopulmonary bypass surgery (CPB). Platelets are known to be activated during passage of blood through extracorporeal circuits (Harker *et al.*, 1980) and therefore these patients serve as a model for platelet activation *in vivo*. Limited increases in P-selectin expression have been reported by Rinder *et al.* (1991a), Corash (1990) and Metzelaar *et al.* (1990), using fixed, washed platelet assays. This contrasts with the reports of George *et al.* (1986) and Dechavanne *et al.* (1987), who saw no increase in P-selectin expression using radiobinding assays. Increased CD63 expression (Nieuwenhuis *et al.*, 1987; Metzelaar *et al.*, 1990) and GMP-33 expression (Metzelaar *et al.*, 1990) was also observed in CPB patients. Abrams *et al.* (1990) used whole blood flow cytometry to analyse CPB patients and found that while little change in P-selectin antigen expression was seen, increased expression of the fibrinogen receptor on GPIIb-IIIa and increased platelet fibrinogen binding, detected by MoAbs PAC-1 and 9F9, respectively, was observed in a proportion of subjects.

Whole blood analysis of platelets from patients undergoing extracorporeal haemofiltration for acute renal failure also showed increased levels of fibrinogen binding and CD63 antigen expression (Janes *et al.*, 1993), consistent with previous observations of platelet activation in such patients. Stimulation of samples from these patients, with ADP, *in vitro* indicated platelet hyporesponsiveness; fibrinogen binding was decreased in the patients while CD63 antigen expression was the same as in the controls (Janes *et al.*, 1993).

Detection of activated platelets in patients with prothrombotic or thrombotic conditions has given variable results. Fixed washed platelet assays have shown elevated P-selectin and CD63 antigen expression in diabetic patients (Tschöpe *et al.*, 1991) but platelets from patients with deep vein thrombosis (DVT) showed no increase in granule membrane antigen expression (CD63, P-selectin and GMP-33) (Metzelaar *et al.*, 1990). Platelets from patients with peripheral vascular disease (PVD) showed no increase in either P-selectin, in a fixed, washed platelet assay (Galt *et al.*, 1991) or in CD63 antigen expression, analysed by whole blood flow cytometry (Mookerjee *et al.*, 1992). In the latter study, however, the whole blood assay allowed analysis of platelet responsiveness to agonists, and the patients were found to have an increased expression of CD63 in response to maximal ADP stimulation (Mookerjee *et al.*, 1992).

Whole blood flow cytometry showed an increase in both CD63 expression and fibrinogen binding in patients with established pre-eclampsia of pregnancy (Janes *et al.*, 1991), and in these patients, CD63 antigen expression was increased further in samples of blood stimulated with ADP (Janes and Goodall, 1992).

Fixed, washed platelet assays, used to analyse platelets from patients with myeloproliferative disease, showed an increase in P-selectin expression in about 25% of cases (Wehmeier *et al.*, 1991), as did a study of essential thrombocythaemia (ET) patients (Metzelaar *et al.*, 1990); however, CD63 antigen expression was not raised significantly in the ET group (Metzelaar *et al.*, 1990).

Changes in the level of expression of GPIIb-IIIa antigen have been observed in CPB patients (Dechavanne *et al.*, 1987), and decreased GPIb has been observed in blood emerging from bleeding time wounds (Michelson *et al.*, 1991), and in normal subjects following strenuous exercise (Kestin *et al.*, 1991).

A number of factors need to be addressed before a coherent picture of platelet activation in different clinical states can emerge. Most of the studies reported so far have been exploratory in nature and have involved relatively few subjects. Patients' status varied considerably, timing of sampling, for example in CPB patients, and the mode of sampling, have all varied. In addition, the different assay protocols used by different groups and even the particular choice of MoAb may have influenced the results. The one clear factor is that activated platelets have been seen in a number of clinical situations where, by other criteria (βTG, aggregometry, etc.) platelet activation has been shown to occur. In addition it would seem that whole blood cytometry, which allows investigation of platelet responsiveness to agonists *in vitro*, can be more informative than fixed assay methods, detecting both hyporesponsive (Janes *et al.*, 1993) and hyperresponsive (Mookerjee *et al.*, 1992) platelets.

Fixed, washed assay methods may, unless performed under the right conditions, actually cause a degree of platelet activation *in vitro*. While this may serve to accentuate differences in platelet responsiveness between patients and controls, it is not clear to what extent different methods of preparation effect such changes and thus lead to variable results. In addition, washing may lead to a preferential loss of subpopulations of platelets.

One situation where all assay methods and all markers give positive findings is the analysis of platelets in concentrates prepared for replacement therapy. Different studies have variously reported elevated P-selectin, CD63 and GMP-33 whether using fixed, washed platelet assays or whole blood analysis (Fijnheer *et al.*, 1990a; Goodall, 1991; Rinder *et al.*, 1991b). In addition, analysis of changes occurring during the preparation of the platelet concentrates has shown a large increase in platelet fibrinogen binding during processing (Goodall, 1991), and a significant increase in platelet degranulation in a percentage of packs, which was greater in platelets prepared by centrifugation of single donor packs than in platelets prepared from buffy coats (Fijnheer *et al.*, 1990b).

George *et al.* (1988) have detected significant levels of platelet microparticles in stored platelet concentrates. Platelet microparticles have also been seen in CPB patients (George *et al.*, 1986; Abrams *et al.*, 1990) and blood emerging from bleeding time wounds (Abrams *et al.*, 1990). In a study of patients with chronic ITP, Wenche *et al.* (1992) have observed significant numbers of platelet microparticles in ITP patients, but only in those patients free of bleeding complications, suggesting a degree of haemostatic protection by the procoagulant microparticles. Warkentin *et al.* (1992) have also observed microparticles in patients with drug-induced thrombocytopenia. In this study microparticles were seen in patients with heparin-induced thrombocytopenia, who exhibit thrombotic complications, but not in those with quinine/quinidine-induced thrombocytopenia, who are at risk of bleeding, again suggesting a pathological, haemostatic mechanism for the microparticles.

Larger clinical studies are under way in many laboratories, which will help to resolve the questions of assay procedure. It is clear, however, that careful preparation of samples is a prerequisite for obtaining meaningful results. It is unclear to what extent the particular disease affects the pattern of expression of platelet activation markers but the different patterns of activation marker expression observed in the different disease states investigated to date, together with the fact that platelets respond differently to different stimuli *in vitro* suggests that a comprehensive analysis of platelet changes may be required to understand the nature of the changes occurring *in vivo*. This has important implications for the design of anti-platelet therapy for different clinical conditions.

Diagnosis of congenital platelet abnormalities

Flow cytometry offers a clear-cut method of diagnosing the rare congenital platelet abnormalities of glycoprotein deficiency.

Glanzmann's thrombasthenia (GT) is caused by a deficiency in the GPIIb-IIIa complex. The patients have a prolonged bleeding time with normal platelet counts and morphology. The platelets do not aggregate in response to ADP and other agonists, and clot retraction is impaired. Patients with type I GT are homozygous for the condition and have a virtual absence (<5% of normal) of GPIIb-IIIa. Patients with Type II GT have 10–20% of the normal level of GPIIb-IIIa, their platelets fail to aggregate, but clot retraction is present, albeit often reduced (George *et al.*, 1990). Variant forms of the disease have also been reported in which the patients' platelets have detectable GPIIb-IIIa but defective fibrinogen binding, and hence fail to aggregate (Nurden *et al.*, 1987).

Bernard–Soulier syndrome (BSS) results from a deficiency in GPIb, the platelet receptor for vWF bound to damaged blood vessel subendothelium. Patients have giant platelets and thrombocytopenia, a prolonged bleeding time and their platelets fail to aggregate with ristocetin (Berndt *et al.*, 1989).

Both conditions show an autosomal, recessive mode of inheritance. Heterozygotes for GT and BSS have approximately 50% of the normal level of GPIIb-IIIa or GPIb, respectively, without bleeding problems.

Other, rarer platelet defects have been reported. For example Nieuwenhuis *et al.* (1985) have documented a patient with a deficiency in GPIa whose platelets failed to bind collagen.

Diagnosis of these conditions has, until recently, relied on Born aggregometry. The presence or absence of the particular glycoproteins has been established by immunoelectrophoresis or SDS-PAGE gel analysis (Clemetson and Lüscher, 1988). Flow cytometry is proving an effective diagnostic method for these patients which allows both the detection and quantitation of antigen expression (Johnston *et al.*, 1984; Adelman *et al.*, 1985; Jennings *et al.*, 1986; Gruel *et al.*, 1986; Fabris *et al.*, 1989). It can also be used to detect heterozygote carriers of these conditions. It lends itself to whole blood assay and so can be performed on very small samples of blood, and thus can be used to analyse neonatal or fetal blood samples (Gruel *et al.*, 1986).

Method

1 Blood should be analysed within 24 hours of collection. Unlike the detection of platelet activation antigens the total expression of GPIIb-IIIa and the GPIb-IX complex is less susceptible to alteration *in vitro*; although prolonged storage of samples can lead to changes in the level of expression of GPIIb-IIIa or GPIb. This can be reduced by addition of PGI_2 (50 µmol/l) to the blood samples.
2 Samples are collected into citrate. Five-microlitre aliquots are added to 50 µl buffer containing FITC-labelled MoAbs to the platelet membrane antigens. Hepes-buffered saline is suitable for this assay but other buffers can also be used (e.g. PBS).
3 Following incubation for 20 min at room temperature, the samples are diluted in 0.5 ml of 0.2% formyl saline and analysed.

This method is suited to patients in whom platelet size is essentially normal (e.g. GT patients) because the platelets can be discriminated from red cells and other blood cells by their light scatter characteristics.

Bernard–Soulier syndrome, in which the patients have giant platelets, usually associated with thrombocytopenia, is better analysed in a two-colour assay. This mode of analysis is also recommended for fetal or neonatal blood samples where the diagnosis may be unclear and the sample size small. In the two-colour assay the blood is diluted in buffer containing a mixture of an FITC-conjugated anti-GPIIb-IIIa MoAb and a biotinylated MoAb to GPIb. Following 15 min incubation at room temperature, streptavidin–phycoerythrin (ST-PE) conjugate is added to identify the biotinylated MoAb. Normal blood samples, incubated with each antibody alone, should be analysed in parallel to enable colour compensation to be set on the flow cytometer. Following a further 15 min incubation, 0.5 ml formyl saline is added and the particles are analysed in the flow cytometer and discriminated by their light scatter characteristics. If the platelet size and morphology are normal, as with thrombasthenic platelets, they appear as a discrete population as shown previously in Fig. 6.3. Expression of both markers can be detected by two-colour analysis, as illustrated in Fig. 6.4, which shows a comparison of normal platelets and platelets from a patient with Type I GT.

Bernard–Soulier platelets, however, are large and thus fall within the area occupied by the red cells (Fig. 6.5). They can be identified by setting a large bit-map to include the platelets and red cells. A fluorescence gate is then set on the enclosed particles so that only those that bear GPIIb-IIIa are analysed for expression of GPIb. In this way, BSS platelets

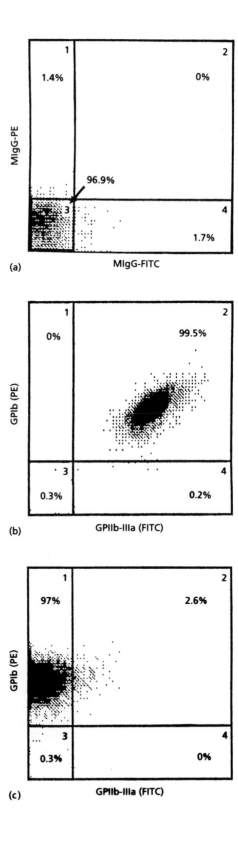

(a)

(b)

(c)

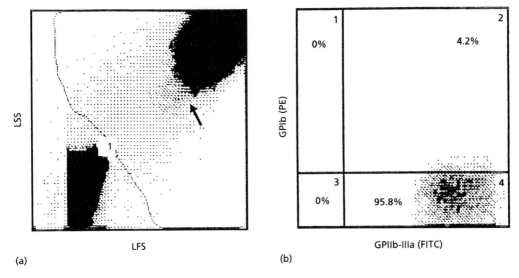

(a) LSS / LFS

(b) GPIb (PE) / GPIIb-IIIa (FITC)

1 0%   2 4.2%
3 0%   95.8% 4

Fig. 6.5 (a) and (b) Analysis of platelets in blood from a patient with BSS. Blood has been incubated with RFGP56-FITC (anti GPIIb-IIIa) and RFGP37-biotin (anti-GPIb) plus ST-PE. The sample is first analysed by light scatter (Fig. 6.5a). The large size of the BSS platelets (arrowed) means they fall within the area occupied by red cells. They are enclosed in a large bit-map (region 1) and analysed for fluorescence on the green channel. Particles positive for green fluorescence (i.e. platelets bearing GPIIb-IIIa) are gated and analysed for expression of both antigens (Fig. 6.5b). More than 95% of platelets express GPIIb-IIIa while GPIb, in this sample, was detectable on less than 5% of platelets.

can be analysed without the need for centrifugation and separation from other blood cells which, in these patients, leads to large losses of platelets which, because of their size and density, tend to sediment with the leucocytes.

Flow cytometry can be also used to analyse functional defects of platelet membrane glycoproteins, as illustrated in two recent publications. Ginsberg et al. (1990) used the binding of PAC-1 and LIBS antibodies to identify patients with defective GPIIb-IIIa receptor function, while Hardisty et al. (1992) reported a case of a patient with a

---

Fig. 6.4 (*opposite*) Analysis of platelets in blood from a normal subject ((a) and (b)) and a patient with Type I Glanzmann's thrombasthenia (c). Platelets are first identified by their light scatter characteristics, as illustrated in Fig. 6.3, then analysed for fluorescence. (a) Normal platelets incubated with negative control reagents (mouse IgG-FITC and mouse IgG-phycoerythrin). More than 95% of platelets are in the negative quadrant. (b) Normal platelets incubated with two MoAbs; an anti-GPIIb-IIIa MoAb conjugated to FITC and an anti-GPIb MoAb conjugated to biotin and visualized with an ST-PE conjugate. More than 99% of platelets fall within the positive quadrant and there is a direct correlation between the level of expression of both antigens on each platelet. (c) Type I GT platelets incubated with GPIIb-IIIa and GPIb MoAbs. Platelets are more than 95% positive for GPIb but have less than 5% expression of GPIIb-IIIa. MoAbs used in this study were RFGP56 (GPIIb-IIIa) and RFGP37 (GPIb), raised in the laboratory of one of us (AHG). The MIgG-FITC negative control was from Coulter Immunology and MIgG-PE and ST-PE were from Becton Dickinson.

lifelong bleeding tendency who displayed a new, variant form of GT in which the platelet surface pool of GPIIb-IIIa was markedly reduced and was unable to bind fibrinogen effectively but the intracellular pools of GPIIb-IIIa were essentially normal.

Patients with congenital storage pool defects (Hardisty, 1989) have also been investigated by flow cytometry. Rosa *et al*. (1987) demonstrated that platelets from patients with α-storage pool disease (SPD), while lacking α-granule contents, still contained α-granule membranes bearing P-selectin antigen, which could fuse with the platelet surface on stimulation with thrombin. In a more recent study, Lages *et al*. (1991) have investigated a patient with severe αδ SPD and found decreased levels of P-selectin and defective expression of the antigen following stimulation.

Calcium flux measurements

Thrombin-induced stimulation of human platelets is accompanied by a dramatic increase in cytoplasmic calcium concentrations followed by a slow decrease (Davies *et al*., 1988). These changes are very rapid, are maximal at 10–15 seconds and may be detected by probes and flow cytometry. Fluo-3 is a recently developed fluorescein chromophore derived Ca^{2+} probe (Minta *et al*., 1989). It combines a high fluorescence intensity upon Ca^{2+} binding with an absorption and emission spectrum very similar to that of fluorescein: its fluorescence intensity increases 40-fold after binding of Ca^{2+} with 506 nm as optimum excitation and 526 as maximum emission wavelength. Fluo-3 has a low affinity for Ca^{2+} with a dissociation constant for Ca^{2+} (K_d) of 400 nmol/l. It does not display significant wavelength shifts after Ca^{2+} binding. The excitation and emission spectra of Fluo-3 is thus optimally compatible with flow cytometers equipped with 488 nm argon laser excitation source and fluorescein filter settings. Moreover, its low affinity for Ca^{2+} makes it theoretically attractive for measuring transient $[Ca^{2+}]_i$ peaks. The method described is for measurement of calcium changes in platelets but may be applied to other cell types (Tsien *et al*., 1982).

Platelet preparation

All procedures are at room temperature.
1   Blood is collected into ACD (citric acid 0.8%, trisodium citrate 2.2%, dextrose 2.45%, pH 4.5) with 1 volume ACD to 9 volumes of blood.
2   The blood is centrifuged at 100 g for 15 min. The PRP is removed and acidified to pH 6.4 with 0.15 mol/l citric acid (usually 30 μl/ml PRP).
3   The acidified PRP is centrifuged at 900 g for 10 min, the plasma removed and the platelet pellet resuspended in modified Tyrodes-Hepes buffer pH 7.35 (0.137 mol/l NaCl, 2.68 mmol/l KCl, 11.9 mmol/l

NaHCO$_3$, 0.146 mmol/l NaH$_2$PO$_4$, 1 mmol/l MgCl$_2$, 0.555 mmol/l dextrose, 5 mmol/l Hepes) to a final concentration of 2×10^8/ml.

Measurement of Ca^{2+}

1 Fluo-3 AM ester (Becton Dickinson) should be prepared as a stock 2 mmol/l solution in dry dimethyl sulphoxide or dimethyl-formamide containing 37.5 g/l Pluronic F-127.
2 The cells are incubated at 37°C with the Fluo-3 for 20 min, then washed three times in modified Tyrodes buffer and resuspended to the original cell count for analysis.

Note. Fluo-3 is supplied as a 50 μg aliquot to which 50 μl of dimethyl-formamide is added. To 5 μl of Fluo-3 add 1.5 μl of Pluronic F-127 non-ionic detergent at 10% and vortex. Add 20 μl modified Tyrodes-Hepes and vortex. The resultant 26.5 μl is sufficient to label 1 ml of cells, although smaller amounts may be used. This gives a final concentration of Fluo-3 of 5 μmol/l.

Flow cytometric analysis

1 Cells should be analysed at a rate of 50 000 cells/min.
2 All experiments are performed in modified Tyrodes-Hepes buffer and any perturbing reagent (e.g. thrombin 0.1–1.0 units/ml final concentration) should be added in as small a volume as possible.
3 Cells should be gated on log forward angle and log 90° light scatter. Excitation is from an argon laser at 488 nm and emission at 525 nm is measured on a linear scale.
4 Thrombin stimulation should be performed at 37°C and discontinuous analysis used.
5 The peak fluorescence for each stimulatory condition is recorded and employed in the analysis described below.

Calculation of calcium concentration

The fluorescence of Fluo-3 labelled cells is measured in arbitrary fluorescence units. To convert these data into absolute [Ca^{2+}]$_i$, a calibration procedure is required. This must be performed at the end of each experiment if absolute [Ca^{2+}]$_i$ are to be obtained.

In order to calculate the exact calcium concentration the following equation (Tsien *et al.*, 1982) is used:

$$[Ca^{2+}]_i = K_d \times (F - F_{min})/(F_{max} - F)$$

where $K_d = 400$ nm (for Fluo-3); F = fluorescence value of experimental cells; F_{max} = calcium saturation level; and F_{min} = calcium-free value.

To calculate F_{max} a sample containing 2 mmol/l Mn^{2+} and 2.5 μmol/l ionomycin (Calbiochem-Behring, Hoechst) are added to cells and allowed to equilibrate for 10–15 min. The fluorescence value obtained is one-fifth of F_{max}. Therefore multiply the value by 5 to five F_{max}. F_{min} is calculated from:

$$F_{min} = (F_{max} - Fbkg)/40 + Fbkg$$

where $Fbkg$ is the fluorescence value for unlabelled cells.

Alternatively, F_{max}, which represents the maximum fluorescence with Ca^{2+}-bound Fluo-3, is obtained by permeabilizing cells for Ca^{2+} in a 1 mmol/l Ca^{2+} containing medium with 5–10 μmol/l of bromo-A23187 (Becton Dickinson) which is a non-fluorescent derivative of the calcium ionophore A23187 (Deber *et al.*, 1985). To obtain F_{min} the method of Hesketh *et al.* (1983) is used. Two millimoles per litre $MnCl_2$ are added to Ca^{2+} ionophore-treated cells. Mn^{2+} displaces Ca^{2+} from Fluo-3. The Mn^{2+}/Fluo-3 complex is eight times as fluorescent as the metal-free dye, but only one-fifth as fluorescent as the Ca^{2+}/Fluo-3 complex (Kao *et al.*, 1989; Minta *et al.*, 1989). F_{min} is calculated as follows:

$$F_{min} = F_{max} - (F_{max} - F_{MnCl_2}) \times 1.25$$
$$= 1.25 \times F_{MnCl_2} - 0.25 \times F_{max}$$

Improved method for measuring intracellular calcium

The accuracy of flow cytometric measurement of intracellular calcium with Fluo-3 is compromised by variation in the basal fluorescence intensity due to heterogeneity in dye uptake or compartmentalization. To overcome this, cells may be loaded simultaneously with Fluo-3 and a second dye (Rijkers *et al.*, 1990). A ratio between the two dyes can then be used to compensate for dye loading heterogeneity. The assumption must be made that the uptake and intracellular conversion of both fluorochromes would be equivalent and that the signal of the second fluorochrome would not vary upon activation. SNARF-1 (seminaphtho-rhodafluor) is a dye which when excited at 488 nm has a pH-independent isoemission point at 610 nm and its fluorescence emission does not change upon cell activation. SNARF-1 and Fluo-3 fluorescence signals have a linear relationship. SNARF-1 has therefore been used with Fluo-3 to provide a ratio of fluorescence intensities to determine calcium flux.

Assay procedure

1   Cells are prepared as above and resuspended in modified Tyrodes buffer with 10 mmol/l Hepes, pH 7.0 to a final concentration of 1×10^6/ml.
2   Fluo-3 and SNARF-1 (Molecular Probes) are dissolved in DMSO (BDH) at a concentration of 1 mmol/l and added directly to the cells.

3 The cells are incubated for 30 min at 37°C, then an equal volume of modified Tyrodes buffer with 10 mmol/l Hepes, pH 7.4 and 5% fetal bovine serum (FBS) is added to the cells.
4 After 10 min incubation at 37°C the cells are washed twice then resuspended in modified Tyrodes buffer with 10 mmol/l Hepes pH 7.2 with 5% FBS and 10 μg/ml DNAase (Sigma) to a final concentration of 1×10^6/ml.

Flow cytometric analysis

1 A laser excitation wavelength of 488 nm is used. Fluo-3 and SNARF-1 emissions are measured at 525 and 610, respectively.
2 Fluorescence intensity data are collected during consecutive five-second increments (approximately 2500 cells/increment per channel) and are depicted as three parameter cytograms of fluorescence intensity *vs* time *vs* cell number. The data from four consecutive increments are analysed.
3 Data analysis may be performed using Chronys (Becton Dickinson).
4 If the Fluo-3/SNARF-1 fluorescence intensity ratio is plotted against time this provides a more reliable measure of cell activation than measurement of Fluo-3 intensity alone.

Megakaryocyte preparation

Megakaryocyte ploidy and platelet production

Circulating blood platelets are heterogeneous in size, density and reactivity. In 1964 McDonald *et al.* suggested that size heterogeneity reflected platelet ageing in the circulation, so that young platelets were large platelets which decreased in size as they aged. Since platelet size and density were found to be linked, Karpatkin (1969) extended the ageing hypothesis of McDonald *et al.* (1964) to suggest that platelet density decreased with platelet age. However, evidence has now been presented by a number of groups suggesting that platelets do not change their size or density as they age in the circulation. It is now widely believed that platelet heterogeneity is determined primarily at thrombopoiesis (Martin, 1990).

Several studies have demonstrated that the mean volume of circulating platelets is altered in a variety of situations. For example, following myocardial infarction or coronary bypass grafting, and in autoimmune thrombocytopenic purpura, platelets have an increased mean platelet volume (Paulus, 1975; Cameron *et al.*, 1983; Martin *et al.*, 1983a, 1987). If platelet changes are determined at thrombopoiesis, such alterations in size might be expected to be preceded by changes in the parent cell, the megakaryocyte. These large, fragile cells, produced in the bone marrow, undergo endoreduplication as they mature, resulting in a marked degree of heterogeneity, in both DNA content and size (Levine *et al.*, 1982).

At times of decreased platelet number in human and animal models, it has been observed that the megakaryocyte population can increase their mean ploidy and size (Martin *et al.*, 1982, 1983b; Trowbridge *et al.*, 1984). In conditions of perturbed thrombopoiesis, it has been observed that changes in mean platelet volume and megakaryocyte ploidy can occur independently or simultaneously. For example, in myocardial infarction, both mean platelet volume and megakaryocyte DNA content and size are increased; however, in secondary thrombocytosis associated with malignant lymphoma, the megakaryocyte size is similarly increased but mean platelet volume is unchanged compared with controls.

It has been proposed (Gladwin and Martin, 1990) that an increased mean platelet volume occurs following an increased rate of platelet destruction and an increased megakaryocyte size and ploidy occurs in association with an increased demand for platelets. Thus it is of clinical interest to determine megakaryocyte ploidy by flow cytometry. Two methods for preparing megakaryocytes have been described (Tomer *et al.*, 1988; Gladwin *et al.*, 1990).

Percoll gradient enrichment of bone marrow

Marrow preparation

1 Bone marrow (6–8 ml) is collected from a single site in the posterior illiac crest. Cells are collected into a 1/10 volume of anticoagulant consisting of ACD formula A containing EDTA (2.5 mmol/l final concentration) and PGE_1 (2.2 µmol/l final concentration).
2 The marrow is gently passed through a 200 µm monofilament nylon gauze filter (Millipore) and diluted with cold Ca and Mg free PBS supplemented with 13.6 mmol/l sodium citrate, 2.2 µm/l PGE_1, 1 mmol/l theophylline, 3% BSA, 11 mmol/l glucose and adjusted to pH 7.3 (supplemented PBS).

Fractionation of marrow

1 The cell suspension is adjusted to 20×10^6 cells/ml, mixed with Percoll (Pharmacia) to a final density of 1.020 g/ml (isotonic 83.1% Percoll diluted with PBS containing 13.6 mmol/l sodium citrate).
2 The bone marrow mixture is layered over 12 ml of Percoll density 1.055 g/ml and the marrow layer is overlain with 10 ml of supplemented PBS.
3 After centrifugation at 400 g for 20 min at 15°C the upper 8 ml of the medium layer is removed and the cells from the upper Percoll layer and the interface collected.
4 The collected cells are washed in cold supplemented PBS containing 6% BSA by centrifugation at 300 g for 10 min at 15°C.

5 The supernatant is discarded and the cell pellet resuspended in the same medium and stored on ice ready for antibody labelling.

The Percoll density fractionation should result in depletion of 96% of the bone marrow cells with a 26-fold enrichment of megakaryocytes that have a characteristic morphology which may be assessed by phase-contrast microscopy (Japa, 1943) or by haematoxylin or Wright-Geimsa staining (Levine *et al.*, 1982).

Immunomagnetic separation method for preparing megakaryocytes

Bone marrow preparation

1 Iliac crest bone marrow (1 ml) is taken into modified PBS containing 7.5 mmol/l glucose, 3 mmol/l EDTA, 2 mmol/l KCl, 0.5 mmol/l Na_2SO_4, 0.1% BSA and 10 µl of PGE_1 (0.4 mg/ml) pH 6.5 at 4°C.
2 The sample is made up to 50 ml in modified PBS and mono-dispersed by gentle pipetting, then filtered through 100 µm nylon gauze.

Megakaryocyte separation

1 Plt-1 (Coulter) is freshly prepared then 500 µl is added to 50 ml of bone marrow suspension, mixed gently by inversion and incubated on ice for 30 min (anti-GpIIIa (DAKO) may also be used).
2 After which 10 µl of magnetizable particles coated with goat anti-mouse (diluted in PBS to give a ratio of one to two beads per cell) (Dynal) are added.
3 The preparation is gently mixed then incubated for a further 30 min at 4°C.
4 At the end of the incubation period cells bound to magnetizable particles are harvested by placing the tube containing the cell suspension in contact with a magnet (Dynal) for 2 min.
5 The supernatant is carefully removed, ensuring that magnetized cells are not disturbed.
6 The magnet is then removed and cells with magnetizable particles attached are resuspended in modified PBS and washed twice by concentrating with the magnet.
7 Harvested cells are resuspended in 1 ml modified PBS ready for antibody labelling.

Antibody labelling

1 Megakaryocytes should be directly labelled with FITC-conjugated

Continued on p. 184

mouse anti-human GpIIIa (DAKO) at saturating concentrations in modified/supplemented PBS containing 6% BSA.

2 An isotype negative control should be included and dead cells, debris and unbound antibody are removed by centrifugation at $100\,g$ for 10 min at 15°C over 10% BSA.

3 The cell pellet is resuspended in modified or supplemented PBS for propidium iodide labelling of the DNA content.

Propidium iodide labelling

1 Following labelling with MoAbs, the cells are fixed by the addition of an equal volume of 2% paraformaldehyde (Sigma) in PBS supplemented with 13.6 mmol/l sodium citrate and incubated at 4°C for 30 min.

2 After which propidium iodide (Sigma) at a final concentration of 50 µg/ml, RNase (50 µg/ml, bovine pancreas, Sigma) and Triton X-100 (Sigma) at a final concentration of 0.05% are added.

3 The suspension is gently mixed for 30 min at 4°C then filtered through a 100 µm nylon mesh to remove aggregates prior to flow cytometric analysis.

4 Cells stained with one fluorochrome only should be prepared to correct for overlap between emitting spectra.

5 Human mononuclear cells or chick erythrocytes (Becton Dickinson) should be propidium iodide stained to determine the fluorescence intensity of cells with diploid DNA.

Flow cytometric analysis

The cells are analysed using a dual parameter histogram of green fluorescence and forward angle light scatter which allows identification of the large highly fluorescent megakaryocytes. This population should be gated and the red fluorescence (<610 nm) analysed.

Summary

Flow cytometry has been used in the study of immune thrombocytopenia to identify PAIg, platelet-specific antibodies and antigen-specific antibodies. More recently, analysis of the activation state of platelets has been assessed in a number of disease states. Future analysis may reveal correlations between platelet activation state and disease progress. In addition whole blood cytometry allows investigation of platelet responsiveness to agonists *in vitro* such that both hypo- and hyperresponsive platelets may be detected. Finally, analysis of megakaryocytes may aid in understanding the cause of perturbed thrombopoiesis.

References

Abrams C, Shattil SJ (1991) Immunological detection of activated platelets in clinical disorders. *Thromb. Haemost.* **65**: 467–473.

Abrams CS, Ellison N, Budzynski AZ, Shattil SJ (1990) Direct detection of activated platelets and platelet-derived microparticles in humans. *Blood* **75**: 128–138.

Adelman B, Michelson AD, Handin RI, Ault KA (1985) Evaluation of platelet glyco-protein Ib by fluorescence flow cytometry. *Blood* **66**: 423–427.

Adelman B, Carlson P, Powers P (1987) von Willebrand factor is present on the surface of platelets stimulated in plasma by ADP. *Blood* **70**: 1362–1366.

Aiken ML, Ginsberg MH, Plow EF (1987) Mechanisms for expression of thrombo-spondin on the platelet cell surface. *Semin. Thromb. Haemost.* **13**: 307–316.

Azorsa DO, Hyman JA, Hildreth JE (1991) CD63/Pltgp40: a platelet activation antigen identical to the stage-specific, melanoma-associated antigen ME491. *Blood* **78**: 280–284.

Beardsley SS, Speigel JE, Jacobs MM, Handin R II, Lux SE (1984) Platelet membrane glycoprotein IIIa contains target antigens that bind anti-platelet antibodies in immune thrombocytopenias. *J. Clin. Invest.* **74**: 1701–1707.

Berman CL, Yeo EL, Wencel-Drake JD, Furie BC, Ginsberg MH, Furie B (1986) A platelet alphagranule membrane protein that is associated with the plasma mem-brane after activation: Characterization and subcellular localization of platelet activation-dependent granule-external membrane protein. *J. Clin. Invest.* **78**: 130–137.

Berndt MC, Fournier DJ, Castaldi PA (1989) Bernard–Soulier syndrome. In: Caen JP, ed., *Baillières's Clinical Haematology: Platelet Disorders*. Baillière Tindall London, pp. 585–607.

Bevers EM, Comfurius P, Zwaal RFA (1983) Changes in membrane phospholipid distribution during platelet activation. *Biochim. Biophys. Acta* **736**: 57–66.

Bevilacqua M, Butcher E, Furie B *et al.* (1991) Selectins: A family of adhesion receptors. *Cell* **67**: 233.

Blumberg N, Masel D, Mayer T, Horan P, Heal J (1984) Removal of HLA-A-B antigens from platelets. *Blood* **63**: 448–450.

Cameron HA, Philips R, Ibbotson RM, Carson PHM (1983) Platelet size in myocardial infarction. *Br. Med. J.* **287**: 449–451.

Capitanio AM, Niewiarowski S, Rucinski B *et al.* (1985) Interaction of platelet factor 4 with human platelets. *Biochim. Biophys. Acta* **839**: 161–173.

Chen JW, Murphy TL, Willingham MC, Pastan I, August JT (1985) Identification of two lysosomal membrane glycoproteins. *J. Cell Biol.* **101**: 85–95.

Cines DB, Schreiber AD (1979) Immune thrombocytopenic purpura. Use of a Coombes antiglobin test to detect IgG and C3 on platelets. *N. Engl. J. Med.* **300**: 106–111.

Clemetson KJ, Lüscher EF (1988) Membrane glycoprotein abnormalities in pathological platelets. *Biochim. Biophys. Acta* **947**: 53–73.

Corash L (1990) Measurement of platelet activation by fluorescence-activated flow cytometry. *Blood Cells* **16**: 97–106.

Cox AD, Goodall AH (1991) Activation-specific neo-antigen on platelet detected by monoclonal antibodies. In: Albertini A, Lenfant CL, Mannucci PM, Sixma JJ, eds, *Current Studies in Haematology and Blood Transfusion*, 58. Karger, Basel, pp. 194–199.

Cox AD, Janes SL, Goodall AH (1991) Fibrinogen and vWF share a common binding site on GPIIb-IIIa: direct evidence in whole blood. *Br. J. Haematol.* **77**: 104 (Abstr.).

Davies TA, Drotts D, Weil GJ, Simons ER (1988) Flow cytometric measurements of cytoplasmic calcium changes in human platelets. *Cytometry* **9**: 138–142.

Deber CM, Tom-Kun J, Mack E, Grinstein S (1985) Bromo-A23187: a nonfluorescent calcium ionophore for use with fluorescent probes. *Anal. Biochem.* **146**: 349–353.

Dechavanne M, Ffrench M, Pages J *et al.* (1987) Significant reduction in the binding of a monoclonal antibody (LYP 18) directed against the IIb/IIIa glycoprotein complex to platelets of patients having undergone extracorporeal circulation. *Thromb. Haemost.* **57**: 106–109.

Dixon RH, Rosse WF (1975) Platelet antibody in autoimmune thrombocytopenia. *Br. J. Haematol.* **31**: 129–134.

Dixon RH, Rosse WF, Ebbert L (1975) Quantitative determination of antibody in idiopathic thrombocytopenic purpura; correlation of serum and platelet bound antibody with clinical response. *N. Engl. J. Med.* **242**: 230–236.

Ejim OS, Powling MJ, Dandona P, Kernoff PB, Goodall AH (1990) A flow cytometric analysis of fibronectin binding to platelets from patients with peripheral vascular disease. *Thromb. Res.* **58**: 519–524.

Fabris F, Casonato A, Randi ML *et al.* (1989) The use of fluorescence flow cytometry in the characterization of Bernard–Soulier syndrome and Glanzmann's thrombasthenia. *Haematologica* **74**: 39–44.

Febbraio M, Silverstein RL (1990) Identification and characterization of LAMP-1 as an activation-dependent platelet surface glycoprotein. *J. Biol. Chem.* **265**: 18531–18537.

Fijnheer R, Modderman PW, Veldman H *et al.* (1990a) Detection of platelet activation with monoclonal antibodies and flow cytometry. Changes during platelet storage. *Transfusion* **30**: 20–25.

Fijnheer R, Pietersz RN, de-Korte D *et al.* (1990b) Platelet activation during preparation of platelet concentrates: a comparison of the platelet-rich plasma and the buffy coat methods. *Transfusion* **30**: 634–638.

Fijnheer R, Modderman PW, Veldman H *et al.* (1990c) Detection of platelet activation with monoclonal antibodies and flow cytometry. Changes during platelet storage. *Transfusion* **30**: 20–25.

Frelinger AL, Lam SC-T, Plow EF, Smith MA, Loftus JC, Ginsberg MH (1988) Occupancy of an adhesive glycoprotein receptor modulates expression of an antigenic site involved in cell adhesion. *J Biol. Chem.* **263**: 12397–12402.

Frelinger AL, Cohen I, Plow EF *et al.* (1990) Selective inhibition of integrin function by antibodies specific for ligand-occupied receptor conformers. *J. Biol. Chem.* **265**: 6346–6352.

Fukuda M, Viitala J, Matteson J, Carlsson SR (1988) Cloning of cDNAs encoding human lysosomal membrane glycoproteins, h-Lamp-1 and h-Lamp-2. Comparison of their deduced amino acid sequences. *J Biol. Chem.* **263**: 18920–18928.

Furihata K, Nugent DJ, Bissonette A, Aster RH, Kunicki TJ (1987) On the association of the platelet-specific alloantigen Pen[a], with glycoprotein IIIa. Evidence for heterogeneity of glycoprotein IIIa. *J. Clin. Invest.* **80**: 1624–1630.

Galt SW, McDaniel MD, Ault KA, Mitchell J, Crowenwett JL (1991) Flow cytometric assessment of platelet function in patients with peripheral arterial occlusive disease. *J. Vasc. Surg.* **14**: 747–756.

George JN, Pickett EB, Saucerman S *et al.* (1986) Platelet surface glycoproteins. Studies on resting and activated platelets and platelet membrane microparticles in normal subjects, and observations in patients during adult respiratory distress syndrome and cardiac surgery. *J. Clin. Invest.* **78**: 340–348.

George JN, Pickett EB, Heinz R (1988) Platelet membrane glycoprotein changes during the preparation and storage of platelet concentrates. *Transfusion* **28**: 123–126.

George JN, Caen JP, Nurden AT (1990) Glanzmann's thrombasthenia: The spectrum of clinical disease. *Blood* **75**: 1383–1395.

Gerrard JM, Lint D, Sims PJ *et al.* (1991) Identification of a platelet dense granule membrane protein that is deficient in a patient with the Hermansky–Pudlak syndrome. *Blood* **77**: 101–112.

Gilbert GE, Sims PJ, Wiedmer T, Furie B, Furie BC, Shattil SJ (1991) Platelet-derived microparticles express high affinity receptors for factor VIII. *J. Biol. Chem.* **266**: 17261–17268.

Ginsberg MH, Frelinger AL, Lam SC-T *et al.* (1990) Analysis of platelet aggregation disorders based on flow cytometric analysis of membrane glycoprotein IIb-IIIa with conformation-specific monoclonal antibodies. *Blood* **76**: 2017–2023.

Gladwin AM, Martin JF (1990) The control of megakaryocyte ploidy and platelet production: Biology and pathology. *Int. J. Cell Cloning* **8**: 291–298.

Gladwin AM, Carrier MJ, Beesley JE, Lelchuk R, Hancock V, Martin JF (1990) Identification of mRNA for PDGF b-chain in megakaryocytes isolated using a novel immunomagnetic separation method. *Br. J. Haematol.* **76**: 333–339.

Goodall AH (1991) Platelet activation during preparation and storage of concentrates: detection by flow cytometry. *Blood Coag. Fibrinolysis* **2**: 377–389.

Gruel Y, Boizard B, Daffos F, Forestier F, Caen J, Wautier JL (1986) Determination of platelet antigens and glycoproteins in the human fetus. *Blood* **68**: 488–492.

Hardisty RM (1989) Disorders of platelet secretion. In: Caen JP, ed., *Bailliére's Clinical Haematology: Platelet disorders*. Bailliére Tindall, London, pp. 673–694.

Hardisty RM, Pidard D, Cox A *et al.* (1992) A defect of platelet aggregation associated with an abnormal distribution of glycoprotein IIb-IIIa complexes within the platelet: the cause of a lifelong bleeding disorder. *Blood* **80**: 696–708.

Harfenist EJ, Packham MA, Mustard JF (1985) Comparison of the interactions of fibrinogen and soluble fibrin with washed rabbit platelets stimulated with ADP. *Thromb. Haemost.* **53**: 183–187.

Harker LA, Malpass TW, Branson HE, Hessel EA, Slichter SJ (1980) Mechanism of abnormal bleeding in patients undergoing cardiopulmonary bypass: acquired transient platelet dysfunction associated with selective alpha-granule release. *Blood* **56**: 824–834.

Harmon DC, Weitzman SA, Stossel TP (1980) A staphylococcal slide test for detection of antineutrophil antibodies. *Blood* **56**: 64–69.

Harrington WJ, Minnich V, Arimura G (1956) Auto-immune thrombocytopenias. *Prog. Haematol.* **1**: 166–172.

Hauch TW, Rosse WF (1977) Platelet bound complement (C3) in immune thrombocytopenia. *Blood* **50**: 1129–1136.

Hegde UM, Gordon-Smith EC, Worlledge S (1977) Platelet antibodies in thrombocytopenic patients. *Br. J. Haematol.* **35**: 113–122.

Hegde UM, Powell DK, Bowes A, Gordon-Smith EC (1981) Enzyme linked immunoassay for the detection of platelet associated IgG. *Br. J. Haematol.* **48**: 39–46.

Hesketh TR, Smith GA, Moore JP, Taylor MV, Metcalf JC (1983) Free cytoplasmic calcium concentration and the mitogenic stimulation of lymphocytes. *J. Biol. Chem.* **258**: 4876–4882.

Hoffman M, Monroe DM, Roberts HR (1992) Coagulation factor IXa binding to activated platelets and platelet-derived microparticles: a flow cytometric study. *Thromb. Haemost.* **68**: 74–78.

Horejsi V, Vlcek C (1991) Novel structurally distinct family of leucocyte surface glycoproteins including CD9, CD37, CD53 and CD63. *FEBS Lett.* **288**: 1–4.

Hourdille P, Heilmann E, Combrie R, Winckler J, Clemetson KJ, Nurden AT (1990) Thrombin induces a rapid redistribution of glycoprotein Ib-IX complexes within the membrane systems of activated human platelets. *Blood* **76**: 1503–1513.

Hsu-Lin S, Berman CL, Furie BC, August D, Furie B (1984) A platelet membrane protein expressed during platelet activation and secretion. Studies using a monoclonal antibody specific for thrombin-activated platelets. *J. Biol. Chem.* **259**: 9121–9126.

Hymes K, Schulman S, Karpatkin S (1979) Solid phase radioassay for bound antiplatelet antibody. *J. Lab. Clin. Med.* **14**: 639–648.

Imbach P, d'Apuzzo V, Hirt A *et al.* (1981) High dose intravenous gammaglobulin for idiopathic thrombocytopenic purpura in children. *Lancet* **i**: 1228–1239.

Israels SJ, Gerrard JM, Jacques YV *et al.* (1992) Platelet dense granule membranes contain both granulophysin and P-selectin (GMP-140). *Blood* **80**: 143–152.

Jackson CW, Jennings LK (1989) Heterogeneity of fibrinogen receptor expression on platelets activated in normal plasma with ADP: analysis by flow cytometry. *Br. J. Haematol.* **72**: 407–414.

Janes SL, Goodall AH (1992) Platelet activation in pregnancy: enhanced degranulation and the pathogenesis of pre-eclampsia. *Br. J. Haematol.* **66** (Abstr).

Janes SL, Cox AD, Hardisty RM, Goodall AH (1991) Flow cytometric detection of platelet activation and hyper-reactivity in clinical conditions: pre-eclampsia as a model. *Thromb. Haemost.* **65**: 680 (Abstr.).

Janes SL, Wilson DJ, Chronos N, Goodall AH (1993) Evaluation of whole blood flow cytometric detection of platelet bound fibrinogen in normal subjects and patients with activated platelets. *Thromb. Haemost.* (in press).

Japa J (1943) A study of the morphology and development of the megakaryocyte. *Br. J. Exp. Pathol.* **24**: 73–80.

Jennings LK, Ashmun RA, Wang WC, Dockter ME (1986) Analysis of human platelet glycoproteins IIb-IIIa and Glanzmann's thrombasthenia in whole blood by flow cytometry. *Blood* **68**: 173–179.

Johnston GI, Heptinstall S, Robins RA, Price MR (1984) The expression of glycoproteins on single blood platelets from healthy individuals and from patients with congenital bleeding disorders. *Biochem. Biophys. Res. Comm.* **123**: 1091–1098.

Johnston GI, Pickett EB, McEver RP, George JN (1987) Heterogeneity of platelet secretion in response to thrombin demonstrated by fluorescence flow cytometry. *Blood* **69**: 1401–1403.

Kao JPY, Harootunian AT, Tsien RY (1989) Photochemically generated cytosolic calcium pulses and their detection by fluo-3. *J. Biol. Chem.* **264**: 8179–8184.

Karpatkin S (1969) Heterogeneity of human platelets. I. Metabolic and kinetic evidence suggestive of young adult platelets. *J. Clin. Invest.* **48**: 1073–1082.

Karpatkin S, Siskind GW (1969) *In vitro* detection of platelet antibody in patients with idiopathic thrombocytopenic purpura and systemic lupus erythematosis. *Blood* **33**: 795–812.

Kelton JG, Giles AR, Neame PB, Powers P, Hageman N, Hirsh J (1979) Comparison of two direct assays for platelet associated IgG (PAIgG) in assessment of immune and nonimmune thrombocytopenia. *Blood* **55**: 424–429.

Kestin AS, Ellis PA, Errichetti A, Barnard MR, Rosner B, Michelson AD (1991) The effect of strenuous exercise on platelet activation state and reactivity: differences between physically trained and untrained subjects. *Thromb. Haemost.* **65**: 1117 (Abstr.).

Kiefel V, Santoso S, Weisheit M, Mueller-Eckhardt C (1987) Monoclonal antibody-specific immobilization of platelet antigens (MAIPA): A new tool for identification of platelet reactive antibodies. *Blood* **70**: 1722–1726.

Kurata Y, Oshida M, Take H *et al.* (1990) Acid treatment of platelets as a simple procedure for distinguishing platelet-specific antibodies from anti-HLA antibodies: comparison with chloroquine treatment. *Vox Sang.* **59**: 106–111.

Lagarden M, Bryon PA, Guichardant M, Dechavanne M (1980) A simple and efficient method for platelet isolation from their plasma. *Thromb. Res.* **17**: 581–588.

Lages B, Shattil SJ, Bainton DF, Weiss HJ (1991) Decreased content and surface expression of alpha-granule membrane protein GMP-140 in one of two types of platelet alpha delta storage pool deficiency. *J. Clin. Invest.* **87**: 919–929.

Langenscheidt F, Keifel V, Santoso S, Nau A, Mueller-Eckhardt C (1989) Quantitation of platelet antigens after chloroquine treatment. *Eur. J. Haematol.* **42**: 186–192.

Larsen E, Celi A, Gilbert GE *et al.* (1989) PADGEM protein: a receptor that mediates the interaction of activated platelets with neutrophils and monocytes. *Cell* **59**: 305–312.

Laudano AP, Doolittle RF (1980) Studies on synthetic peptides that bind to fibrinogen and prevent fibrin polymerization. Structural requirements, number of binding sites, and species differences. *Biochemistry* **19**: 1013–1019.

Lazarchick J, Hall SA (1986) Platelet associated IgG assay using flow cytometric technique. *J. Immunol. Methods* **87**: 257–265.

Leung LLK, Nachman RL (1982) Complex formation of platelet thrombospondin with fibrinogen. *J. Clin. Invest.* **70**: 542–549.

Levine RF, Hazzard KC, Lamberg JD (1982) The significance of megakaryocyte size. *Blood* **60**: 1122–1131.

Lin RY, Levin M, Nygren EN, Norman A, Lorenzana FG (1990) Assessment of platelet antibody by flow cytometric and ELISA techniques: a comparison study. *J. Lab. Clin. Methods* **116**: 479–486.

Lindahl TL, Festin R, Larsson A (1992) Studies of fibrinogen binding to platelets by flow cytometry: An improved method for studies of platelet activation. *Thromb. Haemost.* **68**: 221–225.

Lucas GF, Holburn AM (1987) The effect of anticoagulant on platelet associated IgG. *Br. J. Haematol.* **65**: 111–115.

Martin JF (1990) Platelet heterogeneity in vascular disease. In: Martin JF, ed., *Platelet Heterogeneity: Biology and Pathology*. Springer-Verlag, London, pp. 205–226.

Martin JF, Trowbridge EA, Salmon GL, Slater DN (1982) The relationship between platelets and megakaryocytes volume. *Thromb. Res.* **28**: 447–459.

Martin JF, Plumb J, Kilbey RS, Kishk YT (1983a) Changes in volume and density of platelets in myocardial infarction. *Br. Med. J.* **287**: 456−459.

Martin JF, Trowbridge EA, Salmon GL, Plumb J (1983b) The biological significance of platelet volume: its relationship to bleeding time, platelet thromboxane B$_2$ production and megakaryocyte nuclear DNA concentration. *Thromb. Res.* **32**: 443−460.

Martin JF, Daniels TD, Trowbridge EA (1987) Acute and chronic changes in platelet volume and count after cardiopulmonary bypass induced thrombocytopenia in man. *Thromb. Haemost.* **57**: 55−58.

McDonald TP, Odell TT Jr, Grossless DG (1964) Platelet size in relation to platelet age. *Proc. Soc. Exp. Biol. Med.* **115**: 684−689.

McEver RP, Martin MN (1984) A monoclonal antibody to a membrane glycoprotein binds only to activated platelets. *J. Biol. Chem.* **259**: 9799−9804.

McMillan R, Tani P, Berchtold P, Renshaw L, Woods VL Jr (1987) Platelet associated and plasma anti-glycoprotein autoantibodies in chronic ITP. *Blood* **70**: 1040−1045.

Metzelaar MJ, Clevers HC (1992) Lysosomal membrane glycoproteins in platelets. *Thromb. Haemost.* **68**: 378−382.

Metzelaar MJ, Sixma JJ, Nieuwenhuis HK (1990) Detection of platelet activation using activation specific monoclonal antibodies. *Blood Cells* **16**: 85−93.

Metzelaar MJ, Heijnen HF, Sixma JJ, Nieuwenhuis HK (1992) Identification of a 33-Kd protein associated with the alpha-granule membrane (GMP-33) that is expressed on the surface of activated platelets. *Blood* **79**: 372−379.

Michelson AD, Barnard MR (1987) Thrombin-induced changes in platelet membrane glycoproteins Ib, IX, and IIb-IIIa complex. *Blood* **70**: 1673−1678.

Michelson AD, Ellis PA, Barnard MR, Matic GB, Viles AF, Kestin AS (1991) Down-regulation of the platelet surface glycoprotein Ib-IX complex in whole blood stimulated by thrombin, adenosine diphosphate, or an *in vivo* wound. *Blood* **77**: 770−779.

Minta A, Kao JPY, Tsien RY (1989) Fluorescent indicators for cytosolic calcium based on rhodamine and fluorescein chromophores. *J. Biol. Chem.* **264**: 8171−8178.

Mookerjee RP, Stansby G, Hamilton G, Goodall AH (1992) Platelet activation in peripheral vascular disease patients. *Platelets* **3**: 109.

Morris A, Macey MG, Newland AC (1991) Platelet immunoglobulins, glycoproteins and activation antigens in autoimmune thrombocytopenic purpura (ATP). *Br. J. Haematol.* **71** (Suppl.): 27.

Mueller-Eckhardt C, Mahn L, Schulz G, Mueller-Eckhardt G (1978) Detection of platelet autoantibodies by a radioactive antiimmunoglobulin test. *Vox Sang.* **35**: 357−365.

Mueller-Eckhardt C, Kayser W, Mersch-Baumert K *et al.* (1980a) The clinical significance of platelet associated IgG; a study on 298 patients with various disorders. *Br. J. Haematol.* **46**: 123−131.

Mueller-Eckhardt C, Lechner K, Heinrich D *et al.* (1980b) Post-transfusion thrombocytopenic purpura. Immunological and clinical studies in two cases and review of the literature. *Blut* **40**: 249−257.

Mueller-Eckhardt C, Mueller-Eckhardt G, Kayser W, Voss RM, Weger J, Kenzler E (1982) Platelet associated IgG, platelet survival and platelet sequestration in thrombocytopenic states. *Br. J. Haematol.* **52**: 49−58.

Mueller-Eckhardt C, Keifel V, Santoso S (1989) Recent trends in platelet antigen/antibody detection. *Blut* **59**: 35−43.

Murphy MF, Waters AH (1985) Immunological aspects of platelet transfusions. *Br. J. Haematol.* **60**: 409−414.

Myllyla G (1973) Aggregation of human blood platelets by immune complexes in the sedimentation pattern test. *Scand. J. Haematol.* **Suppl. 19**: 50.

Newland AC, Treleaven JG, Minchinton RM, Waters AH (1983) High dose intravenous IgG in adults with autoimmune thrombocytopenic purpura. *Lancet* i: 84−87.

Nieuwenhuis HK, Akkerman JWN, Houdijk WPM, Sixma JJ (1985) Human blood platelets showing no response to collagen fail to express surface glycoprotein Ia. *Nature* **318**: 470−472.

Nieuwenhuis HK, van Oosterhout JJG, Rozemuller E, van Iwaarden F, Sixma JJ (1987) Studies with a monoclonal antibody against activated platelets: Evidence that a secreted 53,000-molecular weight lysosome-like granule protein is exposed on the surface of activated platelets in the circulation. *Blood* **70**: 838–845.

Nordhagen R, Flaathen ST (1985) Chloroquine removal of HLA antigens from platelets for platelet immunofluorescence test. *Vox Sang.* **48**: 156–159.

Nurden AT, Rosa JP, Fournier D *et al.* (1987) A variant of Glanzmann's thrombasthenia with abnormal glycoprotein IIb-IIIa complexes in the platelet membrane. *J. Clin. Invest.* **79**: 962–969.

Paulus JM (1975) Platelet size in man. *Blood* **46**: 321–336.

Phillips DR, Charo IF, Parise LV, Fitzgerald LA (1988) The platelet membrane glycoprotein IIb-IIIa complex. *Blood* **71**: 831–843.

Rijkers GT, Justement LB, Griffioen AW, Cambier JC (1990) Improved method for measuring intracellular Ca^{++} with fluo-3. *Cytometry* **11**: 923–927.

Rinder CS, Bohnert J, Rinder HM, Mitchell J, Ault K, Hillman R (1991a) Platelet activation and aggregation during cardiopulmonary bypass. *Anesthesiology* **75**: 388–393.

Rinder HM, Murphy M, Mitchell JG, Stocks J, Ault KA, Hillman RS (1991b) Progressive platelet activation with storage: evidence for shortened survival of activated platelets after transfusion. *Transfusion* **31**: 409–414.

Rosa JP, George JN, Bainton DF, Nurden AT, Caen JP, McEver RP (1987) Gray platelet syndrome: demonstration of alpha granule membranes that can fuse with the cell surface. *J. Clin. Invest.* **80**: 1138–1146.

Rubinstein E, Kouns WC, Jennings LK, Boucheix C, Carroll RC (1991) Interaction of two GPIIb/IIIa monoclonal antibodies with platelet Fc receptor (Fc gamma RII). *Br. J. Haematol.* **78**: 80–86.

Shattil SJ, Hoxie JA, Cunningham M, Brass LF (1985) Changes in the platelet membrane glycoprotein IIb.IIIa complex during platelet activation. *J. Biol. Chem.* **260**: 11 107–11 114.

Shattil SJ, Cunningham M, Hoxie JA (1987) Detection of activated platelets in whole blood using activation-dependent monoclonal antibodies and flow cytometry. *Blood* **70**: 307–315.

Shattil SJ, Budzynski A, Scrutton MC (1989) Epinephrine induces platelet fibrinogen receptor expression, fibrinogen binding, and aggregation in whole blood in the absence of other excitatory agonists. *Blood* **73**: 150–158.

Silverstein RL, Asch AS, Nachman RL (1989) Glycoprotein IV mediates thrombospondin-dependent platelet-monocyte and platelet-U937 cell adhesion. *J. Clin. Invest.* **84**: 546–552.

Sims PJ, Faioni EM, Wiedmer T, Shattil SJ (1988) Complement proteins C5b-9 cause release of membrane vesicles from the platelet surface that are enriched in the membrane receptor for coagulation factor Va and express prothrombinase activity. *J. Biol. Chem.* **263**: 18 205–18 212.

Snyder HW, Cochran SK, Balint JP *et al.* (1992) Experience with protein A immunoadsorption in treatment resistant adult immune thrombocytopenic purpura. *Blood* **79**: 1–6.

Stenberg PE, McEver RP, Shuman MA, Jacques YV, Bainton DF (1985) A platelet alpha-granule membrane protein (GMP-140) is expressed on the plasma membrane after activation. *J. Cell Biol.* **101**: 880–886.

Stoolman LM (1989) Adhesion molecules controlling lymphocyte migration. *Cell* **56**: 907–910.

Sutherland DR, Yeo E, Ryan A, Mills GB, Bailey D, Baker MA (1991) Identification of a cell-surface antigen associated with activated T lymphoblasts and activated platelets. *Blood* **77**: 84–93.

Szatkowski NS, Kunicki TJ, Aster RH (1986) Identification of glycoprotein Ib as a target for autoantibody in idiopathic thrombocytopenic purpura. *Blood* **67**: 310–315.

Taaning E, Antonsen H, Petersen S, Svejgaard A, Thompson M (1983) HLA antigens and maternal antibodies in allo-immune neonatal thrombocytopenia. *Tissue Antigens* **21**: 351–359.

Tomer A, Harker LA, Burstein SA (1988) Flow cytometric analysis of normal human megakaryocytes. *Blood* **71**: 1244–1252.

Tomiyama Y, Kurata Y, Mizutani H *et al.* (1987) Platelet glycoprotein IIb as a target antigen in two patients with chronic idiopathic thrombocytopenic purpura. *Br. J. Haematol.* **66**: 535–538.

Trowbridge EA, Slater DN, Kishk YT, Woodcock BW, Martin JF (1984) Platelet production in myocardial infarction and sudden cardiac death. *Thromb. Haemost.* **52**: 167–171.

Tschöpe D, Rösen P, Schwippert B *et al.* (1990) Platelet analysis using flow cytometric procedures. *Platelets* **1**: 127–133.

Tschöpe D, Rösen P, Esser J *et al.* (1991) Large platelets circulate in an activated state in diabetes mellitus. *Semin. Thromb. Haemost.* **17**: 433–438.

Tsien RY, Pozzan T, Rink TJ (1982) Calcium homeostasis in intact lymphocytes: cytoplasmic free calcium monitored with a new, intracellularly trapped fluorescent indicator. *J. Biol. Chem.* **94**: 325–334.

van Leeuwen EF, van der Ven JThM, Engelfriet CP, von dem Borne AEGKr (1982) Specificity of autoantibodies in autoimmune thrombocytopenia. *Blood* **59**: 23–26.

Varon D, Karpatkin S (1983) A monoclonal anti-platelet antibody with decreased reactivity for autoimmune thrombocytopenic platelets. *Proc. Natl Acad. Sci. USA* **80**: 6996–6995.

Veys PA, Gutteridge CN, Macey MG, Ord J, Newland AC (1987) The detection of granulocyte antibodies using flow cytometric analysis of leukocyte immunofluorescence. *Vox Sang.* **56**: 42–47.

von dem Borne AEGKr, Decary F (1990) ICSH/ISBT working party on platelet serology: Nomenclature of platelet specific antigens. *Vox Sang.* **58**: 176.

von dem Borne AEGKr, Helmerhorst FM, van Leeuwen EF, Pegels HG, von Riesz E, Engelfriet CP (1980) Autoimmune thrombocytopenia; detection of platelet autoantibodies with a suspension immunofluorescence test. *Br. J. Haematol.* **45**: 319–327.

von dem Borne AEGKr, Vos JJE, van der Lelie J, Bossers B, van Dalen CM (1986) Clinical significance of positive platelet immunofluorescence test in thrombocytopenia. *Br. J. Haematol.* **64**: 767–776.

Warkentin TE, Powling MJ, Hardisty RM (1990) Measurement of fibrinogen binding to platelets in whole blood by flow cytometry: a micromethod for the detection of platelet activation. *Br. J. Haematol.* **76**: 387–394.

Warkentin TE, Santos AV, Hayward CPM, Boshkov LK, Kelton JG (1992) Heparin- but not quinine/quinidine-induced thrombocytopenia sera produce procoagulant platelet-derived microparticles: an explanation for the differing clinical syndromes. *Br. J. Haematol.* **18**.

Wehmeier A, Tschöpe D, Esser J, Menzel C, Nieuwenhuis HK, Schneider W (1991) Circulating activated platelets in myeloproliferative disorders. *Thromb. Res.* **61**: 271–278.

Wencel-Drake JD, Plow EF, Kunicki TJ, Woods VL, Keller DM, Ginsberg MH (1986) Localization of internal pools of membrane glycoproteins involved in platelet adhesive responses. *Am. J. Pathol.* **124**: 324–334.

Wenche JY, Horstman LL, Arce M, Ahn YS (1992) Clinical significance of platelet microparticles in autoimmune thrombocytopenias. *J. Lab. Clin. Med.* **119**: 334–345.

Woods VL, Kurata Y, Montgomery RR *et al.* (1984a) Autoantibodies against platelet glycoproteins Ib in patients with chronic immune thrombocytopenic purpura. *Blood* **64**: 156–160.

Woods VL, Mason D, McMillan R (1984b) Autoantibodies against platelet glycoproteins IIb/IIIa complex in patients with chronic ITP. *Blood* **63**: 368–375.

Woods VL, Wolff LE, Keller DM (1986) Resting platelets contain a substantial centrally located pool of glycoprotein IIb-IIIa complex which may be accessible to some but not other extracellular proteins. *J. Biol. Chem.* **261**: 15 242–15 251.

Zamarron C, Ginsberg MH, Plow EF (1989) Receptor induced binding sites (RIBS) are exposed in fibrinogen as a consequence of its interaction with platelets. *Blood* **74** (Suppl. 1): 208a (Abstr.).

Zamarron C, Ginsberg MH, Plow EF (1990) Monoclonal antibodies specific for a conformationally altered state of fibrinogen. *Thromb. Haemost.* **64**: 41–46.

Chapter 7
Red Cells and Reticulocytes

T. HOY

Introduction

Flow cytometry has been accepted in the routine haematology laboratory as an efficient means of counting blood cells since the introduction of electronic counters in the 1950s. These have developed into sophisticated instruments performing automatic differential counts. More recently the introduction of laser powered, multiparameter instruments has resulted in many haematology laboratories performing immunopheno-typing using this technology. Although it is commonly understood that one of the major advantages of flow cytometry is the ability to analyse large numbers of cells on a discrete basis, some implications of this aspect may not have been fully appreciated. It offers a means of quantifying minor subpopulations of cells to a degree that has been unobtainable by manual techniques. In the research environment many assays have been adapted for flow cytometry; however, the feasibility of transferring these assays to the routine laboratory has awaited the appearance of 'user friendly' flow cytometers. Now that many routine laboratories possess such a flow cytometer for immunophenotyping, the possibility of conducting other assays by flow has become a practicality.

This chapter covers developments in the field of red cells where some flow cytometric assays are now accepted as the method of choice and others have demonstrated considerable potential in terms of accuracy when compared with manual methods. It is not the intention to suggest that flow is always the method of choice but where accuracy is a prime requirement it should be considered if a suitable cytometer is available.

The majority of topics covered in this chapter have one feature in common in that they are concerned with estimating minor subpopulations of cells. It is therefore worthwhile considering the statistics of this process separately.

Accurate enumeration of minor populations: Poisson statistics

In the process of flow cytometry, particles (events) arrive at the point of analysis at random and their distribution will therefore be described by Poisson statistics. Any subset of cells will also be distributed at random within the parent population and we can consider the statistics of these separately. The essential feature of Poisson distributions is that if n events are observed the standard deviation (s.d.) associated with that count is $\sqrt{n}$. The coefficient of variation (CV) is then given by

$$CV = 100 \times s.d./n \text{ or } 100/\sqrt{n}$$

Two features are obvious. First, if a subset smaller by a factor of S is investigated the total number of events processed must be increased by a factor of S to maintain the same precision; and second, to improve precision by a factor P the number of rare events recorded, and hence the total number of events, must be increased by a factor of P^2.

It is common practice in flow cytometry to collect data on 10 000 events. If a subpopulation exists at the 10% level 1000 of these would be observed with an associated CV of 3.16%, which would be acceptable for many experiments. However, at the 1% level only 100 cells would be expected with a CV of 10% resulting in a dramatic drop in precision. The only solution to this is to count more cells and it is useful to construct a reference chart as shown in Table 7.1 for estimating how many total events to process for a required precision. For practical reasons the table terminates at a total count of 10^7 events, which represents about 20 min per sample at 10 000 events per second. It is limited to a frequency of 1 in 100 000, beyond which only rough estimates can be obtained even after collecting 10^7 events. Naturally, the subset has to be well resolved if these theoretical levels are to be approached. The golden rule for rare event analysis is quite simple, accuracy is determined by the number of rare cells examined.

The enumeration of reticulocytes in peripheral blood

The application of flow cytometric assays to estimate reticulocytes in

Table 7.1 Statistics of rare event analysis (Poisson distribution)

Total events collected	True distribution of rare events			
	1 : 100	1 : 1000	1 : 10 000	1 : 100 000
	EC (CV %)	EC (CV %)	EC (CV %)	EC (CV %)
10^4	100 (10)	10 (32)	1?	—
10^5	1000 (3.2)	100 (10)	10 (32)	1?
10^6	10^4 (1)	1000 (3.2)	100 (10)	10 (32)
10^7	10^5 (0.1)	10^4 (1)	1000 (3.2)	100 (10)

EC, expected count

peripheral blood can be used to illustrate several important considerations, which must be made when transposing assays from one system
to another. Traditionally reticulocytes have been defined by the appearance of stained RNA as reticulum on microscopic examination. This
leads to an immediate problem: all flow cytometric techniques measure
either an integrated or peak signal derived from the total RNA content
of each cell. Obviously, small amounts of highly dispersed RNA could
be detected that would not be apparent as reticulum on visual examination. There are two solutions to this problem: first, to correlate flow
cytometric assays with manual methods; and second, to redefine the
reticulocyte as measured by flow cytometry. No doubt there will be
consideration for the latter as more laboratories adopt flow for this
measurement. Most laboratories attempting to correlate the two methods
have appreciated the inherent weakness of manual reticulocyte count,
i.e. the lack of accuracy associated with the tedious process of counting
as many as 1000 cells. A normal reticulocyte count in the range 0.6–
2.7% of the red cell count makes the estimation one of rare event
analysis. Only six to 30 positive cells would be expected if 1000 cells
were counted with errors approaching 50% at the lower end of the
range. Obviously flow cytometry is ideally suited to counting large
numbers of cells to improve the accuracy of results; however, the
inherent lack of accuracy of the manual method prohibits any serious
attempt at correlating the results.

It is interesting to trace the development of fluorochromes used to
detect the RNA present in red cells. Retrospectively this appears to be
an attempt to find a compound that clearly discriminates between
reticulocytes and mature red cells, which in many respects has been
an impossible task. The RNA that defines reticulocytes is gradually
degraded so no clear demarcation would be expected. The initial
attempts were made by Tanke *et al.* (1980) using pyronin Y which had
the disadvantages of a lengthy fixation stage and very poor discrimination
of positive cells. Tanke *et al.* introduced a mathematical Gaussian fit to
the low fluorescence cells and deduced a reticulocyte count from cells
not accounted for by this fit at higher levels of fluorescence. Since
reticulocyte RNA content is inversely related to maturity, quantifying
the amount of RNA gives a measure of the age distribution of reticulocytes. Tanke *et al.* (1983) attempted this by another mathematical procedure applied to pyronin Y fluorescence. Staining RNA with acridine
orange avoids the lengthy fixation stage, but unfortunately this also
results in high background fluorescence from mature red cells, making
discrimination difficult. This method was eventually optimized by
Schmitz and Werner (1986). They addressed the critical issue of discriminating between reticulocytes and erythrocytes and concluded that
this was only possible after logarithmic amplification of the fluorescent
signal, Tanke *et al.*'s methods having utilized linear amplification. Fixation was avoided as this was known to produce autofluorescence
(Tanke *et al.*, 1980). They also found the concentration of acridine
orange very important and optimal at 0.5 mg/l in unbuffered 0.15 mol/l

NaCl; below this not all reticulocytes were counted and at higher concentrations the discrimination was impaired. With hindsight this might have been expected; 'reticulocytes' with lower RNA content than those detected by the traditional methods were probably being detected. RNA fluorochromes, unlike pyronin Y and acridine orange which are fluorescent stains, increase their fluorescence on binding to RNA and therefore have inherently lower background fluorescence. The first of these to be used for reticulocyte analysis was thioflavin T (Sage *et al.*, 1983). Fluorescence histograms were produced that gave a reasonable discrimination between red cells and reticulocytes without mathematical deconvolution. Phillips *et al.* (1988) utilized this feature to flow sort pure reticulocytes from very small samples of neonatal blood; they then estimated haemoglobin F in these cells in a study designed to investigate the rate of switch-over to adult erythropoiesis. Thioflavin T has some major disadvantages for routine use; the fluorescence is sensitive to both temperature and time and requires excitation at 457 nm, a wavelength not available on benchtop flow cytometers. This was solved by the introduction of thiazole orange (Lee *et al.*, 1986) and being less sensitive to temperature and time it rapidly became the fluorochrome of choice for staining reticulocytes. Its fluorescence increases by a factor of 3000 on binding to RNA, which implies a high signal-to-noise ratio and a reliable reticulocyte count and maturity index can be derived from a comparison with unstained cells (Davis and Bigelow, 1989).

All the methods above could be applied to any commercial flow cytometer with a suitable laser and analytical filters. Thiazole orange (Molecular Probes) can be prepared as a stock solution at a concentration of 1 mg/ml in methanol and stored at 5°C for long periods. Working solutions, prepared by diluting the stock 1 in 10 000 in phosphate-buffered saline (PBS) with 0.002 mol/l EDTA and 0.02% sodium azide, are stable for 1 week if kept in the dark at room temperature. Whole blood (5 μl EDTA or heparin anticoagulated) is mixed with 1 ml working solution and incubated at a fixed temperature for up to 100 min before analysis. An isometric plot of fluorescence *vs* forward scatter for a blood sample stained in this way is illustrated in Fig. 7.1. The reticulocyte count was 1.5% and the continuum of fluorescence from the reticulocytes into the mature erythrocytes is apparent.

There is good evidence that the staining varies with time and temperature of incubation (Bowen *et al.*, 1991) and they should be standardized within the laboratory if accurate, reproducible counts are required. No significant changes were found in blood samples stored for up to 48 hours at 4°C, but storage at room temperature resulted in increased counts over a period of 4 days.

In 1989 a flow cytometer dedicated to measuring reticulocytes, the Sysmex R-1000 (Sysmex-TOA Electronics Company, Kobe, Japan), was introduced. This utilizes another fluorochrome, auramine O, which reacts rapidly with RNA and produces reticulocyte counts in approximately 1 min from a 100 μl sample of well-mixed, EDTA anticoagulated whole blood. This represents a considerable time saving over other

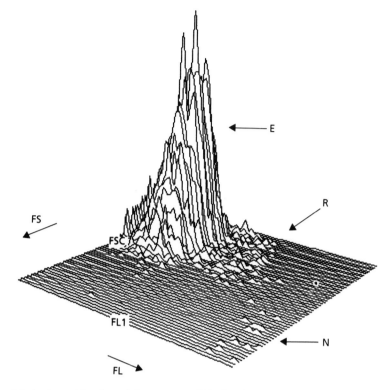

Fig. 7.1 An isometric view of fluorescence (FL) after logarithmic amplification *vs* forward scatter (FS) for a blood sample with a reticulocyte count of 1.5% stained with thiazole orange. Three regions are apparent: mature erythrocytes (E), reticulocytes (R) and highly fluorescent nucleated cells (N). The cells in region N comprised 0.2% of the total.

methods and effectively gives real-time reticulocyte counts. Blood can be stored for up to 4 days at 4°C with no effect on the auramine O reticulocyte count, but at room temperature a small but significant fall during the first 24 hours was apparent before stability was reached (Bowen *et al.*, 1991).

Table 7.2 gives a selection of the more important dyes and fluorochromes used for RNA detection in reticulocytes. As these fluorochromes have been introduced, software has also developed to derive reticulocyte counts and indices of maturity. Perhaps the best known of these is Reticount (Becton Dickinson), which is fully automatic and based on a

Table 7.2 Dyes commonly used for RNA detection

Compound	Absorption maximum	Laser line	Emission maximum	Comments
Acridine orange	492	488	530–640	Metachromic 530 = DNA 640 = RNA
Pyronin Y	545	515	565	Requires fixation
Thioflavin T	422	457	487	Relatively sensitive to time
Thiazole orange	509	488	533	Currently the favoured fluorochrome
Auramine O	460	488	550	Used on the Sysmex R-1000

thiazole orange method. This highlights another problem: given that two assays collect information on sufficient cells to obtain accurate counts (50 000 for 5% CVs at the lower end of the normal range) the effective definition of a reticulocyte is probably different. We would then expect a correlation significant at the 0.05 level but with a correlation coefficient not necessarily unity. It is not always common practice to give this information in publications either commercial or scientific which makes quality control difficult. As an illustration Fig. 7.2 presents the data of Bowen et al. (1991) where the thiazole orange technique was compared with results from a Sysmex R-1000. In the former assay reticulocytes were defined by a marker set to give at 0.3% cells positive on an unstained sample; in the latter a definition is not supplied by the manufacturer. A correlation of 0.805 existed with $P < 0.01$. The same problem of lack of uniformity exists with various methods of calculating the maturity index. The Sysmex software divides the fluorescence scale into three levels and gives the percentage reticulocytes in each, Bowen et al. (1991) calculated the mean fluorescence of the top 10% of the reticulocytes, and Davis and Bigelow (1989) calculated the mean fluorescence intensity of cells above the 99.9% level measured with unstained blood.

Two problems encountered with measuring reticulocytes by flow cytometry are eliminating unwanted cells (platelets and leucocytes) and interference from red cells containing DNA (Howell—Jolly bodies and parasites). Careful attention to gating can eliminate most of these problems (Agrawal and Pentillä, 1992). Nobes and Carter (1990) suggest that Howell—Jolly bodies do not represent a problem at the frequency at which they normally occur and that results are not affected by low red cell counts, high platelet counts or high leucocyte counts. Makler et al. (1987) demonstrate that thiazole orange fluorescence binding to DNA in malarial parasites is easily resolved from the staining associated with

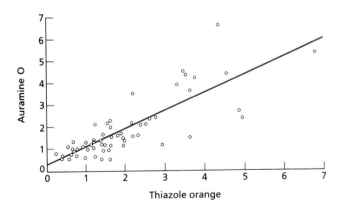

Fig. 7.2 Reticulocyte counts for 59 independent samples showing the good correlation ($r = 0.805$, $P < 0.01$) between thiazole orange and auramine methods when sufficient cells are analysed (100 000). The inherent discrepancy of some 16% results from methodological and analytical variations.

reticulocyte RNA. Conversely, red cells infected with parasites could presumably be gated out from a reticulocyte count.

Accurate determination of reticulocyte numbers has stimulated considerable interest in the field of erythropoietic activity. In the areas of bone marrow transplantation (BMT) Davis *et al.* (1989) have demonstrated that their reticulocyte maturity index calculated from the thiazole orange method is often one of the earliest indicators of engraftment. Davies *et al.* (1992) presented similar findings using the high fluorescence reticulocytes as measured by the Sysmex R-1000 to monitor erythroid activity during the engraftment process following allogeneic and autologous BMT. In both situations increased numbers of highly fluorescent reticulocytes preceded increased counts in both reticulocytes and neutrophils by several days. Graft-*vs*-host disease resulted in a slight transient fall in reticulocyte count but neither infection nor transfusion significantly affected reticulocytes or the highly fluorescent population. A typical response of reticulocytes and neutrophils to BMT is shown in Fig. 7.3.

Detection of malarial parasites

Many DNA fluorochromes have been investigated for detecting the presence of malarial parasites in red blood cells. As early as 1979

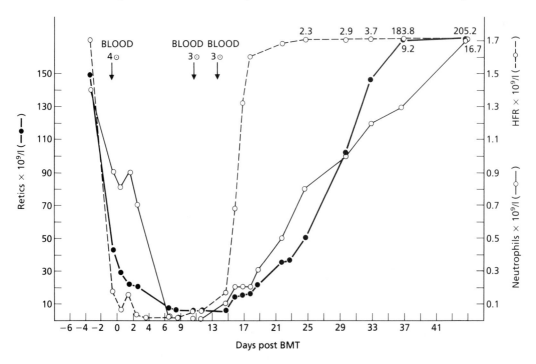

Fig. 7.3 Variations in reticulocyte and neutrophil counts during BMT. Absolute reticulocyte counts and highly fluorescent reticulocytes (HFR) were measured on a Sysmex R-1000. The importance of measuring immature reticulocytes (HFR) as an early indicator of changing marrow activity is apparent. Reproduced with permission from data supplied by Dr. S. Davies.

Howard *et al.* were sorting infected cells stained with Hoechst 33258. This, and some other stains represent a problem for cytometers lacking UV excitation but the RNA fluorochrome used for reticulocyte studies (thiazole orange) may be utilized as it was shown to be independent of the presence of antimalarial drugs (Makler *et al.*, 1987). Approximately 10 million red blood cells are simply suspended in 1 ml PBS pH 7.0 containing 10 µl (10^{-5} mol/l) thiazole orange and incubated in the dark for 15 min at room temperature. Either 0.25% glutaraldehyde or 1% paraformaldehyde can be included in the PBS to fix the erythrocytes with no significant changes to the staining. The parasitized cells are easily resolved from weakly staining reticulocytes.

A recent study by Pattanapanyasat *et al.* (1992) used propidium iodide to stain fixed red blood cells for DNA content in the presence of an immunofluorescent label for the complement regulatory decay accelerating factor (DAF). After normal immunofluorescence procedures were used to stain for various DAF surface antigens the cells were fixed with 0.5% paraformaldehyde for 2 hours at room temperature. This enabled clear discrimination between different stages of the parasite in asynchronous cultures and as discussed earlier, under these conditions, accurate determination of numbers of infected cells can be made if sufficient data are collected. Alterations of membrane proteins in association with invasion and maturation of parasites should be possible using this bivariate technique. Using 0.025% glutaraldehyde fixation followed by treatment with 1% Saponin (Sigma) to permeabilize erythrocytes, Pattanapanyasat *et al.* (1993) were able to detect a parasite-dependent surface antigen (Pf155/RESA) in conjunction with DNA. The antigen (ring-infected erythrocyte surface antigen) was detected by indirect immunofluorescence using human antimalaria antibody (33G2); this reacted weakly with cells containing only schizonts and strongly with ring-infected cells. This antibody in association with DNA staining provides a simple flow cytometric method for determining parasite content and surface density of parasite-associated membrane antigen.

In a study on cattle by Wyatt *et al.* (1991) protozoan haemoparasites present in erythrocytes were observed to convert hydroethidine to fluorescent ethidium. In this way they were able to distinguish between infected, uninfected and erythrocytes containing dead parasites using *Babesia bovis*.

Paroxysmal nocturnal haemoglobinuria (PNH)

In the previous section Pattanapanyasat *et al.* (1992) investigated DAF in association with malarial parasites. A considerable number of publications on DAF and related proteins have resulted from the study of PNH. In this disease erythrocytes and other peripheral blood cells have defects that result in abnormal sensitivity to complement-mediated lysis. A common feature of surface proteins found to be deficient on PNH blood cells is that they are linked to the membrane by a glycosyl-phosphatydylinositol (GPI) anchor. These include DAF or CD55, homologous restriction factor (HRF), membrane inhibitor of reactive lysis (MIRL or CD59), lymphocyte function-associated antigen-3 (LFA-3 or CD58) and acetylcholine-esterase (ACE). As components of the cell surface these proteins are accessible for quantitative and qualitative study by flow cytometry. In an early study Kinoshita *et al*. (1985) demonstrated on normal erythrocytes that although the total amount of DAF was fairly constant the antigen density in any individual ranged over an order of magnitude. This distribution was attributed to hetero-geneity in precursors and/or secondary changes related to red cell ageing. The latter suggestion was confirmed by density gradient frac-tionation showing mean amounts of DAF to be lower on the older, denser erythrocytes. This provides a potential mechanism for the prefer-ential removal of senescent red cells from the circulation by the reticulo-endothelial system, supporting the idea that DAF prevents damage to autologous cells by complement.

Kinoshita *et al*. (1985) were the first to demonstrate the simultaneous existence of DAF-positive and DAF-negative cells in PNH with widely different patterns between individuals. In some patients the abnormal cells were restricted to erythroid, myeloid and megakaryocytic lineages, while in others lymphocytes were involved, giving rise to the idea that PNH cells were of monoclonal origin from a lesion that could occur at different stages of haemopoietic differentiation. Moore *et al*. (1985) flow sorted progenitor cells from PNH patients and conducted clonogenic assays. They were only successful in growing erythroid colonies from DAF$^+$ cells, but a proportion of their progeny acquired the DAF$^-$ phenotype. Ueda *et al*. (1990) used dual fluorescence to examine expression of ACE and DAF and present evidence of ACE$^+$DAF$^-$ cells in PNH. ACE is lost in parallel with LFA-3 as the erythrocytes mature, supporting the hypothesis that this is a common feature of proteins anchored by GPI.

In a larger series of experiments Rosse *et al*. (1991) addressed the problem of erythrocytes with intermediate sensitivity to complement lysis using two-colour immunofluorescence to study DAF, MIRL and ACE. Changes in all three proteins took place in parallel and were inversely proportional to the cells' sensitivity to complement lysis. Plesner *et al*. (1990) made use of calibration beads to standardize measurements of ACE, DAF and LFA-3 in terms of protein molecules per cell. They included samples from normals and patients with PNH, 'non-PNH' haemolytic anaemias and aplastic anaemia. Erythrocytes were diluted 1:100 in 50 µl isotonic PBS containing 10 mmol/l sodium azide 1 g/l bovine serum albumin and labelled with 50 µl of carefully titrated antibody for 30 min at 4°C before washing and labelling with fluorescein isothiocyanate (FITC)-conjugated rabbit anti-mouse immuno-globulin. They comment on the normal findings for one PNH patient with a negative Ham's test suggesting this could result from selective loss of severely affected erythrocytes and highlighting the importance of also studying leucocytes when PNH is suspected. The influence of storage on results with granulocytes and lymphocytes was considerable (increases of up to 120% in a few hours); however, no data were given for erythroid cells.

The association of PNH with aplastic anaemia is well known. Wanachiwanawin and Pattanapanyasat (1991) have studied 20 aplastic anaemia patients; 18 had only DAF$^+$ erythrocytes but two had significant populations of DAF$^-$ cells just before and during haematological recovery without any clinical evidence of haemolysis.

Direct antiglobulin technique

Many of the serological procedures used in immunohaematology have traditionally relied on the presence of visible agglutination as a method of detection. Such methods are not suitable for quantifying amounts of antigen present or detecting minor subpopulations of cells. Flow cytometry is ideally suited to overcome these limitations but it is essential that agglutination is avoided, which implies that many antibodies developed for agglutination assays are unsuitable. However, many new non-agglutinating antibodies have been developed and methods are available for pre-fixing erythrocytes to prevent agglutination taking place (Langlois *et al.*, 1985).

Preparation of erythrocytes for storage

1 Dimethylsuberimidate (DMS) can be used to fix cells after careful washing in Alsever's solution (30 mmol/l Na citrate pH 6.1, 0.07 mol/l NaCl, 0.11 mol/l dextrose).
2 The final cell pellet is resuspended in 10 volumes of 0.1 mol/l Na carbonate, pH 10.3, 0.15 mol/l NaCl, 0.1 mmol/l EDTA with 3 mg/ml DMS at 37°C for 20 min.
3 After further washing three times, the fixed cells can be stored in PBS containing 5 mg/ml lysine and 1.5 mmol/l sodium azide.

A method of producing spheres by Formalin fixation based on that described by Kim and Ornstein (1983) is given and this has subsequently been refined for use in the glycophorin A somatic mutation assay (Langlois *et al.*, 1990). Sphered, fixed erythrocytes have the advantage of producing a uniform scatter profile when examined by flow cytometry as the effects of preferential orientation in the stream are eliminated.

Sphering and fixing erythrocytes

1 At room temperature 0.1 ml of whole blood is added to 1.0 ml of Isolyte S (Kendall McGraw Laboratories, Irvine, CA, USA) containing 50 µg/ml sodium dodecyl sulphate (SDS) and 1 mg/ml bovine serum albumin.

Continued on p. 202

2 After 1 min this is mixed with 9.7 ml of Isolyte S, 0.3 ml of 37% formaldehyde (Formalin), and 10 µg/ml SDS.
3 After 1.5 hours an additional 0.8 ml of Formalin is added and the mixture fixed overnight.
4 The fixed cells are washed twice and preserved in 10 mmol/l sodium phosphate buffer (pH 7.2) containing 0.15 mol/l NaCl, 5 mg/ml BSA, 0.01% Nonidet P-40 (Sigma), and 100 µg/ml sodium azide, after which they can be stored at 4°C for several weeks with minimal effects on antibody binding.

One of the early objectives was to investigate the relationship of *in vivo* haemolysis in autoimmune haemolytic anaemias and levels of IgG bound to red cells. Quantifying IgG by flow cytometry was first attempted by van der Meulen *et al.* (1980) for red cells sensitized with IgG1 auto-antibodies. Although they claimed to demonstrate a level of IgG above which haemolysis would occur, this claim was refuted by Nance and Garratty (1984) and Garratty and Nance (1990). They concluded that for several groups of patients, mean levels of bound auto-antibodies were always higher in those with haemolysis but no clear discriminant was present for the prediction of haemolysis. The flow cytometric test is, however, seen as a simple, reliable, sensitive and reproducible method for the detection of labelled cells (Nance and Garratty, 1987). Red cells sensitized with IgG, IgM and IgA either *in vivo* or *in vitro* are simply incubated at room temperature for 30 min with fluorescent conjugates of anti-IgG, anti-IgM and IgA added in excess. Methods of preparing the sensitized cells *in vitro* are described in Nance and Garratty (1987) and Petz and Garratty (1980). The question of why quantifying auto-antibody is not a predictable index of the severity of haemolysis, is addressed by Chaplin (1990) in terms of the complexity of pathological processes involved in intravascular and extravascular haemolysis.

Several other areas which could be strictly classified as immuno-haematology can be covered individually as independent topics.

Studies on blood group determinants

Blood group-active surface molecules of erythrocytes are reviewed by Anstee (1990). He considers about 20 polypeptides whose abundance varies from 3000 to 1×10^6 copies per cell. Assuming suitable antibodies are available these densities are amenable to flow cytometric studies. Anstee considers minor components below 1.2×10^4 copies per cell to include antigens relating to Fy, Kell, LW, In^a/In^b, Cromer and Lutheran, while the major components are those responsible for ABH, Ii, MN, Ss, Rh and Ge. Of these glycophorin A and the anion transport protein (band 3) are the most abundant glycoproteins on the erythrocyte surface.

Application of flow cytometric methods to study the red cell membrane protein, glycophorin, can serve to illustrate three features.

1   The detection limits that can be achieved with well-resolved populations of rare cells.

2   Survival studies of transfused red cells.

3   The detection of haemopoietic chimeras following BMT.

There are two allelic forms of glycophorin A gene which result in proteins determining the MN blood groups; hence, the genotype of the precursor is reflected in the phenotype of the resulting erythrocyte. Monoclonal antibodies extremely specific for the M and N forms of human glycophorin A were first described by Bigbee *et al.* (1983). They suggested that the greater reliability compared with conventional rabbit polyclonal sera would lead to several potential applications. The combination of specificity, high numbers of glycophorin molecules present on a red cell (approximately 10^6) and the consistency of expression from one individual to another (variations within 10%) resulted in the development of a somatic mutation assay sensitive to a few variant cells per million.

As the difference between the M and N forms is restricted to two amino acids close to the amino terminus of the protein point mutations can result in a molecule that is not recognized by the antibodies or a transformation from one form to the other. Approximately 50% of the population are heterozygous and have equal amounts of M and N glycophorin on each red cell; for these individuals NO and NN mutants can be detected reliably in the ranges 3–13 and 3–34 per million (Langlois *et al.*, 1990).

Staining erythrocytes for the glycophorin assay

1   A 0.15 ml aliquot of cells that have been sphered and fixed (the method has been outlined earlier) are washed and resuspended in staining buffer.

2   These are immunolabelled simultaneously with antibodies specific to the M form (6A7: purified and conjugated with biotin) and the N form (BRIC157: purified and conjugated with FITC) for 1 hour at room temperature with continuous agitation.

3   After two washes the cells are suspended and incubated with streptavadin–phycoerythrin for a further hour.

4   After two washes cells are resuspended in 1 ml of staining buffer containing 10 µg/ml propidium iodide and finally filtered through a 37 µm nylon mesh to give a final concentration of about 8×10^7 cells/ml.

Figure 7.4 was derived from a mixture of unlabelled and stained cells from an individual of the MN blood group. The superior resolution in detecting the M epitope is apparent; essentially this is why NO and NN mutants can be detected in an MN individual but not the MO and MM mutants as these will be much closer to the parent MN peak.

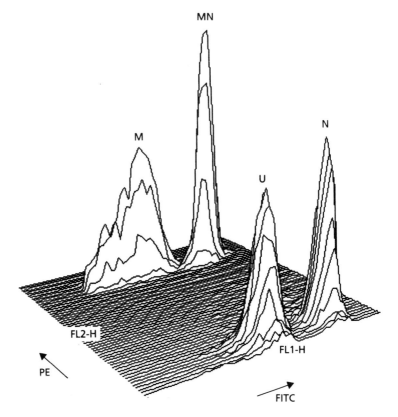

Fig. 7.4 An isometric display of fluorescence after logarithmic amplification for a composite mixture of cells from a heterozygous MN individual. The four peaks are unlabelled cells (U), and cells labelled with anti-N-FITC (N), anti-M-biotin-streptavadin-PE (M), and both anti-N and anti-M (MN). The positions of peak (N) allows the gating of NO variants when a pure MN sample is run in isolation.

In Table 7.1 it can be seen that even after collecting as many as 10^6 events the 10 or so rare events recorded will have an associated CV of the order of 32%. Langlois *et al*. (1990) collected replicate data on 5×10^6 cells and compared the observed CVs with those derived from such a table. They quote figures of 30 and 19 for observed CVs of NO and NN mutants and 18 and 15 as the theoretical values predicted for a Poisson distribution, demonstrating the usefulness of this approach.

Increased levels have been detected in patients who have received cytotoxic therapy (Bigbee *et al*., 1990), patients with ataxia telangiectasia (a defective DNA repair mechanism; Bigbee *et al*., 1989) and atomic bomb survivors (Langlois *et al*., 1987). It seems reasonable to assume that the mutations can occur at the stem cell level since levels related to predicted exposure are reported for atomic bomb survivors after an interval of 40 years (Kyoizumi *et al*., 1989). This is not necessarily always the case since Hewitt and Mott (1992) report levels returning to normal with time in children treated with cytotoxic drugs for leukaemia implying that cells less able to self-replicate, i.e. more differentiated than stem cells, have been mutated. Justification of this sensitive assay

Table 7.3 Recovery of homozygous NN cells seeded into a heterozygous MN sample. Results per million cells

NN cells seeded	NN cells observed	Excess
0	11	—
29	38	27
72	109	98
145	186	175
720	859	848

No significant differences exist between numbers seeded and excess.

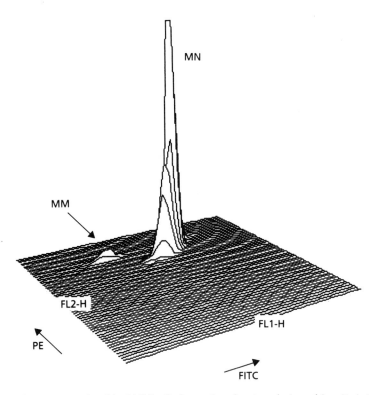

Fig. 7.5 Appearance of residual MM cells 3 months after transfusion of 3 units into a heterozygous MN recipient. Note the increased phycoerythrin fluorescence resulting from the doubling of the M component; 3.3% MM cells were present in this sample.

can be assessed from recovery experiments where cells from an homozygous NN individual are seeded in low numbers into those from a heterozygous MN sample. A sample of such recovery data is presented in Table 7.3.

An assay based on this methodology could obviously be used to monitor survival of transfused cells in the situation of an MN mismatch. An example of a heterozygous (MN) individual previously transfused with three units of homozygous MM cells is shown in Fig. 7.5; the sample was taken approximately 3 months after transfusion and some remaining MM cells are still present.

Pallavicini *et al.* (1992) have utilized this assay to quantify cells in intra- and interspecies haemopoietic chimeras with a reported sensitivity of 1 in 100 000. This compared favourably with DNA-based detection (1 in 10 000) and flow cytometric detection of nucleated leucocytes (1 in 1000). The comparisons given provide a useful guide to the methodologies for assessment of chimerism following transplantation. Presumably other combinations of antigens and antibodies providing similar discrimination could be substituted.

Whereas the glycophorins are fairly uniformly distributed in terms of surface density the ABO phenotype is determined by enzymes modifying a precursor oligosaccharide. Since these enzymes are coded for by allelic genes their abundance will depend on the zygosity of the individual and be reflected in final amounts of detectable A, B and H antigens. Sharon and Fibach (1991) have used dual labelling to investigate quantitative changes in these antigens and found the ratio of A/H or B/H to be a clear discriminator. Homozygotes (A or B) had ratios of more than 200 whereas heterozygotes (AO or BO) had ratios less than 5. The method was also able to distinguish between the A_1 and A_2 phenotypes. The power of flow cytometry over standard agglutination methods for determining zygosity has been recognized for many years (Nance, 1988) and in the case of anti-Fy^a clear discrimination was obtained by the former. This methodology has been applied to cases of disputed paternity using quantitative measurements of several antigens. Hasekura *et al.* (1990) have made quantitative measurements of the D antigen as presented by the rhesus phenotypes and were able to distinguish the rare variants D^u and D_{el} and correlate these findings with genetic studies on transmission of the gene.

Detection of transfused blood: survival studies

Under favourable conditions of an antigen mismatch between donor and recipient cells for which suitable antibodies are available, flow cytometry can be used to study the survival of transfused blood as demonstrated in Fig. 7.5. Given good resolution between the fluorescence of positive and negative cells it is immaterial whether the donor or recipient's cells are labelled. The detection limit under these conditions as we have discussed elsewhere is simply a matter of the number of cells analysed.

The transfusion of autologous red cells labelled with a suitable probe has also proved useful for the non-isotopic determination of total red cell volume (RCV). The ability of biotinylated erythrocytes to survive in animals was reported by Suzuki and Dale (1987), while the same principle was being used to develop a method for measuring the RCV in humans without the use of radio-isotopes (Cavill *et al.*, 1988).

The RCV assay

1 Preparation of the sample for transfusion must be performed under aseptic conditions.

2 For an adult, 16 ml of venous blood is collected into 4 ml acid citrate dextrose (ACD).

3 The cells are pelleted by gentle centrifugation and resuspended to 12 ml with NaCl BP.

4 Biotin in a water soluble form (NHS-LC-Biotin, Pierce Chemical Company, Rockford, IL, USA) is dissolved in NaCl to give a concentration of 0.3 pg biotin/red cell. This concentration is crucial; attempts to bind more biotin result in the rapid clearance of labelled cells by the reticulo-endothelial system.

5 After mixing for 5 min the cells are left at room temperature for 10 min before centrifuging and washing twice and resuspending in 12 ml NaCl.

6 After removing a small sample the remainder is reinjected; the weight of cells injected needs to be recorded with some precision.

7 Samples are taken from the patient after 10 min.

8 1×10^7 cells are taken from the control and both injected and test samples are diluted into 1 ml PBS.

9 To this 10 μl streptavadin—fluorescein (Amersham) is added for 30 min mixing every 10 min.

10 After washing twice the cells are resuspended in 0.5 ml PBS for flow cytometric analysis.

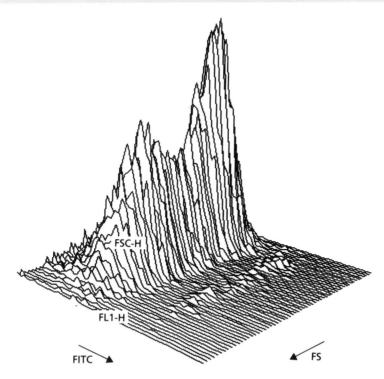

Fig. 7.6 Determination of total RCV. After logarithmic amplification of fluorescence (FITC) biotinylated cells labelled with streptavadin-FITC are clearly resolved from the unlabelled population. The bimodal distribution of forward scatter (FS) results from variations in the orientation of cells to the laser beam. In this sample 0.7% of the cells were labelled.

A small-scale version of this procedure suitable for use with neonates is described by Hudson *et al.* (1990). Dilutions of up to 1 in 1000 can be expected using this procedure and Table 7.1 can be used to establish that 10^6 cells must be examined to provide a precision of 3%. Using the above procedure, positive cells are well resolved from unlabelled cells (see Fig. 7.6 for an example). There is no difficulty in placing markers around the population of labelled cells. Cavill *et al.* (1988) found no significant differences when they compared the method with that recommended by the International Committee for Standardization in Haematology (1980). Several of the preterm infants studied by Hudson *et al.* (1990) required transfusion and the RCV as determined by the biotin method could be checked retrospectively by measuring the dilution of haemoglobin F post-transfusion. An excellent correlation was observed and the data are reproduced in Fig. 7.7. Samples obtained by this method are stable for several days after preparation (Hoy, 1990) avoiding the need for an on-site flow cytometer.

Evidence from samples collected to investigate changes in RCV during pregnancy (J Weiner, unpublished observations) showed that biotinylated cells were still detectable after several months. This indicates that the method may be applicable to red cell survival studies. Read *et al.* (1991) have conducted preliminary experiments with erythrocytes labelled with the fluorescent lipophilic membrane probe PKH-2 (Zynaxis Cell Science). Serial dilution experiments indicated that a sensitivity of 1 in 10 000 was attainable when analysing 50 000 cells. The labelled cells were reported to be 256 times brighter than those unlabelled, from Table 7.1 we could expect even greater sensitivity if more data were collected. Read *et al.* consider that the time taken to collect these data would be excessive; it appears from this, and many other publications, that whereas it is acceptable to spend many hours processing samples for flow cytometry, anything longer than a few seconds for the final acquisition of data is unacceptable! Cells labelled with PKH-2 appear to be stable for 1 month *in vitro* and the label does not interfere with ABO,

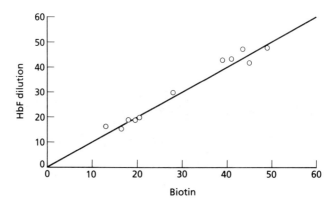

Fig. 7.7 Determination of total RCV in 11 neonates. Correlation between the biotin and haemoglobin F (HbF) dilution methods. There were no significant differences detectable by the ranked pair test ($P < 0.05$).

Rh(D) or common minor antigens. A possible problem might arise from
the echinocytotic appearance of the labelled cells resulting in osmotic
fragility; formal *in vivo* studies will be necessary to resolve whether this
approach is feasible.

Detection of fetal cells in maternal blood

Interest in this area falls into two categories: the first deals with detecting
red cells to elucidate fetal–maternal haemorrhage; and the second ident-
ifies nucleated cells for the purposes of prenatal diagnosis.

The first attempts to measure fetal–maternal haemorrhage by flow
cytometry were made in 1984 (Cupp *et al.*, 1984; Medearis *et al.*, 1984).
These methods were recognized as being more sensitive than standard
methods but required special apparatus and were too time consuming
to be considered. We have now reached the era when many routine
laboratories possess flow cytometers and the flow cytometric methods
have certain advantages in some cases. As already discussed for reticulocytes, analysing rare cells is difficult when they are poorly resolved
from the major population. Cupp *et al.* (1984) used fluorescent immuno-
spheres to maximize the resolution and were able to detect as few as
one cell per 100 000 but this involved lengthy data collection on the flow
cytometer; 5×10^7 events were required to detect one cell in 10^6 with

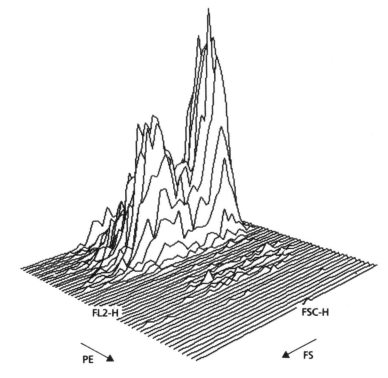

Fig. 7.8 Detection of D^+ cells in a population of D^- cells. Log fluorescence for the
phycoerythrin conjugate (PE) attached to the D^+ cells is shown against forward
scatter (FS); 0.9% of well-resolved D^+ cells are present in this sample.

reasonable accuracy. The underlying problem was one of overlapping background staining from D⁻ cells. As pointed out by Nance (1988) these accurate determinations may answer some basic questions about gestational age and amounts of fetal bleeds but are not necessary in assessment for treatment.

With the inevitable development of new antibodies some assays have benefited and this is a typical case. Patton *et al.* (1990) have reported a two-stage (indirect) immunofluorescent assay which clearly resolves positive from negative cells, they checked the assay to a level of 0.1% Rh(D)-positive cells, this level being adequately covered by a single dose of anti-D immunoglobulin. Figure 7.8 shows the effect of mixing 1% D^+ with D^- cells, incubating with anti-D for 30 min at 37°C, and labelled with goat anti-human-IgG-phycoerythrin. The positive cells are clearly resolved with a recovery of 90%. Results from a similar assay are reported by Bayliss *et al.* (1991) in comparison with the acid elution method (Kleihauer, 1957) and three non-quantitative methods. They conclude that the flow cytometry based method has the advantages of accuracy and reproducibility and offers an acceptable alternative in the clinical laboratory. The assay has been particularly useful for the situation of mothers with hereditary persistence of fetal haemoglobin (Patton *et al.*, 1990). Given the resolution of this assay it should be possible to detect levels as low as 1 in 100 000 with reasonable accuracy in a significantly shorter time than that required by the system described by Cupp *et al.* (1984).

Prenatal diagnosis using fetal cells in the maternal circulation has been an intriguing possibility since the presence of such cells was demonstrated (reviewed by Schroder, 1975). Soon after the introduction of modern flow cytometry this technology was used to investigate fetal leucocytes utilizing differences in HLA antigens between mother and father (Herzenberg *et al.*, 1979; Iverson *et al.*, 1981). The low frequency of these cells makes cytogenetic investigations impractical and early attempts were hampered by high rates of false results. Similar levels were reported using antibodies to detect trophoblasts (Covone *et al.*, 1984). In a subsequent paper Covone *et al.* (1988) reported that most cells bearing the antigen were in fact of maternal origin having simply absorbed the antigen from the serum. The impact of modern molecular biology has renewed the interest in identifying these cells.

Whereas leucocytes and trophoblasts are strictly outside the scope of this chapter, some recent studies have concentrated on nucleated erythrocytes (Bianchi *et al.*, 1990; P. Davies *et al.*, unpublished observations). The majority of fetal red cells are nucleated up to 10 weeks gestational age and considerably outnumber leucocytes, therefore representing a much bigger target for selection. Immunofluorescent labelling, using antibodies to the transferrin receptor, has been used to identify nucleated erythrocytes by Bianchi *et al.* (1990) who detected Y chromosomal material in 75% of male-bearing pregnancies. Transferrin receptors are also present on activated lymphocytes (Pattanapanyasat and Hoy, 1991). These cells can be eliminated by adding a second label identifying erythrocytes from leucocytes (e.g. anti-glycophorin or anti-CD45). The latter approach was used by Bianchi *et al.* (1991) to isolate cells containing Y chromosomal DNA at 10 weeks gestational age but these were no longer present at 20 weeks. This suggests that the nucleated erythrocyte approach is particularly suitable for studies in the early weeks of pregnancy. Some reticulocytes express transferrin receptors (Shumak and Rachkewich, 1984) and these can be excluded by selecting nucleated cells with a third fluorochrome directed against DNA. Preliminary experiments with maternal blood, after selecting mononuclear cells, removing lymphocytes by panning and triple labelling for transferrin receptor, glycophorin and DNA has resulted in very low numbers of positive cells that can be successfully sorted (P. Davies *et al.*, unpublished observations). Other assays have clearly demonstrated the potential of multiparameter flow cytometry for detecting cells at levels approaching one per million (see section on glycophorin mutation assay) and it is apparent that using this approach is more realistic for selecting fetal cells from maternal blood.

Summary

The bench-top flow cytometer is no longer considered as an expensive luxury in the routine haematology laboratory where it has become established as almost essential in the field of immunophenotyping. It is therefore expected that other assays will be adapted from research applications but this is often a lengthy process of justifying new methodologies against traditional techniques. In the field of enumerating reticulocytes it has taken approximately 10 years for a flow cytometric assay to be refined and become acceptable as an alternative in spite of the obvious improvement in accuracy relative to conventional microscopic methods. Many other assays in the haematology laboratory rely upon subjective, visual examinations which are notoriously difficult to quantitate, and those concerned with erythrocytes are no exception. Some pioneering assays have already demonstrated the advantages of flow cytometry in being able to quantitate measurements on a cell by cell basis at high speed. Given that the technology is also available in many clinical laboratories, no doubt the time involved in proving and accepting new assays will be considerably reduced.

Acknowledgement

The author is grateful to J. Fisher, H. Lake and P. Perera for providing data used for many of the figures.

References

Agrawal YP, Pentillä IM (1992) Reticulocyte analysis by flow cytometry using a modified gating procedure. *Eur. J. Haematol.* **48**: 58–60.
Anstee DJ (1990) Blood group-active surface molecules of the human red blood cell. *Vox Sang.* **58**: 1–20.

Bayliss KM, Kueck BD, Johnson ST *et al.* (1991) Detecting fetomaternal hemorrhage: a comparison of five methods. *Transfusion* **31**: 303–307.

Bianchi DW, Flint AF, Pizzimenti MF, Knoll JHM, Latt SA (1990) Isolation of fetal DNA from nucleated erythrocytes in maternal blood. *Proc. Natl Acad. Sci. USA* **87**: 3279–3283.

Bianchi DW, Stewart JE, Garber MF, Lucotte G, Flint AF (1991) Possible effect of gestational age on the detection of fetal nucleated erythrocytes in maternal blood. *Prenatal Diagn.* **11**: 523–528.

Bigbee WL, Vanderlaan M, Fong SSN, Jensen RH (1983) Monoclonal antibodies specific for the M- and N-forms of human glycophorin A. *Mol. Immunol.* **20**: 1353–1362.

Bigbee WL, Langlois RG, Swift M, Jensen RH (1989) Evidence for an elevated frequency of *in vivo* somatic cell mutations in ataxia telangiectasia. *Am. J. Hum. Genet.* **44**: 402–408.

Bigbee WL, Wyrobek AJ, Langlois RG, Jensen RH, Everson RB (1990) The effect of chemotherapy on the *in vivo* frequency of glycophorin A 'null' variant erythrocytes. *Mutat. Res.* **240**: 165–175.

Bowen D, Bentley N, Hoy T, Cavill I (1991) Comparison of a modified thiazole orange technique with a fully automated analyser for reticulocyte counting. *J. Clin. Pathol.* **44**: 130–133.

Cavill I, Trevett D, Fisher J, Hoy T (1988) The measurement of the total volume of red cells in man: a non-radioactive approach using biotin. *Br. J. Haematol.* **70**: 491–493.

Chaplin H (1990) Red cell-bound immunoglobulin as a predictor of severity of hemolysis in patients with autoimmune hemolytic anemia. *Transfusion* **30**: 576–577.

Covone AE, Mutton D, Johnson PM, Adinolfi M (1984) Trophoblast cells in peripheral blood from pregnant women. *Lancet* **ii**: 841–843.

Covone AE, Kozma R, Johnson PM, Latt SA, Adinolfi M (1988) Analysis of peripheral maternal blood samples for the presence of placenta-derived cells using Y-specific probes and McAb H315. *Prenatal Diagn.* **8**: 591–607.

Cupp JE, Leary JF, Cernichiari E, Wood JCS, Doherty RA (1984) Rare-event analysis methods for detection of fetal red blood cells in maternal blood. *Cytometry* **5**: 138–144.

Davies SV, Cavill I, Bentley N, Fegan CD, Poynton CH, Whittaker JA (1992) Evaluation of erythropoiesis after bone marrow transplantation: quantitative reticulocyte counting. *Br. J. Haematol.* **81**: 12–17.

Davis BH, Bigelow N (1989) Flow cytometric reticulocyte quantification using thiazole orange provides clinically useful reticulocyte maturity index. *Arch. Pathol. Lab. Med.* **113**: 684–689.

Davis BH, Bigelow N, Ball ED, Mills L, Cornwell GG (1989) Utility of flow cytometric reticulocyte quantification as a predictor of engraftment in autologous bone marrow transplantation. *Am. J. Hematol.* **32**: 81–87.

Garratty G, Nance SJ (1990) Correlation between *in vivo* hemolysis and the amount of red cell-bound IgG measured by flow cytometry. *Transfusion* **30**: 617–621.

Hasekura H, Ota M, Ito S *et al.* (1990) Flow cytometric studies of the D antigen of various Rh phenotypes with particular reference to D^u and D_{el}. *Transfusion* **30**: 236–238.

Herzenberg LA, Bianchi DW, Schroder J, Cann HM, Iverson GM (1979) Fetal cells in the blood of pregnant women: detection and enrichment by fluorescence-activated cell sorting. *Proc. Natl Acad. Sci. USA* **76**: 1453–1455.

Hewitt M, Mott MG (1992) The assessment of *in vivo* somatic mutations in survivors of childhood malignancy. *Br. J. Cancer* **66**: 143–147.

Howard RJ, Battye FL, Mitchell GF (1979) Plasmodium-infected blood cells analysed and sorted by flow fluorimetry using the deoxyribonucleic acid binding dye 33258 Hoechst. *J. Histochem. Cytochem.* **27**: 803–812.

Hoy TG (1990) Flow Cytometry: Clinical applications in haematology. In: Cavill I, ed., *Advancing Haematological Techniques*. Bailliére Tindall, London, pp. 977–998.

Hudson IRB, Cavill I, Cooke A *et al.* (1990) Biotin labeling of red cells in the measurement of red cell volume in preterm infants. *Pediatr. Res.* **28**: 199–202.

International Committee for Standardisation in Haematology (1980) Recommended methods for measurement of red cell and plasma volume. *J. Nucl. Med.* **21**: 793–800.

Iverson GM, Bianchi DW, Cann HM, Herzenberg LA (1981) Detection and isolation of fetal cells from maternal blood using the fluorescence-activated cell sorter. *Prenatal Diagn.* **1**: 61–73.

Kim YR, Ornstein L (1983) Isovolumetric sphering of erythrocytes for more accurate and precise cell volume measurements by flow cytometry. *Cytometry* **3**: 419–427.

Kinoshita T, Medof ME, Silber R, Nussenzweig V (1985) Distribution of decay-accelerating factor in the peripheral blood of normal individuals and patients with paroxysmal nocturnal hemoglobinuria. *J. Exp. Med.* **162**: 75–92.

Kleihauer E, Braun H, Betke K (1957) Demonstration von fetalen hämoglobin in dem erythrocyten eines blutausstricts. *Klin. Wochenschr.* **35**: 635–637.

Kyoizumi S, Nakamura N, Hakoda M *et al.* (1989) Detection of somatic cell mutations at the glycophorin A locus in erythrocytes of atomic bomb survivors using a single beam flow sorter. *Cancer Res.* **49**: 581–588.

Langlois RG, Bigbee WL, Jensen RH (1985) Flow cytometric characterization of normal and variant cells with monoclonal antibodies specific for glycophorin A. *J. Immunol.* **134**: 4009–4017.

Langlois RG, Bigbee WL, Kyoizumi S *et al.* (1987) Evidence for increased somatic cell mutations at the glycophorin A locus in atomic bomb survivors. *Science* **236**: 445–448.

Langlois RG, Nisbet BA, Bigbee WL, Ridinger DN, Jensen RH (1990) An improved flow cytometric assay for somatic mutations at the glycophorin A locus in humans. *Cytometry* **11**: 513–521.

Lee LG, Chen CH, Chiu LA (1986) Thiazole orange: a new dye for reticulocyte analysis. *Cytometry* **7**: 508–517.

Makler MT, Lee LG, Recktenwald D (1987) Thiazole orange: a new dye for *Plasmodium* species analysis. *Cytometry* **8**: 568–570.

Medearis AL, Hensleigh PA, Parks DR, Herzenberg LA (1984) Detection of fetal erythrocytes in maternal blood post partum with the fluorescence-activated cell sorter. *Am. J. Obstet. Gynecol.* **148**: 290–295.

Moore JG, Frank MM, Muller-Eberhard HJ, Young NS (1985) Decay-accelerating factor is present on paroxysmal nocturnal hemoglobinuria erythroid progenitors and lost during erythropoiesis *in vitro*. *J. Exp. Med.* **162**: 1182–1192.

Nance S (1988) Applications of flow cytometry in blood transfusion science. In: Moore SB, ed., *Progress in Immunohematology*. American Association of Blood Banks, Arlington, VA, pp. 1–30.

Nance S, Garratty G (1984) Correlates between *in vivo* hemolysis and the amount of RBC-bound IgG measured by flow cytometry. *Blood* **64**: 88a.

Nance SJ, Garratty G (1987) Application of flow cytometry to immunohematology. *J. Immunol. Methods* **101**: 127–131.

Nobes PR, Carter AB (1990) Reticulocyte counting using flow cytometry. *J. Clin. Pathol.* **43**: 675–678.

Pallavicini MG, Langlois RG, Reitsma M *et al.* (1992) Comparison of strategies to detect and quantitate uniquely marked cells in intra- and inter-species hemopoietic chimeras. *Cytometry* **13**: 356–367.

Pattanapanyasat K, Hoy TG (1991) Expression of cell surface transferrin receptor and intracellular ferritin after *in vitro* stimulation of peripheral blood T lymphocytes. *Eur. J. Haematol.* **47**: 140–145.

Pattanapanyasat K, Webster HK, Udomsangpetch R, Wanachiwanawin W, Yongvanitchit K (1992) Flow cytometric two-color staining technique for simultaneous determination of human erythrocyte membrane antigen and intracellular malarial DNA. *Cytometry* **13**: 182–187.

Pattanapanyasat K, Udomsangpetch R, Webster K (1993) Two-color flow cytometric analysis of intraerythrocytic malaria parasite DNA and surface membrane-associated antigen in erythrocytes infected with *Plasmodium falciparum*. *Cytometry* **14**: 449–454.

Patton WN, Nicholson GS, Sawers AH, Franklin IM, Ala FA, Simpson AW (1990) Assessment of fetal–maternal haemorrhage in mothers with hereditary persistence of fetal haemoglobin. *J. Clin. Pathol.* **43**: 728–731.

Petz L, Garratty G (1980) *Acquired Immune Hemolytic Anemias*: Churchill Livingstone, New York.

Phillips HM, Holland BM, Jones JG, Abdel-Moiz AL, Turner TL, Wardrop CAJ (1988) Definitive estimate of rate of hemoglobin switching: measurement of per cent hemoglobin F in neonatal reticulocytes. *Pediatr. Res.* **23**: 595–597.

Plesner T, Hansen NE, Carlsen K (1990) Estimation of PI-bound proteins on blood cells from PNH patients by quantitative flow cytometry. *Br. J. Haematol.* **75**: 585–590.

Read EJ, Cardine LL, Yu MY (1991) Flow cytometric detection of human red cells labeled with a fluorescent membrane label: potential application to *in vivo* survival studies. *Transfusion* **31**: 502–508.

Rosse WF, Hoffman S, Campbell M, Borowitz M, Moore JO, Parker CJ (1991) The erythrocyte in paroxysmal nocturnal haemoglobinuria of intermediate sensitivity to complement lysis. *Br. J. Haematol.* **79**: 99–107.

Sage BH, O'Connell JP, Mercolino TJ (1983) A rapid vital staining procedure for flow cytometric analysis of human reticulocytes. *Cytometry* **4**: 222–227.

Schmitz FJ, Werner E (1986) Optimization of flow-cytometric discrimination between reticulocytes and erythrocytes. *Cytometry* **7**: 439–444.

Schroder J (1975) Transplacental passage of blood cells. *J. Med. Genet.* **12**: 230–242.

Sharon R, Fibach E (1991) Quantitative flow cytometric analysis of ABO red cell antigens. *Cytometry* **12**: 545–549.

Shumak KH, Rachkewich RA (1984) Transferrin receptors on human reticulocytes: variation in site number in hematologic disorders. *Am. J. Hematol.* **16**: 23–32.

Suzuki T, Dale GL (1987) Biotinylated erythrocytes: *in vivo* survival and *in vitro* recovery. *Blood* **70**: 791–795.

Tanke HJ, Nieuwenhuis IAB, Koper GJM, Slats JCM, Ploem JS (1980) Flow cytometry of human reticulocytes based on RNA fluorescence. *Cytometry* **1**: 313–320.

Tanke HJ, Rothbarth PH, Vossen JMJJ, Koper GJM, Ploem JS (1983) Flow cytometry of reticulocytes applied to clinical hematology. *Blood* **61**: 1091–1097.

Ueda E, Kinoshita T, Terasawa T *et al.* (1990) Acetylcholinesterase and lymphocyte function-associated antigen 3 found on decay-accelerating factor-negative erythrocytes from some patients with paroxysmal nocturnal hemoglobinuria are lost during erythrocyte aging. *Blood* **75**: 762–769.

van der Meulen FW, de Bruin HG, Goosen PCM *et al.* (1980) Quantitative aspects of the destruction of red cells sensitized with IgG1 autoantibodies: an application of flow cytofluorometry. *Br. J. Haematol.* **46**: 47–56.

Wanachiwanawin W, Pattanapanyasat K (1991) Emerging of DAF-negative erythrocyte clone in aplastic anaemia before and during haematologic recovery. *Br. J. Haematol.* **79**: 123–124.

Wyatt CR, Goff W, Davis WC (1991) A flow cytometric method for assessing the viability of intraerythrocytic hemoparasites. *J. Immunol. Methods* **140**: 23–30.

Chapter 8
The Measurement of DNA Content, Alone or Combined with Other Markers

R. S. CAMPLEJOHN

Introduction

The study of cell proliferation has long been the major part of cell kinetics. However, it should not be forgotten that the size or rate of growth of a cell population depends just as much on the rate of cell loss (Fig. 8.1). Cell loss may occur directly from the pool of proliferative cells or after a process of differentiation has occurred. Although the bulk of this chapter will be concerned with measurements related to cell proliferation, we will later touch on the processes of cell death and differentiation.

Cell proliferation has long been assessed clinically as part of grading systems for various types of tumour. Prior to the late 1950s, the only method available to assess proliferative activity was counting mitoses on tissue sections. For experimental systems, more information could be obtained by using metaphase-arrest agents. These drugs, such as colcemid or vincristine, arrest cells in the metaphase stage of mitosis and by serially sampling a cell population at various times after drug administration, the rate of entry of cells into mitosis can be estimated. In this way information about the rate of cell passage around the cell cycle can be gleaned, as opposed to the static information yielded by a simple mitotic index. Although the metaphase-arrest method was applied to clinical situations (see for example Camplejohn et al., 1973), its relevance to the study of human disease was severely limited by the requirement for multiple serial biopsies (for a review of this technique see Wright and Appleton, 1980).

Following the work of Howard and Pelc (1953), it was realized that proliferating cells go through four discrete phases, namely G_1, S, G_2 and mitosis, in the so-called cell cycle (Fig. 8.1). DNA is replicated in the (S)ynthetic phase, which is temporally discrete from mitosis. Modern

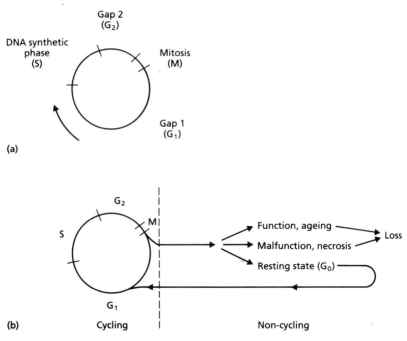

Fig. 8.1 (a) Shows a very simplified version of the cell cycle with the four phases G_1, S, G_2 and mitosis illustrated. (b) Emphasizes that most real cell populations *in vivo* consist of a mixture of cycling and non-cycling cells. In addition, processes which lead to cell loss are shown in (b).

molecular biology has added much detail to this simple cell cycle concept, although important aspects relating to the control of entry of cells into the S and mitotic phases remain to be elucidated (Brooks, 1992). Historically, the synthesis of convenient radioactivity labelled DNA precursors such as tritiated thymidine (^{3}H-TdR) (Taylor *et al.*, 1957; Firket and Verley, 1958) allied to the concept of the cell cycle, led to an explosion of studies of cell proliferation. The administration of ^{3}H-TdR to a cell population allowed an estimate of the labelling index to be made; this is a measure of the number of cells in the S-phase of the cell cycle. However, more sophisticated techniques such as the fraction-labelled mitosis (FLM) method were developed, which in experimental systems can yield detailed kinetic information. For a review of these 'classical' methods of studying cell proliferation see Dover (1992).

Advantages and disadvantages of flow cytometry

All of the 'classical' methods detailed above suffer from a number of disadvantages in relation to the study of clinical disease. All of them depend upon the counting of events (either labelled cells and/or mitoses) on tissue sections. If done properly (Quinn and Wright, 1990), this is a laborious undertaking. Further, methods involving radioactive precursors such as ^{3}H-TdR are limited in application to humans by considerations of safety. Although *in vivo* studies with ^{3}H-TdR have been performed on humans, their application and impact has been limited. Most clinical studies have been restricted to determining a simple labelling index on tissue exposed *in vitro* to ^{3}H-TdR. Such studies may provide useful prognostic information (Silvestrini *et al.*, 1989) but the disadvantages described above apply. More sophisticated techniques such as the FLM method or the metaphase-arrest technique, both of which can yield real kinetic information about the rate of passage of cells around the cell cycle, require serial samples to be taken. In the case of the FLM technique, this would ideally require many samples spread over at least 48 hours. The requirement for multiple samples is clearly a major problem in the study of most clinical diseases.

What then are the potential advantages of flow cytometric techniques to assess proliferative activity in clinical disease? One major advantage is speed; typically 10 000 to 100 000 cells or nuclei can be scanned in a few minutes. This leads to a high degree of statistical precision in the measurements which are made. In addition, multiple parameters, such as DNA content and antibody binding, can be measured simultaneously and quantitatively on individual cells. Further, some measurements can be made on nuclei extracted from Formalin-fixed, paraffin-embedded, archival material as well as from fresh tissue. However, no technique is without its disadvantages. Among the disadvantages of flow cytometry, is that a relatively expensive machine is required. In addition, when studying solid tissues, the need to disaggregate the tissue into a suspension of single cells or nuclei can be a problem. Some solid tissues are difficult to disaggregate and in all cases tissue morphology is lost. Flow cytometric techniques also require a minimum number of cells, usually in the region of 10^5, and this can be a limitation for certain potential applications. As with all techniques the relevance of flow cytometry to a particular clinical situation depends on the question being asked and the amount and quality of material available for study.

DNA flow cytometry

Introduction

The earliest flow cytometrically measured DNA histograms, which showed clearly defined G_1, S and G_2/M phases of the cell cycle seem to have been produced by Van Dilla *et al.* (1969). Since then a vast number of studies have been published, in which DNA content of clinical material has been measured. In this chapter the discussion will be restricted to cancer-related topics.

Two main parameters can be measured from DNA histograms. The first of these relates to the presence of cells with abnormal amounts of DNA (see Fig. 8.2), so-called DNA aneuploid cells. Early studies using both static and flow cytometry tended to show that tumours containing DNA aneuploid cells had a worse prognosis than those containing only DNA diploid cells. The second major parameter to be gleaned from DNA histograms is a crude index of proliferative activity. In general,

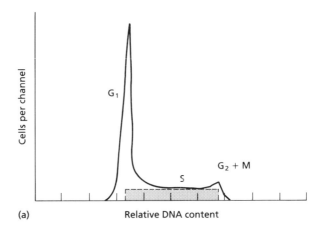

(a)

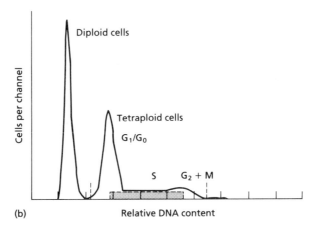

(b)

Fig. 8.2 (a) Shows a diploid histogram. SPF is calculated by fitting a rectangle to represent the S-phase. (b) Shows à DNA histogram for a tetraploid tumour. The tumour G_1 peak has twice the normal amount of DNA (DI = 2.0). SPF is calculated by a modified version of the rectangular method.

where proliferative activity is high there will be many cells in the S and G_2/M phases of the cell cycle and conversely when proliferative activity is low there will be few such cells. Thus, the percentage of cells in the S-phase (the S-phase fraction or SPF) or the combined percentage of cells in the $S + G_2/M$ phases are often used as indices of proliferative activity (Fig. 8.2). SPF is a state parameter with the properties described earlier in relation to labelling or mitotic index; it gives no information about the rate of proliferation.

Production of cell suspensions for flow cytometry

A prerequisite for flow cytometry is a suspension of single cells. If one wants to investigate solid tissues, then these must first be disaggregated. Clearly, disaggregation is not required for peripheral blood cells or cells in suspension culture. Cells growing in monolayer culture can usually be disaggregated by simple enzymic methods such as treating with trypsin plus EDTA.

Disaggregation of fresh solid tumours

For the sake of convenience, disaggregation techniques for fresh tissue can be split into three categories:
1   Those which rely solely on mechanical disaggregation.
2   Those which involve the use of enzymes.
3   Enucleation techniques.

Mechanical disaggregation

The quickest and simplest methods of dissociation involve only mechanical procedures. An example of such a technique is given in Method 1. Cell suspensions can be produced from solid tumour samples in a few minutes by this method, which works extremely well with friable tissue, particularly lymph nodes from which high cell yields can be obtained (Ensley *et al.*, 1987a; Camplejohn *et al.*, 1989). In contrast, attempting to pass fibrous tumours through a steel mesh may yield few cells and those that are released may be badly damaged.

Method 1. Physical dissociation of solid tumours

1   Place tissue sample on stainless steel grid (pore size 0.5 mm) placed over a Petri dish. Cut tissue into small (1–2 mm³) pieces.
2   Moisten the tissue fragments with minimal essential medium (MEM) containing 5% serum and using the rubber plunger from a 5 ml disposable syringe, gently push the tissue through the steel mesh into the Petri dish. Rinse steel sieve thoroughly with 4 ml MEM.
3   Take up the crude suspension from the Petri dish into a 5 ml syringe and pass it sequentially twice through each of a 19-, 21-, 23- and finally 25-gauge needle. (Needle aspirates taken directly from solid tumours can be entered into this method here.)
4   Filter the suspension through a 35 μm mesh nylon filter. Adjust the cell concentration to the desired level.

Fine needle aspiration of solid tumours, including those which are not otherwise easily dissociated, may be an effective method to obtain a crude cell suspension, which can be further disaggregated as described from step 3 of Method 1, or can be entered into an enucleation technique (Method 5). Fine needle aspiration may be performed either *in situ* on tumours from suitable sites such as breast cancer (Levack *et al.*, 1987), or may be taken from excised tumour biopsies (Vindelov and Christensen, 1990). In both cases high success rates were reported.

Enzymic disaggregation

I have not given a detailed method in this section for two reasons. First, there are so many variants of enzymic methods for tissue disaggregation that it is difficult to make a rational choice as to the best one and second, we do not routinely use such a method and thus have limited experience of such techniques. A brief discussion of such methods is given by Pallavicini *et al.* (1990). In addition, a detailed description of a particular method involving a cocktail of collagenase, DNAse and trypsin is given by Ensley *et al.* (1987a,b). In these two papers a detailed comparison with other enzymic and mechanical techniques was made.

Enucleation technique

A variety of methods have been described which release nuclei, usually from tissue which has been partly disaggregated mechanically. This can be done with enzymes (Beck, 1977), detergent (Petersen, 1985) or a combination of the two (Vindelov and Christensen, 1990). The group led by Vindelov in Denmark has developed a detailed scheme for disaggregation, staining, data acquisition and analysis based on the production of nuclear suspensions. The disaggregation and staining method (Method 5) from this group is given as a single method and not split arbitrarily into two parts (i.e. disaggregation/staining). It will be discussed more fully in the section on staining DNA.

Which disaggregation technique to choose?

Clearly, the aim of any disaggregation method is to produce a representative suspension of intact single cells or nuclei with a good yield. However, the choice of a particular technique will depend upon a number of factors such as the type of tissue, size of sample, the precise aims of the study, and perhaps on the speed and cost of the various alternatives. A simple mechanical method such as that described in Method 1, is quick and inexpensive and works very well with lymphoid tissue. It does not work well with tough or fibrous samples. The enzymic technique detailed by Ensley *et al.* (1987a,b) is reported to give reasonable cell yields on a variety of tumours, but it is time consuming and relatively labour intensive.

What then might constitute a good general method of disaggregation? From our own experience and reports in the literature (Levack *et al.*, 1987; Vindelov and Christensen, 1990), the use of fine needle aspiration would seem to be a good technique for obtaining a partially disaggregated suspension of cells, which can be further dissociated as described in steps 3–4 in Method 1 or entered into an enucleation method (Vindelov and Christensen, 1990).

Disaggregation of paraffin-embedded archival material

A method was first published in 1983 (Hedley *et al.*, 1983) which described how DNA flow cytometry could be performed on nuclear suspensions released from paraffin-embedded tissue. We have modified this technique (Method 2) and applied it to a wide variety of tumours. The use of paraffin-embedded tissue has a number of advantages:

1 Large retrospective clinical studies can be made on patients for whom long-term follow-up is already available.

2 Rare lesions can be more easily studied.

3 Multicentre studies in which flow cytometry is performed centrally are facilitated by the ease of transportation and storage of paraffin sections.

The disadvantages of the technique are:

1 Quality of results is generally poorer (Hedley *et al.*, 1983; Kallioniemi, 1988).

2 External DNA standards cannot be used.

Method 2. Dissociation of paraffin-embedded archival material

1 Place one 50 μm tissue section for each sample in a small biopsy cassette (pore size 300 μm) with a label written in pencil.

2 Place up to 12 cassettes in a basket and run the batch of samples on a tissue processing machine such as a Histokinette with the following programme. The samples spend 15 min being agitated in:

Xylene	—	3 changes
100% alcohol	—	×2
90% alcohol	—	×2
70% alcohol	—	×2
50% alcohol	—	×2

This process can be performed overnight (total time taken 2 hours 45 min).

3 Wash the basket of cassettes thoroughly, leaving them to soak for 10 min, in two changes of distilled water.

4 Drain the water from the cassette, open it carefully, then using fine forceps transfer the dewaxed section to a universal container with pepsin solution made up as follows: 0.5% pepsin (Sigma 7012) in 0.9% saline with the pH adjusted to 1.5 using 2 mol/l HCl.

5 Transfer the batch of universals to a 37°C water-bath and incubate for 30 min.

6 Centrifuge at 800 g (typically 2000 r/min) for 3 min at room temperature.

7 Carefully remove and discard the supernatant with a Pasteur pipette.

8 Resuspend the tissue fragments and released nuclei in 2 ml of

Continued on page 222

phosphate-buffered saline (PBS) and agitate vigorously using a vortex mixer.
9 Filter the suspension through a 35 μm pore size nylon filter and adjust the concentration of nuclei as desired.

The quality of results from paraffin-embedded tissue can, however, be improved in prospective studies by minor improvements in the fixation of the tissue (Gillett *et al.*, 1990). A good fixation method is neutral, buffered Formalin at 4°C overnight; alternatively tissue can be fixed in phenol Formalin. Unnecessary heating of the tissue during processing should be avoided, as should over-long fixation. In a comparison of results from fresh and paraffin-embedded lymphoid tissue, we were able to show that results in terms of quality, DNA index and SPF were similar (Camplejohn *et al.*, 1989).

Staining for DNA

The ideal stain for the flow cytometric measurement of cellular DNA content should have a number of properties including:
1 Specificity for DNA.
2 Suitable spectral properties so that it can be excited and its fluorescence detected by commercially available flow cytometers.
3 Reasonably low cost and convenience in terms of solubility, stability, etc.

A number of fluorochromes meet these requirements or come close enough to be of practical use. A detailed description of the properties of these dyes is given in three consecutive chapters of the book edited by Melamed *et al.* (Waggoner, 1990; Crissman and Steinkamp, 1990; Latt and Langlois, 1990). In the brief space available here, details are given for only one DNA stain, propidium iodide (PI). PI is probably the most commonly used DNA stain in flow cytometry even though it is not entirely specific for DNA. PI also stains double-stranded RNA and thus RNAse should be included in all protocols with this dye. The spectral characteristics of PI make it a popular choice for flow cytometry, as it is readily excited by the 488 nm line of the argon-ion laser and it fluoresces with a maximum at about 620 nm which makes it suitable for combination with fluorescein in multi-parametric measurements (see later).

Whatever DNA stain is used, it is necessary to achieve a stain : cell concentration ratio which achieves stoichiometric staining (i.e. where the amount of dye bound is proportional to the amount of DNA in the cell). This involves the dye being present in modest excess so that all available sites on the DNA are bound by dye.

The majority of DNA fluorochromes, including PI, are unable to cross intact cell membranes and thus cells must be permeabilized in some way. This is most commonly done using either alcohol fixation or treatment of unfixed cells with detergent.

A simple method for staining fresh cells

This technique, described in Method 3, can be combined with the disaggregation technique detailed in Method 1, to yield rapid results from solid tissues. The result can be obtained within about 1 hour of receiving the sample. This staining technique can also be used on tissue culture cells, peripheral blood mononuclear cells and other types of cell which do not require disaggregation. The use of lymphocytes as an external DNA standard as described in step 3 of Method 3, allows the ploidy of peaks in the test sample to be checked. The position of the lymphocyte peak is used to define the diploid peak of the test sample and allows the DNA index to be calculated as described in the section on analysis of DNA histograms.

Method 3. Simple staining technique for fresh cells

1 Dilute cells to approximately 5×10^5/ml in MEM containing 5% serum.

2 For each sample label three plastic tubes. Aliquot 2 ml of suspension into each of two of these tubes (A and B) and into the third tube (C) pipette 2 ml of medium.

3 Add 2×10^5 human peripheral blood lymphocytes to tubes B and C in a volume of 0.1 ml, so that for each sample we have three tubes containing:

Tube A	10^6 tumour cells in 2 ml
Tube B	10^6 tumour cells $+ 2 \times 10^5$ lymphocytes in 2.1 ml
Tube C	2×10^5 lymphocytes in 2.1 ml

4 To each tube add 0.5 ml of stain solution containing:
250 µg/ml PI
1 mg/ml RNAse
1% Triton X-100

Final concentrations in the cell suspensions are thus PI-50 µg/ml; RNAse 200 µg/ml; Triton X-100 — 0.2%.

5 Mix the suspensions well and leave for 30 min to stain at room temperature protected from the light.

6 Immediately prior to running on the flow cytometer, pass each suspension through a 25-gauge needle to reduce clumping.

7 Run at least 10^5 cells through the flow cytometer recording DNA fluorescence and forward and right-angled light scatter.

DNA staining of alcohol-fixed cells and nuclei from paraffin blocks

It is often convenient to store samples prior to running on a flow cytometer and a simple way to do this involves fixation. Freezing cells is another alternative (Vindelov and Christensen, 1990). The most common fixative used to preserve cells for subsequent DNA staining is ethanol, though others are used.

Method 4 describes a simple fixation and staining method, which again can be combined with the disaggregation technique described in Method 1. In general, the quality of DNA histograms obtained from alcohol-fixed cells may be slightly poorer in terms of CV, and clumping can be a considerable problem. Clumping can be reduced by careful fixation as described in Method 4.

*Method 4. Simple technique for fixing cells in alcohol
and staining for DNA*

1 Aliquot approximately 10^6 cells in medium or PBS into a plastic centrifuge tube.
2 Centrifuge the samples at $250\,g$ for 10 min at 4°C, remove the supernatant, resuspend in 2 ml PBS and spin again.
3 Resuspend each aliquot in 0.4 ml PBS and pass the suspension twice through a 25-gauge needle to reduce clumping, then add 3.6 ml of cold 70% ethanol dropwise while mixing.
4 Fix for at least 30 min (cells will keep for several weeks) at 4°C.
5 Spin, remove ethanol and wash cells with PBS.
6 Stain cells with PI and run on flow cytometer as described in Method 3, steps 4–7, with the exception that Triton-X-100 is not necessary with alcohol-fixed cells.

Enucleation technique

Such methods have been used by a number of groups and Vindelov and Christensen, (1990) developed a detailed strategy for performing DNA flow cytometry of clinical material based around an enucleation technique. This group claims high success rates with clinical material and good quality results (i.e. low coefficient of variation, CV). Details of this technique are given in Method 5.

Method 5. Enucleation technique

1 Cells are obtained by fine needle aspiration either *in situ* or following surgical removal.
2 Add chicken and trout erythrocytes to the needle aspirate containing approximately 10^6 cells in 200 μl citrate buffer.
3 Add 1.8 ml of solution A containing trypsin to the above suspension, invert the tube to mix. Leave for 10 min at room temperature, mixing two to three times.

4 Add 1.5 ml of solution B containing trypsin inhibitor and RNAse, mix and leave for a further 10 min at room temperature.
5 Add 1.5 ml of ice-cold solution C, containing PI and spermine hydrochloride. Mix the solutions and filter through a 25 μm nylon mesh into plastic tubes protected from the light.
6 Keep samples on ice for a minimum of 15 min (maximum 3 hours)
7 Run on flow cytometer as described in step 7 of Method 3.
Note: For details of the various solutions see Vindelov and Christensen, (1990).

This method is clearly not suitable if one wishes to measure DNA content combined with a surface or cytoplasmic antigen (see later).

Running samples on a flow cytometer

Whatever type of flow cytometer is used to produce DNA histograms certain general principles apply if good quality results are to be obtained, these include:
1 Producing a high quality single cell suspension.
2 Making measurements on a sufficient number of cells/nuclei.
3 Making use of all the information available such as light scatter/volume (Fig. 8.3) and pulse area/width data to reduce the contamination of DNA histograms by clumps (Ormerod, 1990).

Data analysis

Analysis of DNA histograms

There are many, sometimes conflicting, approaches to the analysis of DNA histograms reported in the literature (Ormerod, 1990; Dean, 1990). Some attempts have been and are being made, for example, by the International Society for Analytical Cytometry, to standardize procedures and nomenclature (Hiddeman *et al.*, 1984). Nevertheless, many different methods are used to analyse data, often with the aid of a variety of computer algorithms. In this chapter, discussion will be restricted mainly to the methods used in our laboratory.

Calculation of the CV

The CV, usually of the DNA diploid G_1 peak, is a useful shorthand way of representing the quality of DNA data. The CV is calculated from the equation below, on the basis that the G_1 peak can be represented by a normal distribution.

$$CV = W/(M \times 2.35)$$

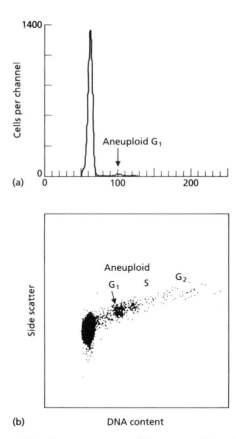

(a)

(b)   DNA content

Fig. 8.3 (a) Shows a DNA histogram prepared from a paraffin-embedded breast
carcinoma sample. A barely discernible aneuploid peak is visible. (b) Shows that by
combining DNA measurement with side scatter, a clearly visible collection of
aneuploid G_1 cells can be seen with the corresponding S and G_2/M-phase cells
present.

where W = full width of the G_1 peak at the half-maximum height and
M = peak channel number of the G_1 peak.

High quality DNA histograms will have a low CV and the G_1 peak
approximates very closely to a normal distribution. Many real DNA
histograms are not so good and it is important in clinical DNA studies
to quote both the average CV and the range of CV seen in the series of
cases reported. This enables readers to judge the quality of the data
presented.

The calculation of the DNA index

The basic principles by which DNA aneuploidy is recognized and by
which the DNA index (DI) is calculated are widely accepted. In histograms
which exhibit two or more G_1 peaks (see Fig. 8.2b) the DI of the DNA
aneuploid peak(s) is calculated by reference to the position of the
diploid G_1 peak. For example in Fig. 8.2b, the tumour G_1 peak has twice
the amount of DNA compared with the DNA diploid G_1 peak and thus

has a DI of 2.0. A DI of 1.5 would mean a DNA aneuploid peak with 50% more DNA than normal. If only DNA diploid cells are present, the DI is reported as 1.0.

DNA aneuploidy should only be recognized in clinical samples when two or more G_1 peaks are evident. For fresh tissue samples, an external DNA standard can be used to confirm which G_1 peak is diploid, in cases where the two peaks are close together. Thus, in Fig. 8.2, the left-hand peak can be confirmed as DNA diploid by comparison with a known diploid cell type such as human peripheral blood lymphocytes. The way in which this can be done is described in Method 3. A report from the Committee on Nomenclature of the Society for Analytical Cytometry (Hiddeman *et al.*, 1984), recommended the use of such DNA diploid cells as external standards. There are, however, other methods used and these mostly involve the use of non-mammalian nucleated red blood cells as DNA standards (Vindelov and Christensen, 1990). This approach is described in Method 5.

When nuclei derived from paraffin-embedded material are used, such external DNA standards cannot be used (Hedley *et al.*, 1983; Schutte *et al.*, 1985). This is due to variability in staining intensity of the DNA in nuclei from different paraffin blocks due to differences in the precise conditions of fixation and processing. With DNA histograms from paraffin-embedded material, the convention is that where two G_1 peaks are seen (as in Fig. 8.2b), the left-hand peak is considered to be DNA diploid. This should not lead to the failure to recognize DNA aneuploidy, as all samples contain internal reference DNA diploid cells (lymphocytes, endothelial cells, etc.) but it will lead to a small percentage of samples being wrongly classified as 'hyperdiploid' when they are really 'hypodiploid'. The clinical significance of such an incorrect classification is unknown but in most instances is likely to be minor.

Two common problems in assessing DNA ploidy status are the difficulties in recognizing either small DNA aneuploid stem lines or even worse, small tetraploid stem lines. These problems can be more easily dealt with if other flow cytometric parameters, which are freely available on most machines, such as 90° light scatter and forward light scatter (or Coulter volume) are used (see Fig. 8.3) in conjunction with DNA content.

Calculation of SPF

For the estimation of SPF we used the method of Baisch *et al.* (1975) for DNA diploid histograms and a modification of this method for DNA aneuploid histograms (Camplejohn *et al.*, 1989). These methods involve fitting a rectangular area to represent the S-phase and calculating the number of cells within this area as shown in Fig. 8.2. We chose this method of calculation for a variety of reasons. First, it is simple and requires only a hand-held calculator to perform. Thus, it can be applied anywhere and does not require any specific computer hardware or software. Second, it gives good agreement with the bromodeoxyuridine

(BrdUrd) labelling index in a series of cell lines we have studied (unpublished data).

Clinical significance of DNA flow cytometry

Much of the early impetus to develop flow cytometers came from a desire to automate diagnostic cytology (Melamed and Staiano-Coico, 1990) but the majority of published studies relate to the prognostic use of the technique. In general, tumours which are DNA aneuploid and have high SPFs are more aggressive and patients with such tumours have a poorer prognosis (Friedlander *et al.*, 1984; Hedley, 1989; Merkel and McGuire, 1990; Macartney and Camplejohn, 1990).

One example of how DNA flow cytometry may help with patient management and add to information available from standard histopathological techniques, is given for node-negative breast cancer. Although survival is better for women with no nodes involved, there is a subgroup of node-negative patients who do badly. It would not generally be acceptable to give all node-negative patients toxic adjuvant therapy but it may be worth giving such treatment to suitable patients with a poor prognosis. How to identify such patients is thus a clinically relevant question. We looked to see whether DNA flow cytometry might be a useful way to do this (O'Reilly *et al.*, 1990). The results suggest that by combining tumour size and SPF a poor prognosis subgroup of node-negative patients can be identified (Fig. 8.4).

Cell loss

The importance of cell loss to the size and growth rate of cell populations was stressed at the beginning of this chapter. Far fewer flow cytometric

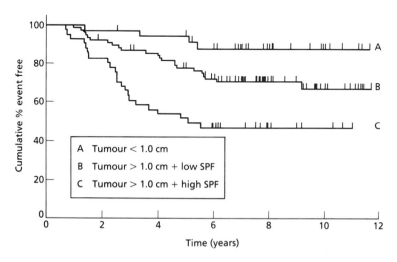

Fig. 8.4 Relapse-free survival for node-negative breast cancer patients: A, tumours < 1.0 cm; B, tumours > 1.0 cm + low SPF; C, tumours > 1.0 cm + high SPF. Data taken from O'Reilly *et al.* (1990).

studies of cell loss have been performed than of cell proliferation. No attempt will be made here to review this topic extensively but a mention of a few examples is made below. Cell loss may occur from tumours by a number of routes, including migration (metastasis) of cells, coagulative necrosis due to nutritional deprivation, apoptosis (controlled cell death) and due to the toxic effects of treatment. Attempts have been made to assess the cell killing effects of treatment, for example radiotherapy (Dyson *et al.*, 1985). This was done by staining cervical tumour cells for RNA and DNA in serial biopsies taken during a course of radiotherapy. The plots produced were, however, complex and such methods have not received wide application.

A potentially more interesting application of flow cytometry is in the study of apoptosis. Apoptosis is defined as a process of controlled cell deletion (Kerr *et al.*, 1972) which occurs widely in embryogenesis but also in many adult normal tissues. In tumours, it may occur spontaneously and as part of the response to therapy. The process involves nuclear condensation followed by the break-up of the nucleus (and cell) into well-preserved membrane-bound particles, which subsequently undergo further degenerative changes. A number of recent studies (Telford *et al.*, 1991; Ormerod *et al.*, 1992) have shown that in experimental systems apoptosis leads to the appearance of discrete peaks to the left of the G_1 peak in DNA histograms. By following the time-course of appearance after an apoptotic stimulus and the size of peaks generated, flow cytometry can provide a rapid means of assessing apoptosis on an individual cell basis.

Multiparametric studies

There are a host of different reasons why combining the simultaneous measurement of DNA content and the binding of antibodies to cells may be of interest. Antibody binding may be used to identify a subpopulation of cells so that the DNA profiles of these cells alone can be studied. This has been done with the aim of distinguishing between tumour and non-tumour cells, for example in non-Hodgkin's lymphoma (Braylan *et al.*, 1984). Combined DNA and marker studies can also be used to investigate the process of cell differentiation. For example, Kirkhus and Clausen (1990), investigated the cell cycle phase specificity of the synthesis of the differentiation-keratin K10 in basal cells of hairless mouse epidermis. These authors also used the BrdUrd method (see Method 7) to investigate cell proliferation in this system. Flow cytometry and cell sorting promise to be of great interest in the study of cell differentiation in skin. Zocchi *et al.* (1990) measured DNA content and the binding of monoclonal antibodies to a series of T-cell specific molecules in a study of human thymocyte development, with interesting results. In this study the antibodies were targeted against cytoplasmic antigens. Our own multiparametric studies have largely been involved with proteins associated with proliferation (Camplejohn *et al.*, 1993; Wilson *et al.*, 1992). Whatever the purpose of the study, techniques exist to label cell surface antigens, cytoplasmic antigens and nuclear antigens. It is difficult to give generalized protocols, particularly for intracellular antigens, as the most appropriate staining method depends upon the precise properties of a given target molecule. A number of simple protocols are given below but, as is made clear, they cannot be considered to have universal application.

Measurement of DNA and cell surface antigens

Method 6 describes a technique for measuring DNA and a cell surface antigen, simultaneously. With all methods involving antibody staining, appropriate negative and positive controls must be used and the correct antibody concentrations for a particular circumstance can be determined by titration (Carter, 1990).

Method 6. Combined measurement of DNA and a surface antigen

1 Dilute cells to 5×10^6/ml in MEM plus 5% serum and aliquot 300 μl of this suspension into the required number of tubes.

2 Incubate on ice for 30 min. (This step is optional but may reduce non-specific binding of antibodies.)

3 Add a suitable amount of monoclonal antibody directed against the desired antigen in a volume of 200 μl and incubate for 30 min on ice.

4 Spin cells at 200 g for 5 min at 4°C, wash cells in MEM plus 5% serum.

5 Resuspend cells in 500 μl of MEM plus serum containing an appropriate concentration of a F(ab')$_2$ fluorescein-linked second antibody (e.g. a rabbit anti-mouse).

6 Mix well and incubate cells on ice for 30 min.

7 Spin down cells and wash twice in MEM (without serum). Fix cells in alcohol as described in Method 4.

8 Spin fixed cells at 800 g for 5 min and wash them twice with PBS.

9 Stain the cells for DNA by resuspending in 2 ml of PBS to which is added PI at a final concentration of 50 μg/ml and RNAse at a final concentration of 200 μg/ml. Incubate at room temperature for 30 min.

10 Pass cell suspensions twice through a 25-gauge needle.

11 Run at least 10 000 cells on a flow cytometer collecting red (PI) and green (FITC) fluorescence and forward and right-angled light scatter.

Measurement of DNA and BrdUrd incorporation

Cells in the S-phase of the cell cycle will incorporate the thymidine analogue BrdUrd, which can thus be used to tag these cells in a manner similar to that of ^{3}H-TdR. Monoclonal antibodies have been developed which bind to DNA containing BrdUrd (Dolbeare *et al.*, 1983). This enables cells which have incorporated BrdUrd to be readily recognized both immunohistochemically and flow cytometrically (Method 7). This method is designed for use with tissue culture cells but can be modified for use with clinical tumours (Wilson and McNally, 1992), when BrdUrd is given by injection to patients in non-toxic doses. By waiting some hours between BrdUrd injection and taking the biopsy, the rate of movement of cells around the cell cycle can be estimated as well as the labelling index. A number of assumptions are necessary to obtain such data from a single biopsy and the estimates obtained cannot be placed within statistical confidence limits. Nevertheless, this approach is the only flow cytometric technique which enables any estimate of the rate of proliferation to be made.

Method 7. Bivariate staining for DNA and BrdUrd

1   Incubate cells with 10 μmol/l BrdUrd at 37°C for 20–30 min.
2   Count cells and divide them into aliquots of 2×10^6 and wash cells in PBS.
3   Fix cells in 70% ethanol as described in steps 3–5 of Method 4.
4   Spin fixed cells down at 800 g for 5 min.
5   Discard the supernatant and resuspend the cells in 2 ml of 1 mol/l HCl. Mix well by vortexing.
6   Incubate samples at 37°C for 20 min. NB: The conditions of acid denaturation may need to be varied depending on the cell type.
7   Spin cells down and wash twice with 5 ml PBS.
8   Add 1 ml PBS containing 0.5% Tween-20 and 0.5% serum. Vortex and incubate at room temperature for 15 min.
9   Spin cells down, discard the supernatant and resuspend in 0.5 ml PBS containing Tween-20, 0.5% serum and 20 μl anti-BrdUrd monoclonal antibody (Becton Dickinson).
10   Spin cells down, discard the supernatant and wash with PBS plus Tween-20 plus serum.
11   Resuspend in 0.5 ml PBS plus Tween-20 plus serum containing 20 μl of a fluorescence-labelled F(ab')$_2$ rabbit anti-mouse monoclonal antibody (DAKO). Mix well and incubate at room temperature for 30 min.
12   Spin cells down and wash in PBS.
13   Resuspend cells in 1 ml PBS and pass gently through a 25-gauge needle (the cells may be fragile at this stage).
14   Add 0.25 ml staining solution containing:
   250 μg/ml PI (final concentration 50 μg/ml)
   1 mg/ml RNAse (final concentration 200 μg/ml)
15   Leave samples to stain for a minimum of 30 min before running on the flow cytometer.
16   Run at least 10 000 cells and collect list mode data for red (PI) and green (fluorescein) fluorescence plus light scatter.

Combined measurement of DNA and nuclear or cytoplasmic antigens

Before cells can be labelled with antibodies to internal antigens, they must first be permeabilized. This can be done as described earlier for DNA stains, by treatment with detergent or by suitable fixation. A generalized method for staining internal antigens is given in Method 8. A method similar to this has been used successfully to stain for the oestrogen-receptor related protein, D5 (Ormerod, 1990) and the protein labelled by the novel proliferation-related antibody Ki-S1 (Fig. 8.5; Camplejohn *et al.*, 1993).

Method 8. Combined measurement of DNA and a cytoplasmic or nuclear marker

1 Fix cells in alcohol as described in Method 4.
2 Wash cells twice with PBS and resuspend in 300 µl of PBS.
3 Add primary antibody at a suitable concentration in a volume of 200 µl and incubate on ice for 30 min.
4 Spin cells down and wash twice with PBS.
5 Resuspend cells in 0.5 ml of PBS containing a suitable concentration of a F(ab')$_2$ fluorescein-linked second antibody (e.g. rabbit anti-mouse) and incubate for 30 min on ice.
6 Spin down and wash cells twice with PBS.
7 Stain with PI and run cells as described in Method 7.

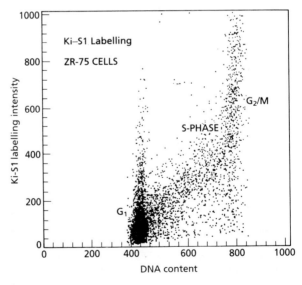

Fig. 8.5 This figure illustrates results from the combined staining of ZR75 cells (a human breast cell line) for DNA content (abscissa) and Ki-S1 (ordinate). It can be seen that labelling with Ki-S1 is relatively weak in G$_1$ but rises linearly through the S-phase, reaching high levels in G$_2$/M. In fact it has been shown that maximal labelling with Ki-S1 is seen in mitotic cells (Camplejohn *et al.*, 1993).

However, the enormous variety of cytoplasmic and nuclear antigens cannot all be labelled with the same method. Some antigens may be destroyed or solubilized by the technique described in Method 8. For example, the nuclear proliferation-related protein labelled by Ki-67 is not preserved by alcohol fixation. We found that the best method of labelling with Ki-67 involved the incubation of unfixed cells with the antibodies (as in step 3 of Method 8) in the presence of a low concentration of detergent (0.1% Nonidet P-40). Interesting results were obtained with an antibody called PC10 targeted against proliferating cell nuclear antigen (PCNA). In this case quite different staining patterns were seen if Method 8 was used or if, prior to fixation, cells were treated with detergent. Detergent-treated cells exhibited S-phase specific staining (Fig. 8.6), while intact cells did not. Thus not only may a staining method for a particular cytoplasmic or nuclear antigen have to be developed specifically for that antigen if simple methods such as Method 8 do not work (Watson, 1990; Darzynkiewicz, 1990), but different protocols may yield different staining patterns with the same antibody.

It may be possible to stain DNA and some nuclear antigens on nuclei extracted from paraffin sections. This has been done, for example, with the protein product of the c-myc gene (Watson, 1990) and the Ki-S1 protein (Camplejohn et al., 1992). To do this, nuclei produced as described in Method 2 are stained as detailed in steps 2–7 of Method 8 (see Watson, 1990). However, caution should be exercised in interpreting results from paraffin-embedded tissue. Changes in specific protein levels

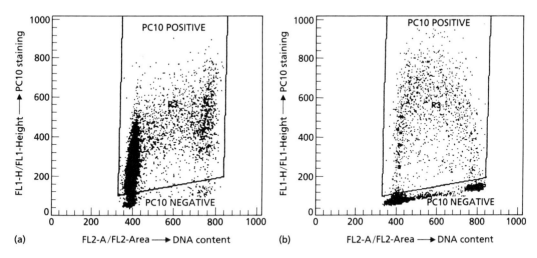

Fig. 8.6 (a) Illustrates the bivariate plot of DNA vs PC10 staining (PC10 is a monoclonal antibody directed against PCNA) on intact ZR75 cells. Virtually all cells are labelled with the average intensity of staining showing a modest increase as cells pass from G₁ through S and into G₂/M. In (b) in contrast, staining with PC10 is restricted to S-phase cells. The results in (b) are for cells treated with detergent prior to fixation to produce a suspension of nuclei. In this case about 75% of PCNA is washed out of the cells, leaving only the PCNA bound tightly to DNA (see Wilson et al., 1992).

due to degradation and/or redistribution during fixation and processing may lead to spurious findings (Lincoln and Bauer, 1989).

Clinical significance of multiparameter methods

Many published studies have demonstrated the feasibility of performing multiparametric measurements combining DNA content with a wide variety of markers. It is quite possible to combine DNA measurement with two antibodies even with a single laser flow cytometer (Landberg *et al.*, 1990). However, the clinical significance of such measurements, though potentially of great interest, remains to be established.

A specific example of the clinical application of a proliferation-related multiparametric technique concerns the BrdUrd method. This technique (see earlier and Wilson and McNally, 1992) is being investigated as a means to select patients for accelerated fractionation schedules in radiotherapy. It is hoped that the proliferative measurement made with this technique (potential doubling time or T_{pot}) may predict those patients most likely to benefit from radiation given three times per day in a period of 12 days.

References

Baisch H, Gohde W, Linden WA (1975) Analysis of PCP-data to determine the fraction of cells in the various phases of cell cycle. *Radiat. Environ. Biophys.* **12**: 31–39.

Beck H-P (1977) Effect of pepsin pretreatment on pulse-cytophotometric DNA histograms. *Cell Tissue Kinet.* **10**: 265–268.

Braylan RC, Benson NA, Nourse VA (1984) Cellular DNA of human neoplastic B-cells measured by flow cytometry. *Cancer Res.* **44**: 5010–5016.

Brooks RF (1992) Regulation of the eukaryotic cell cycle. In: Hall A, Levison DA, Wright NA, eds, *Assessment of Cell Proliferation in Clinical Practice*. Springer-Verlag, London, pp. 1–26.

Camplejohn RS, Bone G, Aherne W (1973) Cell proliferation in rectal carcinoma and rectal mucosa. A stathmokinetic study. *Eur. J. Cancer* **9**: 577–581.

Camplejohn RS, Macartney JC, Morris RW (1989) Measurement of S-phase fractions in lymphoid tissue comparing fresh versus paraffin-embedded tissue and 4′,6′-diamidino-2 phenolindole dihydrochloride versus propidium iodide staining. *Cytometry* **10**: 410–416.

Camplejohn RS, Brock A, Barnes DM *et al.* (1993) Ki-S1, a novel proliferative marker: flow cytometric assessment of staining in human breast carcinoma and an experimental comparison with other proliferative measures (PCNA staining, S-phase fraction, BrdUrd labelling). *Br. J. Cancer* **67**: 657–662.

Carter NP (1990) Measurement of cellular subsets using antibodies. In: Ormerod MG, ed., *Flow Cytometry: A Practical Approach*. IRL Press, Oxford, pp. 45–67.

Crissman AH, Steinkamp JA (1990) Cytochemical techniques for multivariate analysis of DNA and other cellular constituents. In: Melamed MR, Lindmo T, Mendelsohn ML, eds, *Flow Cytometry and Sorting*, 2nd edn. Wiley-Liss, New York, pp. 227–247.

Darzynkiewicz Z (1990) Probing nuclear chromatin by flow cytometry. In: Melamed MR, Lindmo T, Mendelsohn ML, eds, *Flow Cytometry and Sorting*, 2nd edn. Wiley-Liss, New York, pp. 315–340.

Dean PN (1990) Data processing. In: Melamed MR, Lindmo T, Mendelsohn ML, eds, *Flow Cytometry and Sorting*, 2nd edn. Wiley-Liss, New York, pp. 415–444.

Dolbeare F, Gratzner H, Pallavicini MG, Gray JW (1983) Flow cytometric measurement of total DNA content and incorporated bromodeoxyuridine. *Proc. Natl Acad. Sci. USA* **80**: 5573−5577.

Dover R (1992) Basic methods for assessing cellular proliferation. In: Hall A, Levison DA, Wright NA, eds, *Assessment of Cell Proliferation in Clinical Practice.* Springer-Verlag, London, pp. 63−81.

Dyson JED, Joslin CAF, Quirke P, Rothwell RI, Bird CC (1985) Quantitation by flow cytofluorometry of response of tumours of the uterine cervix to radiotherapy. *Br. J. Radiol.* **58**: 41−50.

Ensley JF, Maciorowski Z, Pietraszkiewicz H *et al.* (1987a) Solid tumor preparation for flow cytometry using a standard murine model. *Cytometry* **8**: 479−487.

Ensley JF, Maciorowski Z, Pietraszkiewicz H *et al.* (1987b) Solid tumor preparation for clinical application of flow cytometry. *Cytometry* **8**: 488−493.

Firket H, Verley WG (1958) Autoradiographic visualisation of synthesis of deoxyribonucleic acid in tissue culture with tritium-labelled thymidine. *Nature* **181**: 274−275.

Friedlander ML, Hedley DW, Taylor IW (1984) Clinical and biological significance of aneuploidy in human tumours. *J. Clin. Pathol.* **37**: 961−974.

Gillett CE, Camplejohn RS, O'Reilly SM (1990) Specimen preparation and proliferation markers in human breast cancer. *J. Pathol.* **160**: 173A.

Hedley DW (1989) Flow cytometry using paraffin-embedded tissue: five years on. *Cytometry* **10**: 229−241.

Hedley DW, Friedlander ML, Taylor IW, Rugg CA, Musgrove EA (1983) Method for analysis of cellular DNA content of paraffin-embedded pathological material using flow cytometry. *J. Histochem. Cytochem.* **31**: 1333−1335.

Hiddemann W, Schumann J, Andreeff M *et al.* (1984) Convention on nomenclature for DNA cytometry. *Cytometry* **5**: 445−446.

Howard A, Pelc SR (1953) Synthesis of desoxyribonucleic acid in normal and irradiated cells and its relation to chromosome breakage. *Heredity* **6** (Suppl.): 261−273.

Kallioniemi O-P (1988) Comparison of fresh and paraffin-embedded tissue as starting material for DNA flow cytometry and evaluation of intratumor heterogeneity. *Cytometry* **9**: 164−169.

Kerr JFR, Wyllie AH, Currie AR (1972) Apoptosis: a basic biological phenomenon with wide-ranging implications in tissue kinetics. *Br. J. Cancer* **26**: 239−257.

Kirkhus B, Clausen OPF (1990) Cell kinetics in mouse epidermis studied by bivariate DNA/bromodeoxyuridine and DNA/keratin flow cytometry. *Cytometry* **11**: 253−260.

Landberg G, Tan EM, Roos G (1990) Flow cytometric multiparameter analysis of proliferating cell nuclear antigen/cyclin and Ki-67 antigen: a new view of the cell cycle. *Exp. Cell Res.* **187**: 111−118.

Latt SA, Langlois RG (1990) Fluorescent probes of DNA microstructure and DNA synthesis. In: Melamed MR, Lindmo T, Mendelsohn ML, eds, *Flow Cytometry and Sorting,* Wiley-Liss, New York, pp. 249−290.

Levack PA, Mullen P, Anderson TJ, Miller WR, Forrest APM (1987) DNA analysis of breast tumour fine needle aspirates using flow cytometry. *Br. J. Cancer* **56**: 643−646.

Lincoln ST, Bauer KD (1989) Limitations in the measurement of c-myc oncoprotein and other nuclear antigens by flow cytometry. *Cytometry* **10**: 456−462.

Macartney JC, Camplejohn RS (1990) DNA flow cytometry of non-Hodgkin's lymphomas. *Eur. J. Cancer* **26**: 635−637.

Melamed MR, Staiano-Coico L (1990) Flow cytometry in clinical cytology. In: Melamed MR, Lindmo T, Mendelsohn ML, eds, *Flow Cytometry and Sorting,* 2nd edn. Wiley-Liss, New York, pp. 755−772.

Merkel DE, McGuire WL (1990) Ploidy, proliferative activity and prognosis. DNA flow cytometry of solid tumors. *Cancer* **65**: 1194−1205.

O'Reilly SM, Camplejohn RS, Barnes DM, Millis RR, Rubens RD, Richards MA (1990) Node negative breast cancer: prognostic subgroups defined by tumour size and flow cytometry. *J. Clin. Oncol.* **8**: 2040−2046.

Ormerod MG (1990) Analysis of DNA. In: Ormerod MG, ed., *Flow Cytometry: A Practical Approach.* IRL Press, Oxford, pp. 69−87.

Ormerod MG, Collins MKL, Rodriguez-Tarduchy G, Robertson D (1992) Apoptosis in interleukin-3-dependent haemopoietic cells: quantification by two flow cytometric methods. *J. Immunol. Methods* **153**: 57–65.

Pallavicini MG, Taylor IW, Vindelov LL (1990) Preparation of cell/nuclei suspensions from solid tumors for flow cytometry. In: Melamed MR, Lindmo T, Mendelsohn ML, eds, *Flow Cytometry and Sorting*, 2nd edn. Wiley-Liss, New York, pp. 187–194.

Petersen SE (1985) Flow cytometry of human colorectal tumors: nuclear isolation by detergent technique. *Cytometry* **6**: 452–460.

Quinn CM, Wright NA (1990) The clinical assessment of proliferation and growth in human tumours: evaluation of methods and applications as prognostic variables. *J. Pathol.* **160**: 93–102.

Schutte B, Reynders MMJ, Bosman FT, Blijham GH (1985) Flow cytometric determination of DNA ploidy level in nuclei isolated from paraffin-embedded tissue. *Cytometry* **6**: 26–30.

Silvestrini R, Daidone MG, Valagussa P, Di Fronzo G, Mezzanotte G, Bonadonna G (1989) Cell kinetics as a prognostic indicator in node-negative breast cancer. *Eur. J. Cancer* **25**: 1165–1171.

Taylor JH, Woods PS, Hughes WL (1957) The organization and duplication of chromosomes as revealed by autoradiographic studies using tritium labelled thymidine. *Proc. Natl Acad. Sci. USA* **43**: 122–128.

Telford WG, King LE, Fraker PJ (1991) Evaluation of glucocorticoid-induced DNA fragmentation in mouse thymocytes by flow cytometry. *Cell Proliferation* **24**: 447–459.

Van Dilla MA, Trujillo TT, Mullaney PF, Coulter JR (1969) Cell microfluorometry: a method for rapid fluorescence measurement. *Science* **163**: 1213–1214.

Vindelov LL, Christensen IJ (1990) A review of techniques and results obtained in one laboratory by an integrated system of methods designed for routine clinical flow cytometric DNA analysis. *Cytometry* **11**: 753–770.

Waggoner AS (1990) Fluorescent probes for cytometry. In: Melamed MR, Lindmo T, Mendelsohn ML, eds, *Flow Cytometry and Sorting*, 2nd edn. Wiley-Liss, New York, pp. 209–225.

Watson JV (1990) Nuclear associated antigens. In: Ormerod MG, ed., *Flow Cytometry: A Practical Approach*. IRL Press, Oxford, pp. 209–228.

Wilson GD, McNally NJ (1992) Measurement of cell proliferation using bromodeoxyuridine. In: Hall A, Levison DA, Wright NA, eds, *Assessment of Cell Proliferation in Clinical Practice*. Springer-Verlag, London, pp. 113–139.

Wilson GD, Camplejohn RS, Martindale CA, Brock A, Lane DP, Barnes DM (1992) Flow cytometric characterisation of proliferating cell nuclear antigen using monoclonal antibody PC10. *Eur. J. Cancer* **28A**: 2010–2017.

Wright NA, Appleton DR (1980) The metaphase arrest technique. A critical review. *Cell Tissue Kinet.* **13**: 643–663.

Zocchi MR, Marelli F, Poggi A (1990) Simultaneous cytofluorometric analysis for the expression of cytoplasmic antigens and DNA content in CD3⁻ human thymocytes. *Cytometry* **11**: 883–887.

Chapter 9
Chromosome Analysis and Sorting

L. S. CRAM

Introduction

Mitotic chromosomes can be isolated from plant and mammalian cells, stained with one or more fluorochromes and precisely analysed using flow cytometers. Most, if not all, chromosomes of many mammalian species can be rapidly and quantitatively resolved and separated into as many as 20 distinct populations through the use of one or more fluorescent probes. Both numerical and structural aberrations and shifts in DNA content as small as a few femtograms can be detected. Individual chromosome types can be sorted with high recovery and up to 95% purity.

Flow karyotype analysis, the analysis of a chromosome suspension in a flow cytometer, was first reported in 1975 (Gray *et al.*, 1975; Stubblefield *et al.*, 1975). Since then, further developments include improved instrument design for enhanced resolution (Gray and van den Engh, 1989), two-colour analysis (Langlois *et al.*, 1982), slit scanning (Cram *et al.*, 1985), high-speed sorting (Peters, 1989; Albright *et al.*, 1991), and numerous applications involving chromosome sorting for genome studies (Deaven *et al.*, 1986; Van Dilla *et al.*, 1986).

This chapter focuses on practical applications and the techniques required for pursuing those applications. Applications of flow karyotype analysis include analysing karyotype instability in cells undergoing spontaneous transformation (Cram *et al.*, 1983; Bartholdi *et al.*, 1986), determining the extent of chromosome damage resulting from ionizing radiation (Aten, 1989), identifying normal euploid chromosome(s) in somatic cell hybrids (Gray *et al.*, 1989), and confirming the numerical and structural aberrations suggested by banding analysis of clinical samples (McConnell *et al.*, 1989; Green *et al.*, 1989). Chromosome sorting has been used for gene mapping and is providing an essential capability for the Human Genome Project. Chromosome-specific libraries have been constructed in multiple vectors from sorted chromosomes. These libraries have been distributed to hundreds of research laboratories around the world.

Sample preparation is as important as the analysis and sorting, and it can greatly affect the results. For example, changes in isolation protocols may alter flow karyotype resolution and/or cloning efficiency. Careful evaluation of variables and the adaptation of chromosome-isolation procedures for banding analysis have led to current procedures; new techniques and applications are constantly being developed.

Cell culture, sample preparation and fluorescent staining

Chromosome suspensions prepared for flow karyotype analysis contain individual intact chromosomes, fluorescent nuclei and debris. When sorting chromosomes for cloning purposes, high molecular weight DNA must be maintained. Suitable chromosome preparations have been obtained from a variety of species (human, mouse, Chinese hamster, Indian muntjac, and pig, among others) and tissue sources (primary and established cell cultures, peripheral blood lymphocytes, amniocytes, bone marrow and somatic cell hybrids). Satisfactory procedures have not yet been developed for obtaining high-quality, single intact chromosomes directly from solid tumours.

Cell culture

The efficient production of mitotic cells is required to recover sufficient numbers of chromosomes for sorting experiments. When cells are grown under optimum conditions, they maintain exponential growth, which maximizes the number of mitotic cells in the culture. Although satisfactory preparations can be obtained from cells grown in suspension, monolayer cultures permit the selective recovery of mitotic cells; because mitotic cells round up, maintaining only minimal contact with the tissue culture flask, they can be shaken off the monolayer leaving non-mitotic cells behind. When metaphase-arresting agents such as colcemid are added to growth-synchronized cultures, the fraction of mitotic cells can be as high as 90–95%. However, mitotic indices as low as 5% have produced usable samples. The duration and concentration of colcemid treatment are often varied and depend on the cells' metabolic conditions and proliferation rate. The goal is to increase the proportion of mitotic cells while minimizing chromosome damage caused by hyper-condensation.

Chinese hamster cells with a 14-hour doubling time are maintained at subconfluency for several days and then split at a low split ratio (1:3–1:5). One or two cell divisions later, 0.05–0.1 µg colcemid per ml tissue culture media are added to each flask. After 3–4 hours, the mitotic cells are shaken off and the chromosomes isolated. Most euploid human cell lines growing in tissue culture have a doubling time between 20 and 30 hours. For these cells, 0.1 µg colcemid per ml are added for 12–15 hours. About 10^5 mitotic cells are required for optimum chromosome isolation. As little as 0.5 ml of human peripheral blood has been used to obtain high-quality bivariate flow karyotypes (McConnell *et al.*, 1991). Such specialized procedures require isolating lymphocytes, stimulating them with growth factors such as interleukin-2 (IL-2), and paying careful attention to details. Reproducible results are more easily achieved when 10^6-10^7 mitotic cells are available.

Sample preparation

Most chromosome isolation protocols include: (a) swelling the mitotic cells; (b) stabilizing the chromosomes; (c) disrupting the plasma membrane; and (d) labelling the DNA with one or more DNA-binding fluorochromes. A few laboratories have reported results of chromosome-protein labelling (Stohr *et al.*, 1980; Trask *et al.*, 1984). The preparation methods commonly used are designed to reduce the number of chromosome clumps and broken fragments and to maintain an equal representation of each chromosome type. Final concentrations are between 10^6 and 10^8 chromosomes per ml with concentrations at the higher end of this range preferred. Table 9.1 lists the three most commonly used methods for isolating chromosomes, each of which has its own advantages and variations for use in specific applications. The 'best' method is determined by its intended use: to isolate chromosomes for analysis, identification, or sorting and cloning.

Swelling the mitotic cells and disaggregating their chromosomes are the most critical steps. Hypotonic solutions, such as 50–75 mmol/l potassium chloride, swell the cells without prematurely permeabilizing their plasma membranes. Cell swelling can be easily monitored under

Table 9.1 Common chromosome-isolation buffers

Common name	Buffer components	Chromosome morphology	Protocol choice for:
Propidium iodide	KCl Triton-X-100 Propidium iodide* RNase	Excellent morphology Slightly extended	High resolution, one-colour analysis Fast and easy to reproduce
Magnesium sulphate	MgSO$_4$ Hepes Dithiothreitol RNase Triton-X-100	Slightly contracted Difficult to recognize	High resolution Flexible for different staining protocols Compatible with small sample size
Polyamine	Tris-HCl EDTA EGTA KCl Spermine* Spermidine* Digitonin Mercaptoethanol	Contracted Difficult to recognize	High-resolution, two-colour staining Maintains high molecular weight Method of choice for cloning procedures

* Designates purported stabilizing agent.

the microscope by observing the permeabilization and subsequent transport of propidium iodide (PI) across the lysed plasma membrane. Gradually swelling the cells before permeabilizing their membranes allows the individual chromosomes to disentangle and yields a suspension of well-separated single chromosomes.

Once the cells are swollen, a detergent is added to dissolve their membranes. At this step, chromosome structure must be stabilized. Adding low-ionic-strength divalent cations (calcium or magnesium), PI, or cationic polyamines to the cell suspension stabilizes the chromosomes. Although divalent cations are required for the binding of some fluorochromes (mithramycin and chromomycin), they facilitate nuclease action, which degrades the molecular weight of the sorted chromosomes (Trask, 1989). Chromosomes are next dispersed by either syringing or vortexing; if they do not readily disperse, additional physical force will only fragment the chromosomes and will not separate them further.

Fluorescent staining

PI, Hoechst 33258 (Ho258), and chromomycin A3 (CA3) are the most commonly used fluorochromes. Other options include mithramycin; 4′,6′-diamidino-2 phenylindole (DAPI); ethidium bromide; and, for staining heterochromatin, distamycin with DAPI (Meyne *et al.*, 1984). PI, when used alone, provides excellent resolution and DNA content analysis (Bartholdi *et al.*, 1986). Langlois's development of bivariate (two-colour) staining of human chromosomes (Langlois *et al.*, 1982) provided a breakthrough for resolving a larger number of human chromosome types than was previously possible. Because Ho258 preferentially binds to adenine−thymine ((AT))-rich regions and, similarly, CA3 to guanine−cytosine ((GC))-rich regions, the fluorescence of Ho258 plotted against that of CA3 provides a measure of the differences in the (AT):(GC) ratios between individual human chromosome types. Using this two-colour staining procedure, bivariate analysis of human chromosomes can resolve 18 of the 24 different human chromosome types.

The quality of a chromosome preparation is best determined using a flow cytometer. First, however, the samples should be examined under a microscope so that chromosome clumps and intact nuclei can be counted. High-quality preparations will have less than one nucleus or chromosome clump per field when viewed with a 40× neofluor objective. High-quality flow karyotypes can be characterized by the presence of well-resolved peaks, a minimal debris continuum underlying the peaks and at the origin, and very few events beyond the brightest chromosome peak. The number of nuclei will vary greatly and will depend on whether suspension or monolayer cultures were used.

Chromosome types from univariate or bivariate distributions can be identified by sorting chromosomes on to a microscope slide and then analysing them by Trypsin−Giemsa banding, fluorescent staining, or hybridization (directly on the slide) with chromosome-specific DNA probes. Banding analysis requires relaxing the tight chromosome com-

paction induced by most buffers; diluting the samples in hexylene
glycol or other buffers is sometimes used to loosen the structure of
tightly condensed chromosomes (Trask, 1989).

Instrumentation

Commercial flow cytometers designed for research applications (rather
than those designed for clinical use) are well suited for analysing and
sorting chromosomes. Figure 9.1 illustrates the principles of flow cytometric analysis. Stained chromosomes pass one at a time through one
or two focused laser beams that excite the fluorescent tag on the chromosome; the instrument detects the fluorescent pulse. The decision to sort
a particular chromosome is based on its fluorescent intensity or on the
ratio of its two intensities. Many factors influence the optimum configuration of a flow cytometry system, such as the chromosomes'
relatively dim fluorescence and small size, and the non-fluorescent
extracellular debris in the chromosome suspension.

An analysis of human chromosomes stained with one and two
fluorochromes is illustrated in Fig. 9.2. The univariate flow karyotype
was obtained with chromosomes stained with PI and the bivariate data
are chromosomes stained with Ho258 and CA3. Each peak contains one
or more different types of chromosomes. Chromosome 1 is well resolved,
whereas chromosomes 9 to 12, which are very similar in DNA content,
are all located within a single peak. Twelve to 16 populations of human
chromosomes can be resolved using PI staining. The interpretation of a
flow karyotype can be separated into three components: peak area,
peak intensity and the magnitude of the underlying continuum of
counts. Peak area is proportional to the number of chromosomes. Peak
intensity (brightness) is proportional to DNA content or, for bivariate
analyses, to the relative (AT)-to-(GC) richness. The magnitude of the
underlying continuum of counts is proportional to the amount of debris
in the sample; for irradiated cell populations, it has been used to
measure the extent of chromosome damage (Fantes et al., 1983; Aten,
1989). Additional peak descriptors include the skewness and the coefficient of variation (CV). Peaks consisting of a single chromosome type
should be symmetrical. The CV is a measure of the variability resulting
from both biological and instrumental sources (Holm and Cram, 1973).
All autosome peaks consisting of a single chromosome type will have
the same peak area, if the cell line contains no numerical aberrations
and if the peaks are well resolved. In the case of trisomy 21, the peak
will be three times as large as for single chromosomes (like X and Y)
and 50% again as large as peaks from autosomes.

One application of flow karyotype analysis is the quantitation of
structural and numerical aberrations. Changes in peak area resulting
from numerical aberrations can be detected when at least 10% of the
cells in the population are trisomic for a particular chromosome type.
Shifts in peak position due to structural changes such as insertions or
non-reciprocal translocations usually require a 5% increase or decrease

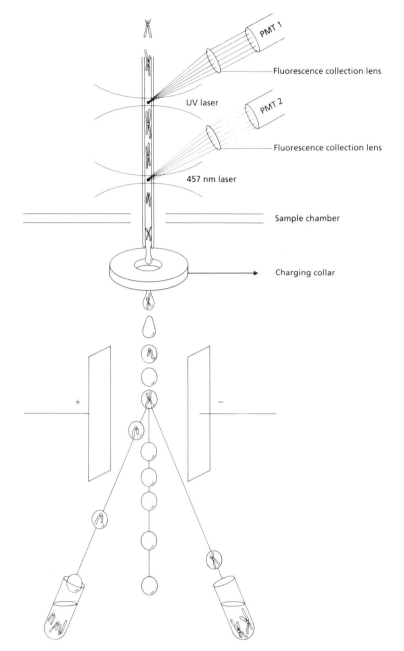

Fig. 9.1 Schematic illustration of a dual-beam chromosome sorter. Single chromosomes traverse first through an ultraviolet laser beam consisting of two laser lines (350 and 360 nm) that excite Hoechst 33258 and, second, through a laser tuned to 457 nm that excites chromomycin A3. The sample stream diameter is reduced to about one or two chromosome diameters (2–4 μm). The sample stream exit orifice diameter is 76 μm. Approximately one droplet out of 40 contains a chromosome. Chromosomes are collected in either silicone-coated tubes, distilled water or tubes containing low-melting-point agarose. Additional details about sorting are in Chapter 1.

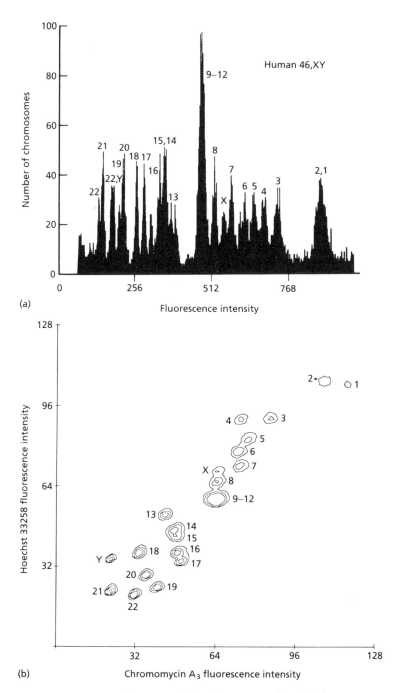

Fig. 9.2 Univariate (a) and bivariate (b) flow karyotypes of euploid human chromosomes. Individual chromosome types are labelled. (a) Chromosomes were isolated in 75 mmol/l potassium chloride and stained with PI. (b) Chromosomes were isolated in polyamine buffer, stained with Hoechst 33258 and chromomycin A3, and analysed as described by Bartholdi (1987).

in fluorescence to be resolved from the unmodified chromosome type. Many factors influence the detectability of structural changes and some changes such as reciprocal translocations cannot be detected by flow karyotype analysis.

Resolution

In contrast with flow cytometric analysis of surface antigens, in which the distributions are very broad and the CVs are often over 20%, flow karyotypes require optimum instrument resolution to resolve multiple populations. The CV of a flow karyotype of human chromosomes ranges from 1.5% for the largest chromosomes to 2.5% for the dim small chromosomes (Fig. 9.2). The CV is larger for the smaller, less-fluorescent chromosomes because they are 'light limited': the statistical variation (the uncertainty) in the number of photons emitted from the smallest chromosome, which contains five times less DNA than chromosome 1, is responsible for the increased CV.

For optimum fluorescent resolution to be achieved, the diameter of the sample stream must be as small as possible, which requires a high sample concentration. At 5×10^7 chromosomes per ml, the sample stream diameter can be reduced to 2−3 μm or even less and still maintain a reasonable count rate. A sample stream diameter about the same size as the chromosome's smallest dimension assures that each chromosome passes through the same region of the focused laser beam and does not drift off the central flow axis. Each chromosome therefore receives the same intensity of illumination. Laser power is important for two reasons: first, uniform light intensity can be maintained across the diameter of the sample stream and, second, at high excitation intensities, all the dye molecules are excited, reducing distributional broadening due to instability of the sample stream trajectory. In addition, low count rates generally improve resolution because the small stream diameter reduces the turbulence caused by nuclei and chromosome clumps passing through the viewing region.

Data acquisition

Linear amplifiers are usually used for flow karyotype analysis because logarithmic amplifiers are electronically less stable and are considered to be 'tricky little devils to work with' by the electronics community. When a logarithmic amplifier is used, the peak height is the same for all chromosome types that have the same number of copies (a peak for a single sex chromosome will be half as high as the peak of a diploid chromosome type and the width of each peak is constant, except for types of chromosomes that are 'light limited'). The resulting shape of the peaks is uniform, and the shape of the distribution appears analogous to the chromosome distribution in a banded karyotype. The type of amplifier used to generate the data does not affect the results; flow karyotypes obtained from both types of amplifiers contain the same essential information.

Electronically gating the fluorescence signal based on the light scatter signal has limited usefulness because of extracellular debris in the samples. Although debris is mostly non-fluorescent, it does scatter light: its heterogeneous size makes it difficult for researchers to distinguish where in the scattering distribution the scattering of small chromosomes leaves off and the scattering of large debris begins.

To modify a commercial flow cytometer so that it can analyse and sort chromosomes one should increase its laser power, match the sheath buffer to the sample buffer, reduce the diameter of the sample stream, select the optimum light filter(s), and align the instrument using fluorescent microspheres that are the same size as the objects being measured. Although PI-stained chromosomes can be excited with 50 mW of laser power, most research applications require 200–300 mW of both ultraviolet and 457 nm light. Matching the principal components of the sheath and sample buffers reduces the differences between their refractive indices and helps maintain chromosome morphology following sorting. An independently operated, motor-driven, non-pulsing syringe pump can produce a small enough sample stream diameter. When a syringe pump is used, the differential pressure control regulates only the sheath pressure. To assure that a maximum amount of the emitted fluorescence reaches the photomultiplier, optical filters must be carefully selected. A single long-pass filter is usually adequate for most systems, including those with two-laser excitation of Ho258 and CA3 in which extensive energy transfer occurs between the two dyes.

The optical and electronic arrangements used to analyse Ho258 and CA3 chromosome binding are considerably different in the Coulter (EPICS and Elite) and the Becton Dickinson (FACS and FACStar Plus) instruments. Becton Dickinson instruments use separate optical paths for the two signals, spatially separating the two emitted beams with a carefully positioned mirror. Coulter instruments take advantage of the energy transfer between the two fluorochromes: 70–80% of the Ho258 emission is absorbed by CA3 and re-emitted as CA3 fluorescence. The fluorochromes produce two signals that are separated in time by a factor proportional to the distance between the two laser beams. These signals have nearly equivalent emission wavelengths; the intensity of each is proportional to the concentration of one of the two fluorochromes. The two fluorescence signals are processed through the same optical path and use the same photomultiplier. A gated amplifier module delays the first signal by 7 μs, which aligns the two signals in time. Both commercial systems give equivalent resolution.

Univariate analysis

Univariate analysis is used primarily in research applications: monitoring karyotype instability (Kraemer *et al.*, 1987), detecting new marker chromosomes (Ray *et al.*, 1986a), analysing polymorphisms (Ray *et al.*, 1986b) and rapidly assessing progressive karyotype changes over long periods of time (Bartholdi *et al.*, 1987). Once the peaks of a flow karyotype have been identified, changes that occur as a result of spontaneous effects or of some type of insult can be easily monitored. For example, univariate flow karyotypes have been used to assay the cytogenetic heterogeneity of tumours arising from cells with a known karyotype.

The advantage of univariate analysis lies in its simplicity: simplicity in instrumentation, data collection and data analysis. Its versatility results from the elegant control a cell maintains over the highly reproducible amount of DNA in a chromosome (Cram *et al.*, 1989).

Single-fluorochrome staining is often used to analyse and sort chromosomes isolated from rodent cells, which contain less chromosome-to-chromosome variation in their (AT)-to-(GC) ratio than human chromosomes do. Figure 9.3 presents a univariate flow karyotype of Chinese hamster cells; in this plot, all 10 autosomes and the sex chromosomes are completely resolved. Human cells contain twice as many chromosome types (24) as Chinese hamster cells, which results in several peaks containing more than one chromosome type (Fig. 9.2).

Because of the high precision afforded by univariate analysis of chromosome DNA content, the technique has been used to detect and characterize chromosome polymorphisms that are as small as 0.15% of the Chinese hamster genome. Variations in DNA content between the two number 9 homologue chromosomes were shown to result from constitutive heterochromatin present on one or, in some cases, both

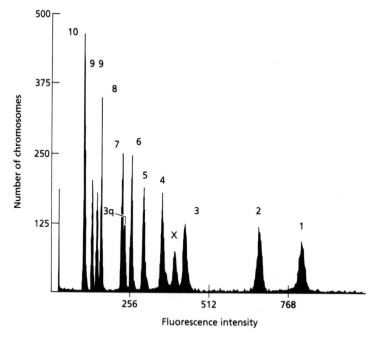

Fig. 9.3 Univariate flow karyotype of CCHE cells 16 passages after the culture was initiated from embryonic material. Chromosomes were isolated using hypotonic potassium chloride, stained with PI and analysed with the high-resolution flow karyotype flow cytometer at Los Alamos National Laboratory. One X chromosome and a marker chromosome (3q) are uniformly represented in most cells. The two 9 chromosome homologues are resolved as two separate peaks due to slightly different amounts of centromeric DNA.

homologues (Ray *et al.*, 1986b). These chromosomal polymorphisms were not previously detected by banding analysis. Similar polymorphisms have been measured in the human chromosomes known to contain more heterochromatin (1, 9, 15, 16 and Y). Additional applications of univariate analysis include measuring the cellular damage that results from radiation or chemical agents and assaying for karyotype instability.

To illustrate how a flow karyotype can quickly provide quantitative karyotype information, low-passage Chinese hamster cells initiated from embryonic tissue (CCHE cells) were injected into preimplanted surgical sponges in athymic mice at a stage when the cells were first becoming aneuploid (passage 28). The tumours from different animals were flow-karyotyped to determine their cytogenetic heterogeneity.

Figure 9.4 illustrates the karyotypes of both the cells that were injected (at passage 28) and two of the tumours that formed in the mice (after *in vivo* cell selection). The initial population of CCHE cells was nearly euploid and contained very few structural or numerical aberrations. The first signs of aneuploidy were an isochromosome 3q, an extra chromosome 6 (trisomy 6) and two marker chromosomes. Tumour 1 (T1) also contained two marker chromosomes and tumour 2 (T2), a deletion of chromosome 3 (3p⁻). When flow karyotypes from several tumours are compared, it is clear that there are very few, if any, common marker chromosomes in different tumours arising from the low-passage cells.

When the CCHE cells were carried in culture to high passage (passage 83) and then injected into the mice, they were found to be highly tumorigenic: tumours rapidly appeared. Furthermore, the flow karyotypes of the tumour cells were identical to those of the cells that were injected. The high-passage cells were less aneuploid than the low-passage cells; the high-passage cells contained fewer marker chromosomes and much less cell-to-cell karyotype heterogeneity. This example illustrates how a flow karyotype can provide quantitative karyotype information in a fraction of the time it takes to analyse a minimum of 50 banded-karyotypes for each of eight to 10 tumours.

Bivariate analysis

The advantage of bivariate analysis is the increased resolution achieved when two independent variables are measured. If the ratio of these variables varies within a population, then the subpopulations can be distinguished. Figure 9.2b illustrates the differences in the relative amounts of (AT) and (GC) base pairing in human chromosomes. A remarkable difference in Ho258 fluorescence can be observed in chromosomes 13–17; these five chromosomes are positioned almost vertically in a bivariate flow karyotype of Ho258 *vs* CA3. Although they have a relatively uniform amount of (GC)-rich regions, they have large variations in their numbers of (AT) base pairs. The reverse situation exists for chromosomes 1 and 2, which have equal numbers of (AT) base pairs and a significant difference in their numbers of (GC) base pairs.

When the data illustrated in Fig. 9.2b are plotted in three dimensions,

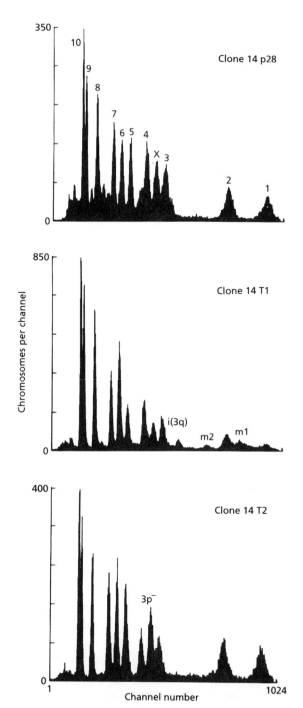

Fig. 9.4 Univariate flow karyotypes of clone 14 CCHE cells (see Fig. 9.3).
Chromosomes were isolated using hypotonic potassium chloride and stained with
PI. Passage 28 cells were injected into surgical sponges implanted in athymic mice.
Two of the resulting tumours (T1 and T2) were removed, the cells placed in short-
term culture, and the chromosomes isolated. Extensive karyotype instability occurs
during the several months between inoculation and tumour appearance. Intertumour
karyotype heterogeneity is easily detected by flow karyotype analysis. The so-called
marker chromosomes (m1, m2, i(3q), and 3p⁻, for example) differ in the two
tumours.

each population appears as a cone positioned on top of the underlying continuum of counts. (The axes on the plane of the page are the number of events caused by each fluorochrome — one fluorochrome on each axis; the third axis is the cumulative number of events at each coordinate.) Interpreting this type of data is complex; because the background continuum is spread in two dimensions, it is difficult to eliminate its effects when calculating the areas of the peaks. The karyotype information from bivariate distributions is analogous to that from univariate distributions.

Limitations of bivariate chromosome analysis include: (a) the problem of chromosome polymorphisms; and (b) the loss of intracellular information. Chromosome polymorphisms result from the inheritance of two homologues of slightly different DNA content. Such polymorphisms result either in an asymmetrically shaped peak or in two peaks, similar to what is shown for chromosome 14 in Fig. 9.5. As a result, interpreting small shifts in peak shape in clinical samples has limited usefulness unless prior analysis has been done on the patient's parents or on the same patient before karyotype instability began. Cell-to-cell cytogenetic heterogeneity is lost in flow karyotypes, since chromosomes isolated from all cells are mixed together.

Figure 9.5 illustrates a representative bivariate flow karyotype obtained from a patient with a 15;22 translocation [45,XX,rob t(15;22)].

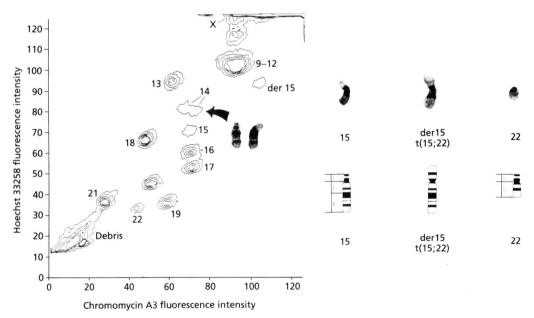

Fig. 9.5 Bivariate flow karyotype of peripheral lymphocytes from a female carrier with a 15;22 translocation [45,XX,rob t(15;22)]. The chromosomes were isolated in polyamine buffer and stained with Hoechst 33258 and chromomycin A3. The der 15 chromosome and the peaks for chromosomes 15 and 22 have volumes approximately one-half that of normal disomic peaks (such as the chromosome 19 peak). The two homologues of chromosome 14 contain slightly different amounts of satellite DNA, which results in a larger-than-normal contour area. An ideogram and a partially banded karyotype are to the right of the flow karyotype (McConnell, 1991).

Peripheral lymphocytes were obtained from 1 ml of blood and were stimulated with phytohaemagglutinin and/or IL-2 to obtain at least 50 000 mitotic cells. The chromosomes were isolated using polyamines and stained with Ho258 and CA3. The contour bivariate plot, a partial ideogram, and a banded karyotype are shown. Three distinct differences from a normal karyotype are noted: an extra peak, designated derivative (der) 15, is present; the chromosome 14 peak is unusually shaped; and the peaks for both chromosomes 15 and 22 are monosomic. The der 15 peak is monosomic and contains the t(15;22) chromosome. Chromosomes 15 and 22 lie to the right of a 45° line drawn through the bivariate distribution, indicating that they are (GC)-rich. The peaks for chromosomes 15 and 22 are monosomic, as expected, and the chromosome 14 peak, while disomic, is spread out much more than normal because of heteromorphic differences in the DNA content between the homologues inherited from the patient's two parents. Except for the slightly enlarged satellites on one of the banded chromosome 14s, the homologues do not appear significantly different.

DAPI and distamycin, when used together, preferentially stain the heterochromatin-rich regions of human chromosomes 1, 9, 15, 16 and Y. However, because this technique reduces the resolution of the remaining chromosome types, its application has been limited to sorting chromosome 9 from normal human chromosome preparations (Meyne *et al.*, 1984).

Chromosome sorting

Chromosome sorting dominates current flow cytogenetic applications. Sorted chromosomes are used for constructing chromosome-specific libraries and *in situ* hybridization probes and for mapping genes. Chromosome-specific libraries continue to expand as vectors capable of accepting larger and larger DNA inserts are developed. Vectors accepting small inserts are constructed using 100−200 ng of sorted chromosomes. At current cloning efficiencies, sorting for yeast artificial chromosomes requires 2−5 µg of sorted chromosomes (McCormick *et al.*, 1992).

Two important factors influencing chromosome sorting are sorting purity and chromosome recovery. As has already been discussed, sorting purity is directly affected by how well individual chromosome types can be resolved. In addition to enhancing the system's resolution, cooling the sample and sheath reservoirs and the recovery tube can improve system stability and, hence, sorting purity. Sorting purity can be determined by fluorescence *in situ* hybridization (FISH), by molecular characterization of individual libraries, or by mathematical analysis of the bivariate distributions. FISH involves hybridizing a fluorescently labelled chromosome-specific or species-specific probe to chromosomes sorted onto a coated microscope slide. This technique is particularly useful for analysing single human chromosomes isolated from somatic cell hybrids; researchers use species-specific probes to distinguish between the desired chromosomes (human) and any rodent (mouse or

Chinese hamster) contaminants. Sorting purity can be as high as 95%
when assayed by the FISH technique. The availability of directly labelled
chromosome-specific probes from Imagenetics and Integrated Genetics,
has simplified FISH. Techniques for generating 'reverse chromosome-
specific painting probes' using polymerase chain reaction (PCR) amplification of small numbers of sorted chromosomes have been described
by Carter *et al.* (1992) and Telenius *et al.* (1992).

Chromosome recovery is the number of chromosomes isolated from
a known number of mitotic cells. Recovery of chromosomes from the
sorter (post-sorting recovery), is the number of chromosomes recovered
following sorting *vs* the numbers of 'sorting events' processed by the
electronics. The number of chromosomes recovered from a known number of mitotic cells averages approximately 20%. Unfortunately, no one
has quantitatively determined where the remaining 80% are lost. Post-
sorting recovery averages approximately 80−90%.

Chromosome recovery depends on the stability of the system. Stability is hindered by: (a) clumps of nuclei and debris; (b) flow rate
fluctuations (caused by changing buffer levels in the sheath during long
sorting sessions); and (c) gradual laser power drift. Because temperature
fluctuations have a noticeable effect on chromosomes' fluorescence, the
temperatures of the sample and the sheath are carefully controlled. In
studies for which it is necessary to recover high molecular weight
DNA, polyamine buffer is preferred to magnesium sulphate buffer.
Sorting into low-melting-point agarose also helps maintain high molecular weight DNA. In the absence of divalent cations such as magnesium,
which increases nuclease activity, it is possible to recover DNA more
than 2 megabases long (McCormick *et al.*, 1992).

Analysis rates and sorting rates are closely linked to chromosome
concentration. Sample concentration is targeted to be at 10^7 chromosomes
per ml. Analysis rates are about 1200−1500 chromosomes per second,
which results in a sorting rate of 50 chromosomes per second when
chromosomes from a normal human euploid cell line are sorted. Between
1.0 and 1.5 million chromosomes can be sorted in a successful day.
Sorting rates from somatic cell hybrids will be somewhat higher because
of the larger fractional representation of the chromosome type being
sorted. Normal human euploid cells contain 24 different types of chromosomes (22 autosomes, X, and Y); therefore, for every 24 events analysed,
only one chromosome type will be sorted. Sorting rates equal analysis
rates only when 100% of the events being analysed are sorted − an
unrealistic situation to be sure.

Conclusions

Flow cytogenetics refers to the techniques and technologies necessary
to classify and purify mammalian chromosomes in a rapid and quantitative manner. These developments are helping us to better understand
karyotype instability and its role in carcinogenesis; to quantitate chromosome damage induced by ionizing radiation; to map genes; to construct

recombinant, chromosome-specific libraries; and to detect numerical and structural aberrations associated with certain genetic diseases.

Two instrumentation developments designed to improve chromosome sorting for the Human Genome Project that have not been discussed are high-speed sorting and slit scanning. By increasing the pressure and droplet-generation frequency, investigators have increased analysis and sorting rates by a factor of five (Peters, 1989; Albright *et al.*, 1991). Morphological information such as chromosome length and centromeric index can be measured in a flow cytometer using the slit-scanning technique (Lucas *et al.*, 1983; Bartholdi *et al.*, 1989). This procedure involves hydrodynamically stretching out chromosomes, focusing the laser beam to its diffraction limit, and recording the resulting waveform of each chromosome as it traverses the laser beam. This technique is useful for detecting dicentric chromosomes and chromosomes containing non-reciprocal translocations that have an altered centromeric index. Especially when combined with FISH on chromosomes prepared in suspension, slit-scanning analysis will become a powerful technology. So far no robust procedures have been developed that maintain chromosome morphology when DNA probes are hybridized to chromosomes in suspension.

As mentioned earlier, information on the chromosomes from individual cells is lost when suspensions of chromosomes from mitotic cells are analysed, Poletaev (1991) has described a system in which the chromosomes from single cells can be analysed; in this method, individual mitotic cells are introduced into a flow-based system and lysed just before they arrive at the laser intersection point.

Future developments in flow cytogenetics will include new probes for distinguishing chromosome types; faster sorting speeds through the use of non-droplet-based techniques, such as those being developed for cells by Herweijer *et al.* (1988); and new clinical applications that will integrate chromosome sorting with molecular biology techniques such as PCR. Reverse chromosome-specific painting as described by Carter *et al.* (1992) is already being routinely used in the clinical arena to identify the origin of translocated chromosome fragments. In this procedure, a few hundred chromosomes of unknown origin are sorted, amplified using a degenerative oligonucleotide primer and hybridized using FISH to yield a normal karyotype. Such advances will continue to be developed and will contribute to the growing importance of flow cytogenetics in both clinical and research applications.

Acknowledgement

The excellent technical editing assistance of Amy Reeves is gratefully acknowledged along with support from the Office of Health and Environmental Research of the US Department of Energy and the National Center for Research Resources of the NIH (RR01315).

References

Albright KL, Cram LS, Martin JC (1991) Separation techniques used to prepare highly purified chromosome populations: sedimentation, centrifugation, and flow sorting. In: Kompala DS, Todd P, eds, *American Chemical Society Symposium Series Cell Separation Science and Technology*. American Chemical Society, Washington DC, pp. 73–88.

Aten JA (1989) Relation between radiation-induced flow karyotype changes analyzed by Fourier analysis and chromosome aberrations. In: Gray JW, ed., *Flow Cytogenetics*. Academic Press, London, pp. 151–160.

Bartholdi MF, Travis GL, Cram LS, Porreca P, Leavitt J (1986) Flow karyology of neoplastic human fibroblast cells. *Ann. N. Y. Acad. Sci.* **468**: 339–349.

Bartholdi MF, Ray FA, Cram LS, Kraemer PM (1987) Karyotype instability of Chinese hamster cells during *in vivo* tumor progression. *Somatic Cell Mol. Genet.* **13**: 1–10.

Bartholdi MF, Meyne J, Johnston RG, Cram LS (1989) Chromosome banding analysis by slit scan flow cytometry. *Cytometry* **10**: 124–133.

Carter NP, Ferguson-Smith MA, Perryman MT *et al.* (1992) Reverse chromosome painting: A method for the rapid analysis of aberrant chromosomes in clinical cytogenetics. *J. Med. Genet.* **29**: 299–307.

Cram LS, Bartholdi MF, Ray FA, Travis GL, Kraemer PM (1983) Spontaneous neoplastic evolution of Chinese hamster cells in culture: Multistep progression of karyotype. *Cancer Res.* **43**: 4828–4837.

Cram LS, Bartholdi MF, Wheeless LL, Gray JW (1985) Morphological analysis by scanning flow cytometry. In: Van Dilla MA, Dean PN, Laerum OD, Melamed MR, eds, *Flow Cytometry Instrumentation and Data Analysis*. Academic Press, London, pp. 163–194.

Cram LS, Bartholdi MF, Ray FA, Cassidy M, Kraemer P (1989) Univariate flow karyotype analysis. In: Gray JW, ed., *Flow Cytogenetics*. Academic Press, London, pp. 113–133.

Deaven LL, Van Dilla MA, Bartholdi MF *et al.* (1986) Construction of human chromosome-specific DNA libraries from flow-sorted chromosomes. In: *Cold Spring Harbor Symposium on Quantitative Biology*. Cold Spring Harbor Laboratory of Quantitative Biology, Cold Spring Harbor, Long Island, New York, pp. 159–168.

Fantes JA, Green DK, Elder JK, Malloy P, Evans HJ (1983) Detecting radiation damage to human chromosomes by flow cytometry. *Mutat. Res.* **119**: 161–168.

Gray JW, van den Engh GJ (1989) Instrumentation for chromosome analysis and sorting in flow cytogenetics. In: Gray JW, ed., *Flow Cytogenetics*. Academic Press, London, pp. 17–32.

Gray JW, Carrano LL, Steinmetz MA *et al.* (1975) Chromosome measurement and sorting by flow systems. *Proc. Natl Acad. Sci. USA* **72**: 1231–1234.

Gray JW, van den Engh GJ, Trask BJ (1989) Bivariate flow karyotyping. In: Gray JW, ed., *Flow Cytogenetics*. Academic Press, London, pp. 137–149.

Green DK, Fantes JA, Evans JH (1989) Detection of randomly occurring aberrant chromosomes as a measure of genetic change. In: Gray JW, ed., *Flow Cytogenetics*. Academic Press, London, pp. 161–170.

Herweijer H, Stokdijk W, Visser JW (1988) High speed photodamage cell selection using bromo-deoxyuridine/Hoechst 33342 photosensitive cell killing. *Cytometry* **9**: 143.

Holm DM, Cram LS (1973) An improved flow microfluorometer for rapid measurements of cell fluorescence. *Exp. Cell Res.* **94**: 464–468.

Kraemer PM, Ray FA, Bartholdi MF, Cram LS (1987) Spontaneous *in vitro* neoplastic evolution: Selection of specific karyotype in Chinese hamster cells. *Cancer Genet. Cytogenet.* **27**: 273–287.

Langlois RG, Yu LC, Gray JW, Carrano AV (1982) Quantitative karyotyping of human chromosomes by dual beam flow cytometry. *Proc. Natl Acad. Sci. USA* **79**: 7876–7880.

Lucas JN, Gray JW, Peters DC, Van Dilla MA (1983) Centromeric index measurement by slit-scan flow cytometry. *Cytometry* **4**: 109–116.

McCormick MK, Campbell E, Deaven L, Moyzis R (1992) Non-chimeric yeast artificial chromosome libraries from flow sorted human chromosomes 16 and 21. *Proc. Natl Acad. Sci. USA* **90**: 1063–1067.

McConnell TS, Cram LS, Baczek N, Fawcett JJ, Luedemann ML, Bartholdi MF (1989) The clinical usefulness of chromosome analysis by flow cytometry. *Semin. Diagn. Pathol.* **6**: 91–107.

McConnell TS, Fawcett JJ, Baczek NA, Cram LS (1991) Chromosome analysis by flow cytometry. *Appl. Cytogenet.* **17**: 1–4.

Meyne J, Bartholdi MF, Travis G, Cram LS (1984) Counterstaining human chromosomes for flow karyology. *Cytometry* **5**: 580–583.

Peters DC (1989) Chromosome purification by high-speed sorting. In: Gray JW, ed., *Flow Cytogenetics*. Academic Press, London, pp. 211–224.

Ray FA, Bartholdi MF, Kraemer PM, Cram LS (1986a) Spontaneous *in vitro* neoplastic evolution: Recurrent chromosome changes of newly immortalized Chinese hamster cells. *Cancer Genet. Cytogenet.* **21**: 35–51.

Ray FA, Bartholdi MF, Kraemer PM, Cram LS (1986b) Chromosome polymorphism involving discrete heterochromatic blocks in Chinese hamster number nine chromosome. *Cytogenet. Cell Genet.* **38**: 257.

Stohr M, Hutter KJ, Frank M, Futterman G, Goerttler K (1980) A flow cytometric study of chromosomes from rat kangaroo and Chinese hamster cells. *Histochemistry* **67**: 179–190.

Stubblefield E, Cram S, Deaven L (1975) Flow microfluorometric analysis of isolated Chinese hamster chromosomes. *Exp. Cell Res.* **94**: 464–468.

Telenius H, Pelmear AH, Tunnacliffe A *et al.* (1992) Cytogenetic analysis by chromosome painting using degenerate oligonucleotide-primed-polymerase chain reaction amplified flow-sorted chromosomes. *Genes Chromosomes Cancer* **4**: 1–7.

Trask B (1989) Chromosome isolation procedures. In: Gray JW, ed., *Flow Cytogenetics*. Academic Press, London, pp. 43–60.

Trask B, van den Engh G, Gray J, Vanderlann M, Turner B (1984) Immunofluorescent detection of histone 2B on metaphase chromosomes using flow cytometry. *Chromosoma* **90**: 295–302.

Van Dilla MA, Deaven LL, Albright KL *et al.* (1986) Human chromosome-specific DNA libraries: Construction and availability. *Bio/Technology* **4**: 537–552.

Chapter 10
Developing Techniques

M. G. MACEY

Introduction

The use of flow cytometry to measure cell surface antigens, DNA and RNA content and chromosomal analysis and sorting are now well-established techniques. In this chapter a number of other techniques employing flow cytometry will be discussed. These include bioassays for cell-mediated cytotoxicity, measurement of multidrug resistance (MDR), hybridoma analysis, *in situ* hybridization, *in vivo* studies of cell migration and detection and analysis of bacteria and parasites.

Bioassays for cell-mediated cytotoxicity

Cytotoxicity is one of the major effector functions of cell-mediated immunity. Two major types of cell-mediated cytotoxicity have been described. First, that mediated by major histocompatibility complex (MHC) restricted cytotoxic T lymphocytes (CTL; Hubbard *et al.*, 1990); and second that mediated by non-MHC restricted natural killer (NK) and lymphokine-activated killer (LAK) cells (Trinchieri, 1989). Assays for measuring cell-mediated cytotoxicity usually involve the incubation of target cells with effector cells, at various target:effector ratios for several hours. The degree of target lysis or death is then determined. Single cell cytotoxicity may be measured by tryphan blue dye exclusion using microscopy (Bonavida *et al.*, 1983). This is, however, subjective and after a short period of time the dye itself becomes cytotoxic. Alternatively target cells may be labelled with radioactive chromium (^{51}Cr), incubated with effector cells and the release of ^{51}Cr from the target cells measured. However, this also has its limitations (Pross *et al.*, 1986), notably the need to use a radioactive compound.

In 1986 McGinnes *et al.* described a fluorescence NK assay using flow cytometry. In this assay the target cells were labelled with carboxyfluorescein diacetate (c′FDA) in place of radioactive chromium. The dye c′FDA is a non-fluorescent, non-polar fatty acid ester that is membrane permeable and so easily enters the cell. In the cytoplasm the c′FDA is hydrolysed by esterases to produce free polar carboxy fluorescein, a fluorescent compound which due to its polarity is retained within the cell. Thus only viable cells with intact enzyme systems and cell membranes are capable of fluorescence when labelled with c′FDA. The fluorescence intensity of c′FDA labelled cells has been shown to be linearly proportional to dye content (Persidsky and Baillie, 1977). The fact that viable cells fluoresce while dead cells do not is the basis of the use of c′FDA in viability assays (Ross *et al.*, 1989a).

Fluorescence NK assay

1 A working solution of c′FDA (Molecular Probes) is prepared by diluting 7.5 µl of a stock solution (20 mg/ml in acetone, stored at −20°C) in 1 ml Hank's balanced salt solution calcium and magnesium free (HBSS⁻) to give a final concentration of 150 µg/ml. The working solution should be used within 15 min to avoid flocculation.

2 After two washes in HBSS⁻, target cells (K562) are labelled with c′FDA by resuspending to 1 ml in the working solution and incubated at 37°C for 10 min.

3 The cells are then washed three times in ice-cold (4°C) HBSS⁻ containing 1% bovine serum albumin (BSA) (Sigma) and resuspended in RPMI1640 supplemented with 10% fetal calf serum (FCS) (ICN Biomedicals) to a concentration of 2×10^5/ml.

4 Target cells (2×10^4/ml) are incubated with effectors (peripheral blood mononuclear cells prepared by Ficoll-Paque density centrifugation, see Chapter 3) in 200 µl RPMI1640-FCS in 5 ml round bottom polystyrene tubes (Bibby) at a range of target to effector ratios. A ratio of 1 : 25 gives consistent results.

5 The cells are centrifuged together (200 g for 5 min) to enhance conjugate formation, then incubated at 37°C for 1 hour.

6 Following incubation the cells are filtered through 30 µm nylon mesh, then held on ice prior to flow cytometric analysis.

7 Control target cells are incubated in parallel in medium alone to monitor spontaneous leakage of c'FDA during incubation.
8 Targets may be distinguished from effectors on the basis of their light scattering properties when analysed by forward and 90° light scatter. Target cells (K562) are considerably larger and more granular than effector cells.
9 Target killing by effectors is measured by determining the fluorescence of the targets examined under standard conditions at 488 nm. The log green fluorescence associated with the cells is measured and specific lysis of the targets is determined by:

$$\% \text{ specific lysis} = \frac{CT - TE}{CT} \times 100$$

where CT = mean number of fluorescent target cells in control samples and TE = mean number of fluorescent target cells in target + effector samples.

This assay compares favourably with the conventional ^{51}Cr release assay; however, it has several advantages. First, it may be used at lower target : effector ratios. Second, it is more sensitive and requires a shorter (1 hour) target/effector incubation period compared with the radioactive assay (3–4 hours). Third, it may be adapted for use in a cell-free cytotoxicity assay in which target cells (L929) are incubated with tumour necrosis factor (TNF)-α instead of effector cells (Macey *et al.*, 1992). In this assay there is a bell-shaped dose–response curve to TNF in the range 25–125 pg/ml (Fig. 10.1). The effect of TNF is abrogated by anti-TNF and in culture supernatants the per cent lysis has been found to correlate with the amount of TNF present as determined by enzyme-linked immunosorbent assay (ELISA) (Fig. 10.2).

An alternative method for the flow cytometric evaluation of cell-mediated cytotoxicity has been described by Jacobs and Pipho (1983)

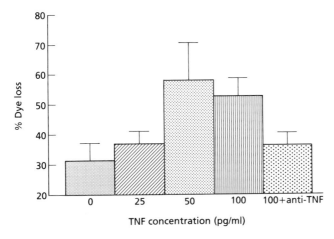

Fig. 10.1 Dose–response curve for TNF α-mediated cytotoxicity of L929 cells.

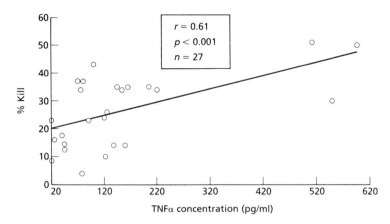

Fig. 10.2 Correlation between TNF α-concentration (pg/ml) and cell cytotoxicity.

and Zarcone *et al*. (1986). In this assay non-viable target cells, following their interaction with effector cells, are identified by exclusion of the dye propidium iodide and expressed as a percentage of the total target cell population. The target cell population is distinguished from the effectors by difference in volume and light scattering properties as in the assay above. In this study the distinction between a single cell cytotoxicity assay (SCCA) and total cell cytotoxicity assay (TCCA) is made. For cell-mediated cytotoxicity target−effector conjugate formation must occur. Following delivery of a lethal hit to the target (SCCA), the effector is freed and under appropriate conditions binds to and kills other targets (TSSA). This is termed effector cell recycling (Bonavida *et al.*, 1983).

SCCA method

1 Effector cells $(2 \times 10^9/l)$ are mixed with target cells $(5 \times 10^9/l;$ effector : target ratio $= 40:1)$ and centrifuged at $200\,g$ for 7 min.
2 The cell pellet is incubated for 10 min at 37°C to allow conjugate formation then gently resuspended in RPMI1640 supplemented with 10% FCS at a concentration of 5×10^4 cells/ml. This prevents recycling (Velardi *et al.*, 1985).
3 Cell suspensions are incubated at 37°C for 1−4 hours, centrifuged and the cell pellet maintained on ice until stained with propidium iodide and analysed by flow cytometry.

TCCA method

1 Effector cells and target cells are mixed at effector : target ratios ranging from 40:1 to 2.5:1 in 200 µl RPMI1640-FCS in 96 well U-bottom microtitre plates.
2 The plates are centrifuged for 1 min at $200\,g$ and the cell pellets incubated for 1−4 hours at 37°C.
3 The cells are then resuspended and washed with medium and the cell pellet kept on ice until stained and analysed.

Cell viability

To determine the cell viability of the target cells, cell pellets are resuspended in propidium iodide (Sigma) at a final concentration of 40 µg/ml in phosphate-buffered saline (PBS). Target cells are identified by their light scatter properties on dual parameter plots of forward angle and 90° light scatter. The number of red fluorescent (590 nm) cells within this population is then determined. Controls for background cell death are provided by analysis of target cells incubated in the absence of effector cells, at the same concentration as the test populations.

This assay again compares favourably with ^{51}Cr release assays and may be used for analysis in both the SCCA and TCCA. A modification of this assay has been reported by Slezak and Horan (1989) in which two fluorochromes are employed. One fluorochrome, PKH-1, is used to distinguish target cells from effectors and propidium iodide is used to measure target cell lysis. The combination of two fluorochromes allows the distinction of four populations in a given sample. The per cent cytotoxicity may be calculated together with the enumeration of the effector to target ratio. Also the viability of the effector population may be determined and phenotypic analysis of the effector population may be made. In long-term cytotoxicity assays it is possible to monitor cytostasis of target cells.

PKH-1 labelling of target or effector cells

1 PKH-1 (Zynaxis Cell Science) is a fluorescent lipophilic dye which is stably incorporated and retained in the plasma membrane of labelled cells. It has an excitation wavelength of 488 nm and emits at 525 nm.
2 For labelling either effector or target cells, $1-5 \times 10^6$ cells/ml are incubated with PKH-1 at a final concentration of 5 µmol/l.
3 After 10 min an equal volume of assay medium is added to the cells which are centrifuged at 300 g then washed four times with 10−20 ml assay medium.
4 The cells are then resuspended to a final concentration of 1×10^5 cell/ml for target cells and 5×10^6 cells/ml for effector cells.
5 The target and effector cells are then incubated together at a range of target : effector ratios for 1−4 hours at 37°C.
6 After incubation, propidium iodide (stock 5 mg/ml in PBS, Sigma) is added for identification of dead cells.
7 The cells are then analysed by flow cytometry. The green fluorescence associated with PKA-1 is measured at 525 nm and the red fluorescence of propidium iodide is measured above 590 nm.
8 For each sample the log green *vs* log red histograms are analysed.

Continued on page 260

This allows analysis of live and dead target cells together with live and dead effector cell populations. If for example the target cells are labelled with PKA-1 then live targets will be green only; dead targets will be green and red; live effectors will be non-fluorescent while dead effectors will be red only.

This method also has been shown to compare with ^{51}Cr release assays and has the advantage that either effector or target cells may be labelled and the actual live effector cell to target cell ratio can be calculated.

Alternative procedures

Mitochondrial dehydrogenase activity may also be used as a test of cytotoxicity. This assay relies on reduced nicotinamide adenine dinucleotide (NADH)-dependent dehydrogenase activity to reduce the substrate 3-(4,5-dimethylthiazolyl-2-yl)-2,5-diphenyltetrazolium bromide (MMT). This enzymic reaction produces dark blue granules of formazan, which increase cell refringency that may be detected as a change in 90° light scatter (Huet *et al.*, 1992).

The MTT assay was originally described, along with other tetrazolium salts, for use in assays to determine its coupling with the respiratory chain, and it has been used to study lactate, malate and succinate dehydrogenase activities in mitochondria (Lippold, 1982). These properties have been applied to the study of cell activation and proliferation (Niks *et al.*, 1990), viability (Green *et al.*, 1984) and cytotoxicity (Carmicheal *et al.*, 1987).

MTT assay

1 Stimulated and unstimulated cells (1×10^6/ml; e.g. by cytokines, cytotoxic factors or mitogens) are incubated for 3 hours at 37°C with MTT at a final concentration 0.6 mmol/l then analysed by flow cytometry at 4°C.
2 The 90° light scatter at 488 nm is determined to follow cell refringency increases due to MTT reduction.
3 Forward angle light scatter is used to detect cells according to size and cell subpopulations may be identified by fluorochrome-labelled antibodies.

Analysis of CTL, NK and LAK target conjugates

In the past few years a number of investigators have reported that flow cytometry can be used to enumerate lymphocyte target conjugates involving CTL (Perez *et al.*, 1985), NK (Storkus *et al.*, 1986) and LAK (Roberts and Lotze, 1988). A technique to identify the effector cell subtypes involved in target conjugation has been described, but requires dual laser excitation (Vitale *et al.*, 1991, 1992). For single laser techniques target cells are labelled with the red dye hydroethidine (HE), which does not significantly influence their conjugation with or lysis by the effector cells. HE is converted to ethidium within cells, which then intercalates into DNA (Luce *et al.*, 1985). Surface labelling of effector cells may influence their interaction with the target. However, the cytoplasmic fluorochrome, calcein, does not alter effector — target conjugation. The acetoxymethyl ester of calcein (Calcein-AM) is hydrolysed by intracellular esterases to highly polar calcein, which does not appear to react with intracellular components and is retained for several hours.

Assay procedure

1 Mononuclear cells in peripheral blood anticoagulated with heparin are isolated by Ficoll-Paque gradient centrifugation (see Chapter 3).
2 The cells are washed with RPMI1640, resuspended in medium, then incubated on polystyrene culture dishes for 1 hour at 37°C.
3 Non-adherent cells are removed (>98% lymphocytes) for use in subsequent assays alone (NK) or with interleukin (IL)-2 activation (LAK).
4 For IL-2 activation, lymphocytes are cultured in RPMI1640 supplemented with 20% FCS and 600−1000 IU/ml recombinant IL-2 (Cetus) for 24−48 hours at 37°C in an atmosphere of 5% CO_2.

Conjugate formation assay

1 Effector cells (NK, LAK) are washed three times in RPMI1640 at 4°C, then resuspended in 1 ml PBS containing 1% BSA, pH 7.4, and incubated with Calcein-AM (acetoxymethyl ester of calcein, Molecular Probes) for 1 hour at a final concentration of 1 μg/ml.
2 Target cells (K562 for NK effectors, Daudi for LAK effectors) are labelled with HE (Molecular Probes) in PBS-1% BSA at a final concentration of 40 μg/ml for 1 hour.
3 After labelling both target and effector cells are washed three times with ice-cold PBS and resuspended in PBS containing 5 nmol/l $MgCl_2$ and 1 mmol/l EGTA (Sigma) at 4°C.
4 Conjugate formation is performed by mixing effector and target cells at a ratio of 1:1. The cells are centrifuged at 100 g for 3 min in round bottom tubes, then incubated at 37°C for 10 min.
5 The cells are resuspended in ice-cold medium and held on ice until analysed. These conditions result in optimal conjugation for E:T = 1:1 with over 90% of conjugates involving one lymphocyte and one target (Storkus *et al.*, 1986). The conjugates are stable for at least 30 min after resuspension.
6 Conjugates and unconjugated cells are analysed by dual colour

Continued on page 262

fluorescence flow cytometry. The percentage of cells conjugated is determined by:

Total number of dual fluorescent positive cells
Total number of green and red fluorescent cells

This method has been shown to correlate very well with standard microscopic techniques (Callewaert *et al.*, 1991).

Clinical significance

Recently, a number of studies of NK cell function in a variety of disease states have been reported. NK cell function has been found to be reduced following allogeneic small bowel transplantation (Tice, 1992); during HIV infection (Lane, 1992); during hypothermia (Yang *et al.*, 1990); and in patients with anorexia nervosa (Schattner *et al.*, 1990), common variable immune deficiency (Duarte *et al.*, 1990), xeroderma pigmentosa (Mariani *et al.*, 1992), primary IgA nephropathy (Antonaci *et al.*, 1992) and primary Sjögren's syndrome (Oxholm *et al.*, 1992). Increased function has also been described during anaesthesia (Hseuh *et al.*, 1992) and in patients with Down's syndrome (Morale *et al.*, 1992), Behçet's disease (Suzuki *et al.*, 1992) and autoimmune thyroid disease (Hidaka *et al.*, 1992). These findings suggest that NK cells play an important role in the control of disease activity and their function requires further investigation.

Measurement of MDR

MDR is a major problem in the treatment of cancer (Deuchars and Ling, 1989; Rothenberg and Ling, 1989) and haematological malignancies (Chaudhury and Roninson, 1991; Jiang *et al.*, 1991; Haber, 1992; Berman and McBride, 1992). Many patients develop resistance to the drugs used in treatment of their condition. This resistance is often effective against a range of chemotherapeutic agents, hence the term multidrug resistance. During the past 10 years the mechanisms underlying the development of MDR have become better understood (Beck, 1990; Hayes and Wolf, 1990). MRD is multifactorial and is the result of decreased intracellular drug accumulation. This is partly due to the presence of a 170 kD plasma membrane protein now termed *p*-glycoprotein. This glycoprotein has been shown to be an energy-dependent efflux pump which has increased expression on drug-resistant cells (Gerlach *et al.*, 1986b). Its presence allows cells to efflux molecules faster than they influx, thus in the case of chemotherapeutic agents they do not accumulate within the cell.

The presence of *p*-glycoprotein may be determined in a number of ways. First, the presence of the *mdr*-genes may be identified by Southern blotting (Kane *et al.*, 1990); however, not all these genes have the ability to produce the multidrug-resistant phenotype (Hayes and Wolf, 1990). Second, the presence of p-glycoprotein may be identified by monoclonal antibodies (MoAbs) (Krishan *et al.*, 1991). Problems also exist with regard to the correlation of p-glycoprotein analysis and *in vivo* resistance profiles. This may be due to the fact that most of the p-glycoprotein molecule resides in the plasma membrane and only a small part is on the cell surface. Thus assays may not be sufficiently sensitive to detect p-glycoprotein expression. Also some commercially available antibodies have been found to cross-react with the heavy chain of myosin and with other proteins containing adenosine triphosphate (ATP) binding sites as well as several types of non-malignant cells (Thiebaut *et al.*, 1989), including normal bone marrow cells (Noonan *et al.*, 1990). For these reasons techniques have been developed to measure the functional ability of cells to efflux drugs (Ross *et al.*, 1988, 1989a; Herweijer *et al.*, 1989; Gheuens *et al.*, 1991).

The measurement and analysis of drug influx and efflux using radio-isotope labelled drugs are technically difficult (Gerlach *et al.*, 1986a). However, the anthracyclines such as doxarubicin and daunorubicin which are commonly used in chemotherapy (Young *et al.*, 1981) are intrinsically fluorescent (Krishan and Ganapathi, 1980). The cellular fluorescence intensity may therefore be used as a measure of drug accumulation and hence sensitivity. Daunorubicin and adriamycin can be excited at 488 nm and have maximum emission at 585 nm; they are therefore ideal for use with standard flow cytometers.

Drug uptake and efflux assay

1 Cells to be studied (leukaemic blasts, multidrug-resistant cell lines and normal drug-sensitive cells) are washed twice with HBSS (with Ca^{2+} and Mg^{2+} but without phenol red) then resuspended in the same to a final concentration of 5×10^5/ml.

2 For drug uptake, the cells are incubated with daunorubicin (Sigma) (0.25 µg/ml final concentration) at 37°C and samples are removed at intervals (0–180 min) and the intracellular drug saturation level (SL) measured by determining the fluorescence intensity by flow cytometry.

3 To measure efflux the cells are incubated with daunorubicin for 60 min, washed in ice-cold HBSS, resuspended and assayed as above.

4 A plot of fluorescence intensity (mean channel fluorescence plotted against time) shows the relative uptake and efflux of different cells (Figs 10.3 and 10.4).

The uptake and efflux of daunorubicin by sensitive and resistant cells is multicomponent (Luk and Tannock, 1989); however, the time (in min) to reach 90% saturation level (SL90) can be used as a measure

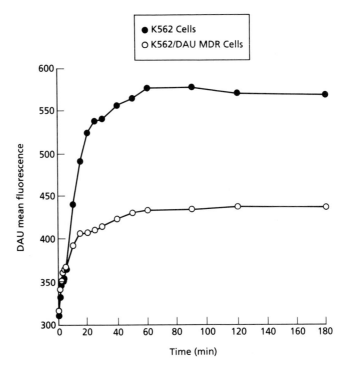

Fig. 10.3 Daunorubicin (DAU) uptake by drug-sensitive and drug-resistant K562 cell lines.

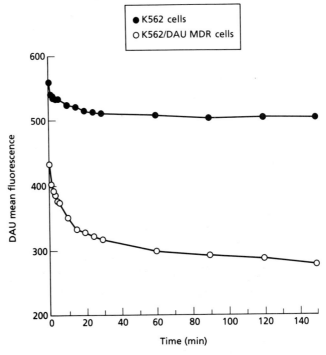

Fig. 10.4 Daunorubicin (DAU) efflux by drug-sensitive and drug-resistant K562 cell lines.

of the rate of drug accumulation. The effect of metabolic inhibitors such as azide (10 mmol/l final concentration) in the presence or absence of glucose (10 nm) may be examined (Table 10.1).

The frequency of drug-resistant cells in human neoplasia may be less than 0.1%. Thus uptake and efflux studies in these situations would not be possible. Ross et al. (1989b) considered the predictive value of intracellular daunorubicin content in distinguishing multidrug-resistant cells. They examined the effect of cell volume on intracellular daunorubicin content and showed that heterogeneity of cell volume did account for some variance of measured intracellular daunorubicin content and the predictive value of the assay was improved when intracellular daunorubicin was normalized for cell volume. However, volume normalization is still limited in accuracy in detecting resistant cell frequencies less than 0.1%. Therefore the measurement of p-glycoprotein expression and cellular daunorubicin content has been suggested to enhance the predictive value of flow cytometry for detecting multidrug-resistant cells. This was studied by Gheuens et al. (1991) in an ovarian carcinoma cell line. The expression of p-glycoprotein was detected by fluorescein isothiocyanate (FITC) indirect labelling and mean channel fluorescence was measured for daunorubicin content. Daunorubicin dim and p-glycoprotein highly positive cells were considered to be multidrug resistant. The method was found to be satisfactory for analysis of clinical samples with high numbers of malignant cells but was not used to detect minimal residual disease.

The dye rhodamine 123 (Rh123) has also been used to examine drug uptake. Rh123 preferentially accumulates in mitochondrial membranes; its uptake has been shown to correlate with p-glycoprotein expression (Chaudhury and Roninson, 1991). These authors also showed the CD34[+] cells within normal bone marrow express high levels of p-glycoprotein and had reduced accumulation of Rh123.

In addition to rapid drug efflux, glutathione (GSH)-dependent cellular detoxification and altered DNA topoisomerase II activity may also contribute to cellular anthracycline resistance. Nair et al. (1991) have developed a flow cytometric assay to measure GSH content in relation to drug resistance. Monochlorobimine (MBCL, Molecular Probes) was

Table 10.1 Multidrug resistance: metabolic and kinetic studies

	Controls mean (n = 7)		With azide (n = 3)		With azide and glucose (n = 3)	
	SL	SL90	SL	SL90	SL	SL90
K562_{Sensitive}	536	14.9	521	16.8	504	14.0
K562_{Resistant}	432	3.9	430	23.5	370	0.6
CEM_{Sensitive}	535	30.4	478	22.0	481	22.0
CEM_{Resistant}	417	15.1	421	22.0	363	10.0

SL, saturation level, maximum fluorescence intensity; SL90, time (in minutes) to reach 90% saturation level.

used as the fluorochrome to quantitate cellular GSH content. MBCL is excited at 351–364 nm and has maximum emission at 465–505 nm. Thus analysis of MBCL content and daunorubicin retention requires a dual laser flow cytometer. Although this assay allows analysis of two parameters of drug resistance, caution must be exercised when interpreting the results because GSH-MBCL staining may be influenced by GSH activity and the presence of other sulph-hydryl groups.

Fluorescent *in situ* hybridization

In 1969 Gall and Pardue introduced the technique of *in situ* hybridization. Since then its use has been refined and developed (Harris and Wilkinson, 1990; Lichter and Ward, 1990; Mitchell *et al.*, 1992) but perhaps the most exciting development has been that of flow cytometric analysis of fluorescent *in situ* hybridization in cells in suspension.

The basis of the *in situ* hybridization technique depends on the specific genetic code that lies within all nucleated cells. Nucleic acids (DNA and RNA) are the 'substrate' of this code, and by virtue of their particular purine (guanine, adenine) and pyrimidine (cytosine, thymine) base composition, every type of protein synthesized by a prokaryotic or eukaryotic cell can be specified. In protein synthesis, RNA molecules are transcribed which are complementary to one strand of the uncoiled DNA molecules in the nucleus. This cleaves from the DNA and passes to a ribosome in the cytoplasm where translation into protein occurs. By applying specially synthesized and labelled (by fluorochrome or radio-isotope) DNA, RNA or oligonucleotide molecules (probes) to a section containing target nucleic acids immobilized (by fixation) in a tissue section, cell smear or cells in suspension, under appropriate (stringent) conditions, complementary binding of the labelled nucleic acids (hybridization) occurs. This enables the presence or absence of the target to be determined. There are a number of factors that should be considered: (a) the preservation and processing of tissue and target; (b) the type of probe used; (c) the probe labelling methodology; (d) the hybridization conditions; and (e) detection of the hybridization. Ideally, cells should be fixed by cross-linking agents such as formaldehyde, oligonucleotide probes should be used, which have non-radioactive labels and the hybridization conditions should not disrupt the cell morphology.

Preservation and processing of tissue and target

Effective fixation is one of the most important steps towards obtaining satisfactory *in situ* hybridization results. Either cross-linking or precipitative fixatives, or combinations of the two types may be used (Angerer *et al.*, 1987; Table 10.2). It is essential to fix cells with minimum delay (30 min is a safe limit) following collection. Loss of target may occur during protease digestion when a precipitative fixative is used. Conversely, protease digestion may fail to expose target sequences masked

	Fixation time	
Fixative	Cells	Tissue
Paraformaldehyde 4%	30 min, RT	60 min, RT
Glutaraldehyde 2%	30 min, RT	60 min, RT
Bouin's	30 min, RT	60 min, RT
Ethanol/acetic acid (95/5)	15 min, RT	30 min, RT
Methanol/acetone (50/50)	4 min, $-20°C$	20 min, $-20°C$

by strong cross-linking during fixation. When RNA is the target, special care should be taken. All specimen handling procedures should be carried out using gloved hands and sterile instruments to avoid ribonuclease activity. All solutions should be treated with 0.1% di-ethyl-pyrocarbonate (DEPC) (Sigma) for 12 hours at 37°C followed by autoclaving to inactivate RNAse.

Pre-hybridization treatments

A number of procedures are commonly employed to treat specimens after fixation to increase accessibility to probe and reduce non-specific binding during hybridization (see Fig. 10.5).

Specimen rehydration and detergent permeabilization is recommended for all cells, especially those recovered from paraffin sections after de-waxing.

Procedure

Cells are incubated in 0.3% Triton-X-100 in PBS for 15 min at RT, then washed twice in PBS.

Pronase digestion is advisable to improve probe penetration following fixation when cross-linking reagents (formaldehyde or glutaraldehyde) have been used. It is optional when precipitative fixatives or small oligonucleotide probes are used.

Procedure

1 Pronase (Sigma) should be prepared as a stock solution in water at 10 mg/ml. The enzyme should be predigested at 37°C for 2 hours to remove nucleases, cooled and stored in small aliquots at $-70°C$.
2 Resuspend cells to be treated in warm (37°C) 100 mmol/l Tris-HCl pH 8.0 containing 50 mmol/l EDTA.
3 Add pronase, 10 μg/ml final concentration to the cells and incubate at 37°C for 30 min.

Continued on page 268

4 Halt the pronase activity by addition of 0.1 mol/l glycine in PBS for 5 min at RT.
5 Centrifuge and resuspend the cells in 4% paraformaldehyde in PBS for 3 min at RT, this prevents possible target diffusion.
6 Then wash and resuspend the cells in PBS.

Acetylation of amino groups reduces non-specific electrostatic binding of probe.

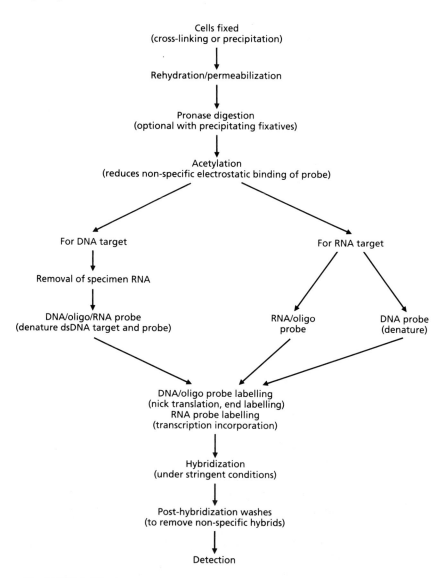

Fig. 10.5 Hybridization treatments.

> *Procedure*
>
> Resuspend cells in 0.1 mol/l triethanolamine pH 8.0 then mix while adding acetic anhydride to a concentration of 0.25% and incubate for 10 min, wash in PBS.

Removal of specimen RNA is necessary when nuclear DNA is the target, to avoid hybridization to mRNA derived from the target sequence.

> *Procedure*
>
> 1 Pancreatic RNAse (RNAse A, Sigma) is prepared as a stock solution at 1 mg/ml in 10 mmol/l Tris-HCl (pH 7.5) and 15 mmol/l NaCl. This is boiled for 15 min to denature DNAse activity and allowed to cool slowly to RT before aliquoting and storage at −20°C. Dilute before use.
> 2 Treat cells with 100 µg/ml RNAse in 2 × SSC (0.3 mol/l NaCl, 0.3 mol/l trisodium citrate pH 7.0) for 1 hour at 37°C.
> 3 Wash cells twice in 2 × SSC.

Choice of probe

In principle either RNA or DNA probes may be used to localize either RNA or DNA sequences. DNA probes may be double-stranded or single-stranded (M13 vector; Sambrook *et al.*, 1989) or synthetic oligonucleotides. RNA probes are single-stranded RNA produced by phage polymerases (Pardue, 1985). The advantages and disadvantages of the different probe types are given in Table 10.3 and guide-lines for which probe to choose are given in Fig. 10.6.

The selection of oligonucleotide probe sequences should be made using the following guide-lines:

1 The probe length should be between 18 and 50 bases. Longer probes will result in longer hybridization times and low synthesis yields, shorter probes will lack specificity.

2 Base composition should be 40−60% G-C. Non-specific hybridization may increase for G-C ratios outside of this range.

3 It is important that no intraprobe complementary regions are present. These may result in 'hairpin' structures, which will inhibit hybridization of the probe.

4 Sequences containing long stretches (more than four) of a single base (i.e. -GGGGG-) should be avoided.

5 Once a sequence meeting the above criteria has been identified, computerized sequence analysis is highly recommended (UK Human Genome Mapping Project). The probe should be compared with the sequence region or genome that it was derived from, as well as the

Table 10.3 Advantages and disadvantages of probes for *in situ* hybridization

	Advantages	Disadvantages
RNA probe	RNA–RNA hybrids have high stability Probe denaturation is not required Probe is strand specific and may be sense or antisense Probe is free of vector Template removal is easy RNase treatment after treatment removes non-hybridized probe	Subcloning of probe into dual promoter vector required RNase degradation of probe must be avoided Some probes have narrow optimum hybridization temperatures
dsDNA probe	No subcloning required Choice of labelling techniques available Hybridization temperature is critical	Probe denaturation needed Re-annealing required in the hybridization reaction Hybrids less stable than RNA probes Gel purification required to remove vector sequence
ssDNA (M13)	Probe free of vector sequence No probe denaturation required No re-annealing during hybridization	Subcloning into M13 required Hybrids less stable than RNA probes Technically cumbersome
Oligo probe*	No cloning required No self-hybridization Small, so good target penetration Can be constructed with deduced sequence from amino acid sequence Multiple probes may be used to overcome most of the disadvantages Stable	Limited labelling methods but new techniques developing Small size limits the amount of label carried Subject to 'design' errors Only short sequences can be used for hybridization Hybrids less stable than RNA probes

* Oligo, oligonucleotide.

reverse complement of the region. If the homologies to non-target regions are greater than 70% or eight or more bases in a row are found, the sequence should not be used. Following these guide-lines does not guarantee that a useful oligonucleotide probe will result, but it greatly enhances the chance of success. The final test is to synthesize, label and hybridize the probe to specific and non-specific target nucleic acids over a range of hybridization temperatures.

Probe labelling

Probes may be labelled in a number of ways: (a) by incorporation of biotinylated nucleotides (Gibco), which are then visualized by addition of FITC avidin or antibiotin antibodies; (b) by incorporation of digoxigenin-conjugated nucleotides (Boehringer-Mannheim) followed by FITC anti-digoxigenin; (c) by incorporation of FITC-conjugated nucleotides (Boehringer-Mannheim).

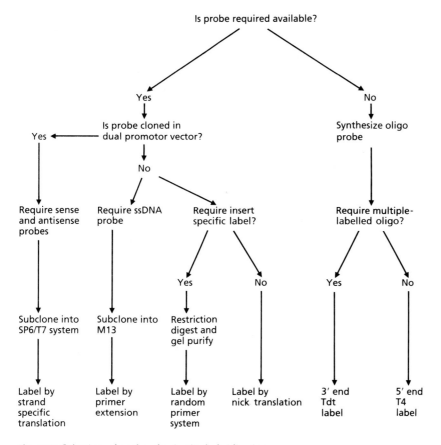

Fig. 10.6 Selection of probes for *in situ* hybridization.

RNA probes are labelled by incorporation of labelled nucleotides during the *in vitro* transcription of cloned DNA by RNA polymerase (SP6 Gibco). Double-stranded DNA probes may be labelled by nick translation with *Escherichia coli* polymerase 1. Starting at a nick in the DNA, the enzyme removes nucleotides from the 5' side of the nick while adding nucleotides to the 3' side. If this replacement synthesis is carried out in the presence of labelled precursors, the DNA becomes labelled. The amount of label depends on the number of nicks, which is directly related to the amount of DNAse in the reaction. M13 based single-stranded DNA probes may be labelled by primer extension by polymerases (Pardue, 1985).

Oligonucleotide probes may be end-labelled either at the 5' terminus with T4 polynucleotide kinase or at the 3' terminus with terminal deoxynucleotidyl transferase (TdT). These enzymes ligate labelled nucleotides to the probe. TdT may be used to form a tail of several nucleotides. In addition RNA and DNA may be labelled with a photo-activatable form of biotin.

Fortunately, commercial kits are available for most of these label-ling procedures. Boehring-Mannheim produce an RNA labelling kit (SP6/T7) for labelling with digoxygenin-UTP by *in vitro* transcription with SP6 and T7 polymerases. A protocol for 3′end-labelling oligo-nucleotides with digoxygenin-11-2′-deoxy-uridine-5′-triphosphate (dUTP) by TdT is also available from Boehring-Mannheim. Gibco have developed a system for labelling DNA with biotin-14-dATP by nick translation to produce biotinylated DNA probes ranging from 50 to 200 base pairs in length. Photoactivatable biotin labelling procedures are available from Gibco and Vector Laboratories.

Pre-hybridization treatment of probes

To develop optimal hybridization conditions several factors should be considered. The size of the probe will influence its access to the target. RNA probes are most efficient when used as smaller fragments of 50–200 nucleotides. RNA probes may be reduced in size by limited alkaline hydrolysis. Hydrolysis time is calculated by:

$$t = \frac{L_o - L_f}{kL_oL_f}$$

where t is the time in minutes and L_o and L_f are the initial and final probe lengths in kilobases. The rate constant for hydrolysis (k) is 0.11 scissions/kb per min. Optimum probe size for DNA probes is usually in the range of 400–600 nucleotides. When using DNA probes labelled by nick translation it is possible to vary probe size by altering the amount of DNAse 1 in the reaction mixture. M13 DNA probes may be produced in a variety of sizes by cutting the probe with various restriction enzymes (Berger, 1986).

It is recommended that before hydrolysis of RNA probes, template DNA is removed to prevent the template annealing to the probe and/or target during hybridization.

Procedure

1 The RNA is incubated with RNAse free DNAse (Sigma) and RNAse inhibitor (Sigma) both at a final concentration of 1 U/ml for 10 min at 40°C in RNAse-free water to a final volume of 100 μl.

2 To this is added 50 μl ammonium acetate 7.5 mol/l and 375 μl ethanol, which is held at −20°C for at least 30 min before centrifugation at 10 000 g for 15 min.

3 The supernatant is removed and the pellet washed with 70% ethanol, which is also removed.

4 To hydrolyse the RNA, dissolve the probe in 50 μl DEPC-treated water and add an equal volume of 0.2 mol/l carbonate buffer, pH 10.2 (80 mmol/l $NaHCO_3$, 120 mmol/l Na_2CO_3), which is made fresh or stored frozen in small aliquots.

5 Incubate at 60°C for the time calculated from the above equation.

6 Neutralize by adding 3 μl 3 mol/l sodium acetate (pH 6.0) and 5 μl 10% (v/v) glacial acetic acid.

7 To precipitate the RNA add 0.1 volume 3 mol/l sodium, potassium or ammonium acetate (pH 5.5) or 0.1 volume 8 mol/l LiCl followed by 2.5 volumes of ethanol.
8 Mix by vortexing and stand at $-20°C$ for at least 30 min.
9 Centrifuge for 15 min at 10 000 g in a microcentrifuge. Carefully remove the ethanol supernatant from the pellet. In general only pellets greater than 10 μg are visible.
10 Add 100 μl 70% ethanol ($-20°C$) to the sample, vortex, re-sediment the precipitate by centrifugation at 10 000 g and remove the supernatant.
11 The probe is redissolved in a small volume of water (20 times the concentration for hybridization) and stored frozen ($-20°C$) until required.

The size of the hydrolysed RNA may be determined by electrophoresis in denaturing formaldehyde or methylmercuric hydroxide 2–2.5% agarose gels (Ogden and Adams, 1987). To check for probe labelling, a bio-dot procedure may be used (Leary *et al.*, 1983; French *et al.*, 1986). The probe is dotted onto nitrocellulose filters and visualized by a colorimetric method, e.g. detect biotin-labelled probes with enzyme-conjugated avidin plus substrate (alkaline phosphatase plus diaminobenzidine (DAB) or peroxidase plus DAB tetrahydrochloride (Vector Laboratories)).

If dsDNA probes or targets are to be hybridized they must be denatured. The probe is denatured immediately prior to use.

Procedure

1 Prepare probe solution in water at 10 times the concentration required for hybridization, then heat in a water-bath at 90°C for 10 min.
2 Transfer the probe to an ice water-bath for 5 min, then add directly to the hybridization mix prewarmed to the hybridization temperature.

Denaturation of DNA targets is performed during the hybridization procedure (see below).

Hybridization rate

The rate of hybridization depends on the length of the probe: the longer the probe the greater the incubation time required, hence the importance of using relatively short probes (18–30 nucleotides) and the usefulness of hybridization accelerators (see below). In general, the hybridization rate increases with probe concentration. Also the sensitivity increases with probe concentration. For *in situ* hybridization optimum probe concentrations are in the range 0.5–5.0 μg/ml (Keller and Manak, 1989). Factors that affect the stability of hybrids determine the stringency of the hybridization conditions. Since hybridization occurs most readily at 25°C below the melting temperature (T_m) of the hybrids, the calculation of T_m is a necessary first step. T_m may be calculated as follows:

$$T_m = \frac{81.5°C + 16.6\log M + 0.41(\%G + C) - 500}{n - 0.61(\%\text{formamide})}$$

where $M = [\text{Na}^+]$ in mol/l, $n =$ length of the shortest chain in the duplex, and

$$T_{hyb} = T_m - 25°C.$$

Other factors that affect T_m are:

1 T_m decreases 1.5°C for each 1% decrease in homology. This effect is much more pronounced for oligonucleotide probes of 15–150 bases.

2 The T_m of RNA : DNA hybrids is 10–15°C higher.

3 The T_m of RNA : RNA hybrids is 20–25°C higher.

Clearly, formamide is necessary when using RNA as probe or target to keep the hybridization temperature reasonably low.

For oligonucleotide probes, the hybridization temperature is usually 5°C below the T_m. In addition a different and more empirical formula is required for oligonucleotides of 14–20 bases:

$$T_m = 4°C \text{ per G-C pair} + 2°C \text{ per A-T pair}$$

Bear in mind that the estimation of T_m is more complex in hybridization systems employing more than one probe. In practice the optimum hybridization temperature for oligonucleotide probes must be empirically determined by performing the hybridization at a range of temperatures and selecting that which provides strong binding to the specific but not to the non-specific target.

Hybridization accelerators

Inert polymers may be used to accelerate the hybridization rate of probes longer than 250 bases. Dextran sulphate and polyethylene glycol are the most commonly used agents (Amasino, 1986; Thompson and Gillespie, 1987). However, short probes do not need acceleration.

Hybridization

The hybridization buffer is prepared by adding the following components in the order shown.

Component	Final concentration
Deionized formamide 5 ml	50%
20 × SSPE (3.6 mol/l NaCl, 200 mmol/l NaH$_2$PO$_4$, 20 mmol/l EDTA pH 7.4)	5×
Warm to 37°C and add:	
Dextran sulphate 1.0 g	10%
Poly-vinyl-pyrolidine (PVP) 0.1 g	1%
Mix until both polymers are dissolved before adding:	5×
100 × Denhardt's solution 500 µl (2% Ficoll, BSA, and PVP in water)	
10% sodium dodecyl sulphate (SDS) 500 µl	2%
10 mg/ml denatured sheared herring sperm DNA 100 µl	100 µg/ml
DEPC-treated water 400 µl	

Note. Keep buffer at 37°C until probe is added.

Formamide is deionized by stirring with mixed bed ion-exchange resin 10 g resin/100 ml formamide (Bio-Rad) for 30 min, then filter twice through No.1 filter paper (Whatman) to remove resin and store formamide in aliquots at −20°C. Herring sperm DNA is denatured by heating to 95°C for 5 min, cooled on ice, then added directly to the buffer.

Add 1 volume of probe to 9 volumes of hybridization buffer to achieve the required probe concentration. For most applications this is 0.5 ng/µl for RNA probes and 1.0 ng/µl for DNA probes. Add the diluted probe to cells. Make sure the cells are as dry as possible to avoid dilution of the hybridization buffer. If the target sequence is DNA, denature DNA by heating the cells to 95°C for 5 min. Incubate the cells with agitation in a damp environment at the required hybridization temperature for 1−2 hours. With hybridization buffer containing 50% formamide the optimum temperature is usually: 42°C for DNA probes; 50−55°C for RNA probes; 37°C for oligo-probes.

Factors influencing the hybridization

Depending on the probe sequence, size and specimen preservation, the stringency (probe/target matching) of the reaction may be altered by varying the temperature. Factors affecting the hybridization temperature have been discussed above. Dextran sulphate increases hybridization fivefold, independent of the hybridization time, by volume exclusion which increases the effective probe concentration. Using a fixed hybridization time hybridization increases linearly with probe concentration until saturation is reached. Formamide is a helix destabilizer which decreases the melting temperature of hybrids and so allows lower hybridization temperatures and so better specimen morphology. Each 1% increase in the formamide concentration reduces the melting temperature by 0.61°C for DNA : DNA hybrids and 0.35°C for RNA : RNA hybrids. Increased ionic strength (sodium ion concentration) of the hybridization buffer stabilizes the hybrids. Hence by varying the salt concentration it is possible to alter the stringency of the reaction. However, increasing the ionic strength above 0.4 mol/l NaCl has little effect on hybridization or hybrid stability.

Post-hybridization washing

Once the hybridization reaction has proceeded to completion, it is necessary to wash off any mismatched or non-specifically bound probe. By controlling the salt concentration of the washing solutions it is possible to promote dissociation of mismatched probe/target sequences. When RNA probes are used, non-specific binding of probe can be reduced by including RNAse, which degrades selectively single-stranded RNA but not hybrid molecules. A typical washing procedure is as follows.

Procedure

1 Wash twice in 2 × SSPE containing 0.1% SDS at RT, wash twice in 0.1 × SSPE containing 0.1% SDS at the hybridization temperature.
2 Wash twice in 2 × SSPE to remove SDS.
3 Incubate cells with 10 µg/ml RNAse A in 2 × SSPE at 37°C for 15 min.
4 Wash twice in 2 × SSPE.

For oligonucleotide probes lower stringency washes may be needed. This may be achieved by either increasing the salt concentration or lowering the temperature of the washes.

Visualization

This will depend on the label used. FITC directly labelled probes can be visualized immediately. Indirect labelling should be carried out according to standard protocols and/or manufacturers' guide-lines.

Experimental controls

Hybridization reactions may lead to misleading results due to unexpected homologies or short regions within a probe hybridizing to unknown target sequences. Similarly, hybridization between G-C rich regions of probe and unrelated target sequences may give spurious positive results. When DNA probes are used, such non-specific hybridization may be identified by using subfractions of the probe sequence to avoid G-C interactions or patchy cross-hybridization. When using RNA probes the use of sense transcripts allows control probes to be of identical specific activity, base composition and fragment length and so allow hybridization observed with antisense probes to be assigned only to specific hybridization arising from the probe sequence and not any other properties of the probe. Pre-hybridization treatment with RNAse and DNAse may be used as controls to confirm the target nucleic acids as DNA and RNA. Care should be taken, however, that reduction in hybridization signal after nuclease treatment is truly due to removal of target and not to destruction of probe by residual enzyme. When DNA is the target, hybridization in the absence of denaturation usually abolishes the signal.

Several *in situ* hybridization methods have been described that allow detection of specific nucleic sequences with non-radioactively labelled probes (Landgent *et al.*, 1984; Pinkel *et al.*, 1986; Lichter and Ward, 1990), and a flow cytometric technique was described by Bauman and Bentvelzen in 1988. In this procedure they used a biotinylated cloned RNA probe of 100–150 nucleotides to detect ribosomal RNA. The optimal hybridization temperature in 50% formamide and $5 \times$ SSC was found to be 45°C, about 8–10°C lower than for the unmodified probe. This is a result of biotinylation, which lowers the melting temperature and efficiency of hybridization. Flow cytometric *in situ* hybridization has also been used to detect nuclear organization (Trask *et al.*, 1988) and messenger RNA (Bayer and Bauman, 1990).

In situ hybridization in suspension for flow cytometry

Procedure

1 Cells to be studied are washed in HBSS without phenol red, Hepes buffered (pH 7.2) and resuspended in HBSS at a final concentration 2.5×10^7/ml.

2 The cells are fixed by addition of an equal volume of 2% Formalin in HBSS for 5 min at RT then centrifuged ($300\,g$) at 4°C for 10 min.

3 The cell pellet is resuspended in 70% ethanol (in water) ready for hybridization.

4 To obtain reproducible results it is essential to block endogenous RNAse activity in fixed cells before rehydration, by the addition of 0.2% DEPC (1 µl of 10% DEPC in ethanol per 50 µl fixed cell suspension in 70% ethanol). In addition all reagents and equipment should be kept RNAse free.

5 After 15 min at RT the cells are centrifuged at $1500\,g$ for 5 min, the fixative is removed and the cell pellet resuspended in HBSS containing 0.5% Tween-20 (HBSS-T) for 5 min at RT. After which one volume of $20 \times$ SSC is added ($1 \times$ SSC is 0.15 mol/l NaCl, 15 mmol/l trisodium citrate, pH 7.0), the cells mixed and two volumes of deionized formamide added (Merck Sharp & Dohme; after deionization with AG501-XB Bio-Rad, stored at −20°C).

Continued on page 278

6 The cells are then aliquoted $(1-2 \times 10^5)$ into Eppendorf tubes now in 50% formamide and $5 \times$ SSC.

7 The cells are pelleted and resuspended in 10 µl of hybridization mixture (50% formamide, $5 \times$ SSC, 0.5 mg/ml *E. coli* tRNA, 0.5% SDS) containing the probe (25 µg/ml).

8 The cells are incubated with a biotinylated probe under the appropriate stringent conditions (see above).

9 The cells are agitated during the incubation period, then excess probe is removed after hybridization by addition of 100 µl of hybridization mixture followed by a further incubation under stringent conditions.

10 The cells are then pelleted as above, resuspended in 100 µl $0.1 \times$ SSC and incubated under stringent conditions to remove mismatched hybrids (stringent washing).

11 The cells are centrifuged and resuspended in HBSS-T and FITC-streptavidin (Amersham) is added (5 µg/ml).

12 After incubation for 30 min under stringent conditions, 400 µl of HBSS-T are added. The cells are washed once and analysed by flow cytometry.

Primer-initiated *in situ* hybridization (PRINS)

One of the most innovative developments of *in situ* hybridization has been that of primer-induced *in situ* hybridization. This is a technique that was first described by Koch *et al.* (1989). In this procedure short, specific, synthetic oligonucleotides are hybridized to DNA or mRNA and act as primers for the *in situ* incorporation of biotin or fluorescein-labelled nucleotides as substrate; the reaction is catalysed by a polymerase or reverse transcriptase, using the target as template. The reaction can be conducted on cells in suspension and the reaction product can be visualized directly when fluorescein-conjugated nucleotides are used or after addition of fluorescein-conjugated avidin or antibiotin antibodies in indirect methods. The main advantages of labelling the site of hybridization rather than the probe are: (a) high concentrations of probe can be used and so reaction times are short and PRINS is an order of magnitude faster than *in situ* hybridization; (b) the high amount of probe is not likely to increase background staining significantly because unhybridized probe is unlabelled; (c) signal intensity is unaffected by probe (primer) size; and (d) the short incubations together with inclusion of divalent cations which stabilize chromatin, result in better preservation of chromosomes and other cellular structures. The method described is based on the incorporation of nucleotides conjugated with fluorescein.

PRINS of mRNA

1 Cells are washed twice in HBSS, pH 7.2, then fixed for 5 min at RT in freshly prepared 2% paraformaldehyde in HBSS, pH 7.2.

2 The cells are pelleted by centrifugation at 4°C and resuspended in ice-cold HBSS, then fixed in ethanol at a final concentration of 2×10^6 cells/ml.

3 All following procedures are performed in Eppendorf tubes.

4 10^6 cells are rehydrated in $5 \times$ SSC, 0.5% Tween.

5 Cellular DNA is denatured and quenched by resuspending the cells in $5 \times$ SSC, 50% deionized formamide for 10 min (SSC: 150 mmol/l NaCl, 15 mmol/l sodium citrate, pH 7.0) and heating at 50°C for 30 min followed by rapid cooling by the addition of ice-cold $5 \times$ SSC, 0.5% Tween-20.

6 The cells are then washed twice in nick translation buffer (50 mmol/l Tris/HCl pH 7.5, 10 mmol/l $MgSO_4$, 100 µmol/l dithiothreitol, 50 µg/ml BSA (Fraction V, Sigma).

7 After this, all the supernatant is removed and the PRINS reaction mix with and without primer is added to 10^6 cells. The conditions for a 37-mer oligonucleotide primer are given and reagents should be added in the order given.

PRINS reaction mix

Reagent	Primed µl	Unprimed µl	Final concentration
H_2O	29.5	34.5	0.5 mmol/l
dATP 10 mmol/l	3.2	3.2	0.5 mmol/l
dGTP 10 mmol/l	3.2	3.2	0.5 mmol/l
dCTP 10 mmol/l	3.2	3.2	0.05 mmol/l
dTPP 1 mmol/l	3.2	3.2	0.078 mmol/l
FITC 12-dUTP 1 mmol/l	4.7	4.7	$1 \times$
* $10 \times$ NT Buffer	6.0	6.0	0.02 U/µl
RNAse block 1 U/µl	1.0	1.0	0.48 U/µl
AMV 29 U/µl	1.0	1.0	0.16 µg/µl
Primer 1.9 µg/µl	5.0	0.0	

* $10 \times$ NT [0.5 mol/l Tris-HCl, pH 7.5, 0.1 mol/l $MgSO_4$, 1 mmol/l dithiothreitol, 500 µg/ml Fraction V (Sigma) aliquoted stored at −20°C].

8 The cells are then incubated at 42°C for 2 hours. The reverse transcriptase is then terminated by washing twice in $2 \times$ SSC. The cells are then analysed. A poly-T oligonucleotide or actin primer should be used as a positive control.

This procedure has been used to detect mRNA for the κ light chain promotor in a mouse myeloma cell line (X63Ag8). Although the PRINS technique has been applied to DNA in cell spreads (Koch *et al.*, 1989; Kolvraa *et al.*, 1991; Mogensen *et al.*, 1991), it has not as yet been applied for the detection of DNA sequences in cells in suspension.

Hybridoma studies

MoAbs have become major constituents of the field of biotechnology-related products. It has become apparent that for the development of MoAb diagnostic and therapeutic products, large-scale production techniques will be required. This may be achieved by mass culture of hybridoma cells. However, to achieve this, it is first necessary to select and maintain hybridoma starter cultures capable of secreting high concentrations of MoAbs. Also, genetic and phenotypic variations exist in monoclonally derived cultures (Andreef *et al.*, 1985) and continued observation and reselection of optimal clones from these strains is desirable. There are a number of ways in which flow cytometry may be employed to aid hybridoma selection: (a) high immunoglobulin-secreting hybrids may be distinguished from poor immunoglobulin secreters and sorted (Marder *et al.*, 1990); (b) hybrid hybridomas may be distinguished from non-fused parental cells and sorted (Koolwijk *et al.*, 1988; Shi *et al.*, 1991); (c) antibody secretion in the culture supernatant may be screened (Durrant *et al.*, 1989).

Selection of high immunoglobulin-secreting hybridomas

Essentially, hybridomas of interest are labelled with FITC-conjugated F(ab')$_2$ fragments of goat anti-mouse isotype antisera and those cells which exhibit high fluorescence intensity at 525 nm when excited at 488 nm are sorted under sterile conditions. Sterile sort conditions are obtained by passing absolute alcohol through the sample tubing and flow cell for 30 min, followed by exhaustive rinsing with sterile PBS pH 7.2 as sheath fluid and the use of sterile PBS during sorting. Propidium iodide (1 μg/ml final concentration, Sigma) may be added to cell preparations immediately prior to sorting to help define and select viable cells (Jacobs *et al.*, 1983).

Selection of hybrid hybridomas

Hybrid hybridomas produce bi-specific MoAbs (bs MoAb), which combine the characteristics of two parental antibodies in one molecule. This molecule is structurally bivalent but functionally univalent. These antibodies have potential applications in immunocytochemistry and immunoassays (Suresh *et al.*, 1986), in the cross-linking of effector and target cells (Wong and Colvin, 1987; Brissinck *et al.*, 1991; Shalaby *et al.*, 1992). The selection of hybrid hybridomas by flow cytometry is based on the fusion of two parental hybridomas labelled with two different dyes. Fused cells are dual fluorescent and may be distinguished from single fluorescence cells and sorted. In the method described rhodamine 123 (Rh123) and HE are used to internally label the fusion partners. These dyes have a strong fluorescent signal, short labelling time and low cytotoxicity. Verapamil is used to block rhodamine efflux via *p*-glycoprotein (see above).

Cell labelling and fusion

1 One hybridoma is labelled by incubation in HBSS (Sigma) with 4 µg/ml HE (Polysciences) at RT for 20 min, then washed three times in Iscove's medium containing 2 mmol/l L-glutamine and without FCS (Gibco).

2 The second hybridoma is labelled in Iscove's medium containing 2 mmol/l L-glutamine and 10% FCS with 0.4 µg/ml Rh123 (Kodak) and 20 µmol/l verapamil (Sigma) in a 37°C water-bath for 10 min.

3 The cells are then washed three times with serum-free medium containing 20 µmol/l verapamil.

4 10^7 hybridoma cells of each line are then fused in 1 ml of 40% (w/v) polyethylene glycol (PEG; Sigma) solution in Iscove's medium.

5 The same number of unfused labelled cells are retained as control suspensions. Both populations are then diluted in 70 ml of complete medium and allowed to recover for at least 4 hours at 37°C before sorting.

Analysis and sorting

1 The cells are excited at 488 nm and three-dimensional histograms correlating log red and log green fluorescence are collected from each sample.

2 Fluorescence from Rh123 and ethidium bromide is measured at 525 and 610 nm, respectively.

3 The control suspensions are used to establish compensation levels and then dual fluorescent cells from PEG fusions are sorted under sterile conditions into culture medium and cultured.

Screening culture supernatants for specific immunoglobulin

In this procedure the antigen to which the MoAb has been raised is covalently coupled to carboxylate modified polymer beads (Polybeads; Polysciences; McConway and Chapman, 1986; Durrant *et al.*, 1989). The antigen-coupled beads are incubated with antibody containing culture supernatants, washed and then bound antibody is visualized with FITC-conjugated anti-mouse antisera. The procedure for antigen labelling of beads is as follows.

Procedure

1 Both 5.29 and 9.67 µm beads may be used. Beads (0.5 ml, 5.29 µm beads) of the initial polybead suspension is added to 0.5 ml of 0.1 mol/l PBS, pH 5.0.

Continued on page 282

2   The suspension is centrifuged at 8000 g for 10 seconds in a microfuge.

3   The supernatant is removed and the beads resuspended in the residual buffer. This procedure is repeated twice with 1.0 ml of PBS.

4   After this, 0.5 ml of PBS and 50 μl of freshly prepared ethyl carbodimide (1 mg/ml, Sigma) in water are added.

5   The mixture is then incubated at 4°C with agitation for 1 hour.

6   After this, 150 μl of antigen is added in solution at 500 μg/ml and the mixture incubated for a further 12 hours.

7   The labelled beads are then washed three times in PBS as above by adding 1.0 ml of PBS per wash.

8   The polybeads are then resuspended in 0.5 ml of PBS containing 0.2% sodium azide (Sigma). For 9.67 μm beads 0.2 ml of the initial bead suspension is labelled and resuspended to 2.0 ml.

Determination of antigenic density of labelled beads

1   Antigen-labelled beads (10 μl) are washed twice in PBS containing 1% FCS by centrifugation as above.

2   FITC anti-antigen is then added and the mixture incubated for 1 hour at 4°C with agitation to prevent the beads settling.

3   Unconjugated beads incubated with FITC antiserum are used as a negative control.

4   The fluorescence intensity at 525 nm of the beads excited at 488 nm is then assessed.

Supernatant screening

1   Antigen-labelled beads (10^5) are incubated with 100 μl of culture supernatant, washed in PBS then incubated with FITC goat anti-mouse antiserum.

2   After a further wash the beads are analysed and the fluorescence intensity recorded.

3   Those hybridomas which produce supernatants with high fluorescence intensities when incubated with antigen-coated beads should be retained and cultured.

Fluorescent *in vivo* tracking of cells

The study of cellular trafficking *in vivo* is important for understanding disease processes such as the migration of leucocytes in inflammation (Zimmerman *et al.*, 1992) and the homing of lymphocytes to specific tissues and organs (Oiszewski, 1987). To evaluate cellular trafficking patterns with respect to a particular disease state, it is necessary to: (a) identify and label cells of interest; (b) be able to define their final location; (c) assess their current state of functional integrity; (d) determine their proliferative activity post-injection; and (e) ensure that viability or functional capability has not been altered. In addition it is necessary that the label: (a) will not be eluted; (b) is not metabolized; and (c) has a sufficiently high signal-to-noise ratio to permit detection of low frequency cells. Radiolabels have been used extensively; however, these have been shown to have cytotoxic effects (Balaban *et al.*, 1987). Experiments using FITC, rhodamine isothiocyanate, carboxy fluorescein diacetate and Di-I-C18-(3) have shown diminished cell lifetimes, altered cell function and elution of label from the cells (Butcher and Weissman, 1980; Honig and Hume, 1986; Jacobs *et al.*, 1986). More recently, Horan and Slezak (1989) have extensively investigated the use of lipophilic probes (PKH-1, 2 and 3) that avidly bind to the membrane, are non-toxic and may be used to identify cells undergoing replication.

Fluorescent cell membrane labelling for cell survival studies

This method may be used for the labelling of erythrocytes, white blood cells, platelets and bone marrow cells (Slezak and Horan, 1989). Cells to be infused should be labelled under sterile conditions.

Procedure

1 Blood is collected into acid citrate dextrose ACD (1 part to 9 parts blood) (ACD contains 14.6 g trisodium citrate, 5.3 g citric acid and 16 g dextrose/l).

2 The cells to be studied are then partially purified. Platelet-rich plasma may be collected by centrifugation at 80 g for 20 min. Buffy coat cells may be collected after centrifugation at 100 g for 5 min. Alternatively the buffy coat may be removed and the erythrocytes retained for labelling.

3 The sample to be labelled is centrifuged at 400 g (800 g for platelets) to pellet the cells. The plasma is removed and centrifuged at 1000 g for 10 min to prepare platelet-poor plasma, which is retained.

4 The cells are washed twice in PBS (PBS-EDTA for platelets, see Chapter 6) to remove residual plasma.

5 Cells 2×10^6/ml are resuspended in PBS containing PKH-1, 2 or 3 (Zynaxis Cell Science) at a final concentration of 1 μmol/l.

6 The cells are incubated at RT for 10 min, then diluted with an equal volume of PBS, centrifuged, then washed five times and the pellet resuspended in autologous platelet-poor plasma.

7 The resulting cell preparation is reinjected and at desired time points 1.0 ml samples are removed from the opposite side to the reinjection and collected into ACD.

8 Cells to be examined are prepared as in step 2 above prior to labelling.

9 For flow cytometric analysis the cells are gated on forward and 90° light scatter and for PKA-1 and 2 the amount of green fluor-

Continued on page 284

escence (log amplification) is determined (these dyes are excited at 488 nm and have maximum emission at 525 nm). While for PKH-3 the amount of red fluorescence (log amplification) is determined (this dye is excited at 595 nm with maximum emission at 610 nm). Data are collected on 100 000 gated events.

The method described may be used for cell survival studies. It may also be used to determine blood volume. Injection of a known volume of cells followed by enumeration of the percentage of cells after injection allows determination of the dilution factor and calculation of blood volume. This method may also be used to monitor cell growth. In contrast to the constant fluorescence intensity of non-dividing cells, a decrease in fluorescence intensity may be monitored in dividing cells. Thus not only specific cell types may be identified but determination of whether division of these specific cell types has occurred *in vivo* can be made. *In vivo* labelling of cells is also possible and a number of studies on phagocytic cells have been reported (Meinicoff *et al.*, 1988, 1989). The technique could also be extended to study cell types such as bacteria, yeast and fungi.

Analysis of bacteria and parasites

During the past few years flow cytometry has been increasingly used for the study of bacteria (Nelson *et al.*, 1991; Kell *et al.*, 1992; Yeaman *et al.*, 1992) and parasites including: *Plasmodium* species (Janse *et al.*, 1987; Makler *et al.*, 1987; Pattanapanyasat *et al.*, 1992), *Leishmania* (Kiderlen and Kaye, 1990; Butcher *et al.*, 1992), and *Trypanosoma* (Jacobson *et al.*, 1992). The use of fluorogenic and chromogenic substrates for rapid and sensitive detection of bacteria has proved a powerful alternative to traditional methods (Boye and Lobner-Olesen, 1990; Manafi and Kneifel, 1991; Molenaar *et al.*, 1991).

Specific bacteria have been identified: (a) by differential labelling of guanine−cytosine and adenine−thymine nucleotides in DNA (Van Dilla *et al.*, 1983; Sanders *et al.*, 1990); (b) by cell size and DNA content (Robertson and Button, 1989); (c) by dual staining of DNA and protein (Miller and Quarles, 1990); (d) with MoAbs (Obernesser *et al.*, 1990; Yeaman *et al.*, 1992); (e) by tetramethylrhodamine and digoxigenin-labelled rRNA-targeted oligonucleotides (Amann *et al.*, 1990; Zarda *et al.*, 1991); and (f) by β-galactosidase activity (Nir *et al.*, 1990). Techniques for counting bacteria have also been described (Pinder *et al.*, 1990; Monfort and Baleux, 1992). A technique for identifying bacteria in blood was first reported by Mansour *et al.* (1985) and is described here.

Detection of bacteria in blood

Blood containing bacteria (1 ml), freshly drawn and anticoagulated with sodium polyanthetholesulphonate (SPS) is added to 1 ml

of lysing agent (2.5% Rhozyme 41 (Corning), 4% Tween-20 (Sigma), in 0.01 mol/l Tricine pH 8.5) and incubated at 42°C for 60 min. This lysing reagent is very effective at lysing eukaryotic cells, while maintaining the morphology and viability of bacteria.
2 Following lysis 1.6 ml of staining buffer is added (100 mmol/l sodium borate, 60 mmol/l EDTA, 0.05% Formalin, 0.05% Triton X-100 pH 9.2) and 0.4 ml of ethidium bromide (Sigma; 100 µg/ml in H_2O) is added.
3 This mixture is incubated for 15 min at RT then centrifuged at 9000 g for 2 min on to a cushion of Fluourinert FC-40 (ISCO) and the pellet resuspended in 2 ml sterile-filtered normal saline.
4 The sample is then analysed. Sample flow rate should be maintained at 70 µl/min with 500 mW excitation energy at 488 nm.
5 Red fluorescence is measured at 580 nm and green fluorescence at 520 nm. The forward scatter and the ratio of green to red fluorescence for each sample is recorded.

Note. Green fluorescence is recorded as a measure of particulate autofluorescence due to debris, while red fluorescence is due to autofluorescence and also the specific emission from ethidium bromide labelled bacteria. Measurement of the fluorescence ratio thus compensates for autofluorescence signals of cellular debris.

The sensitivity of this technique is 10−100 bacteria/ml of blood. However, in bacteraemia the number of bacteria is frequently less than 10/ml. The use of additional bacterial probes such as antibodies to bacteria, fluorogenic substrates for bacterial enzymes or other discriminating factors such as scattering of polarized light will further enhance detection sensitivity.

Detection of bacteria in body fluids and exudates

This method was described by Cohen and Sahar (1989) and is suitable for detecting bacteria in bile, pleural and peritoneal fluid as well as from swabs.

Procedure

1 For recovery of specimen from swabs: the swab transport medium is suspended in 8 ml of sterile PBS and shaken vigorously with a vortex mixer.
2 The test-tube is then placed on ice for 10 min until agar is deposited at the bottom.
3 The supernatant is recovered and retained for subsequent analysis.
4 Body fluids and exudates are diluted 1 : 1 in PBS and centrifuged

Continued on p. 286

at 900 g for 10 min to remove by pelleting any contaminating red cells and leucocytes.

5 All samples are then filtered through a 25 mm diameter sterile disposable polysulphonate filter (Gelman Sciences) to remove anti-microbial agents.

6 The particulate matter deposited on the filter from the sample is resuspended in 1 ml of PBS.

7 Each sample is then divided in two.

8 One sample is heated at 65°C for 10 min to terminate bacterial growth without cell lysis and allow uptake of ethidium bromide.

9 Of the second sample, 10 µl is inoculated into tryptic soya broth (TSB) (Oxoid) supplemented with 10% FCS (Gibco) and incubated for 90–120 min at 37°C. Then it is heat shock treated as above.

10 Both samples are then stained with ethidium bromide (Sigma; 100 µg/ml in H_2O) for 15 min at RT.

11 Fluorescent polystyrene microspheres, with diameter 1.55 µm (Polysciences) are added to each sample at a final concentration of 10^6/ml. These beads serve to quantitate the bacterial concentration in the sample. They are also used to monitor optical alignment.

12 The number of particles with fluorescence and light scatter properties of bacteria are determined after the sphere count has reached a predetermined number (usually 2000). The red fluorescence associated with bacteria is determined in the samples at 600 nm.

When measuring clinical samples, background noise due to particles other than bacteria is encountered. This is overcome in this procedure by analysing cultured samples together with the fresh sample. If the number of red fluorescent particles in the cultured sample per 2000 beads is greater than in the uncultured sample this provides dynamic evidence of bacteria in the specimen.

To reduce background noise the following are advisable: (a) ensuring that the flow cell is as clean as possible by rinsing with filtered chlorine bleach followed by distilled water and cleaning with dichromate solution regularly; (b) using filtered (0.1 µm) distilled water as sheath fluid for analysis; (c) sample flow rate should be minimal (5 µl/min); (d) the corresponding sheath flow rate should also be high (3.1 ml/min; very slow flow rates result in slow data acquisition but the sensitivity of detection is increased sixfold); and (e) reducing the width of the laser beam (if possible) thereby also reducing the volume of illuminated sheath fluid, which is the main source of background scatter signal.

Detection of intra-erythrocytic malaria parasites

Various flow cytometric methods using nucleic acid binding fluoro-chromes have been described for detection of intra-erythrocytic malarial parasites (Whaun *et al.*, 1983; Franklin *et al.*, 1986; Makler *et al.*, 1987).

Similarly, red blood cell antigens are routinely identified by immuno-fluorescence techniques (Raphael and Eitan, 1991). A simple method for simultaneous two colour staining of red cell membrane determinants and parasite nucleic acids has been described (Pattanapanyasat *et al.*, 1992). This method employs a single 488 nm laser and the simultaneous measurement of malaria parasite DNA and red blood cell membrane determinants enables the investigation of red blood cell membrane protein changes in association with invasion and maturation of the parasite (see also Chapter 7).

Assay procedure

1 Two million infected red blood cells in 50 μl PBS, pH 7.2, containing 1% BSA are incubated with 20 μl antibody (e.g. CD43, CD44, CD55) on ice for 30 min.

2 Cells may be incubated with CD2 and CD19 antibodies to determine the percentage of contaminating lymphocytes.

3 Control samples are set up with 20 μl PBS-BSA and mouse isotype IgG.

4 The cells are then washed twice in PBS containing 0.02% sodium azide. After this they are resuspended in 50 μl PBS-BSA and mixed with 20 μl FITC goat (F(ab')$_2$ anti-mouse immunoglobulin G (Becton Dickinson).

5 After incubation on ice for a further 30 min the cells are washed in PBS azide and resuspended in 50 μl for subsequent fixation and parasite DNA staining.

6 The cells are first fixed in 1 ml of 0.5% paraformaldehyde (Sigma) in PBS for 2 hours at RT. Paraformaldehyde is used to cross-link protein and immobilize cell surface fluorescein-labelled antigens, so preventing capping or internalization, it also increases the strength of the surface fluorescein signal (Lanier and Warner, 1981).

7 The cells are then centrifuged at 400 g for 5 min, the paraformaldehyde is decanted and the cells resuspended in 1 ml of 0.25% (w/v) glutaraldehyde (Sigma) for 10 min on ice. Glutaraldehyde is used to permit propidium iodide to enter the cell and to maintain cellular morphology.

8 The cells are centrifuged at 400 g for 5 min then washed in PBS to remove residual fixative and finally resuspended in 2 ml PBS containing propidium iodide (Molecular Probes) at a final concentration of 10 μg/ml and incubated for 1 hour prior to flow cytometric analysis. Logarithmic forward and 90° light scatter are used to gate the red blood cells.

9 For each sample, 50 000 cells are analysed for log fluorescence intensity at 530 nm for green fluorescence and 585 nm for red fluorescence. FITC and phycoerythrin calibration beads (Becton Dickinson) are used to calibrate the instrument fluorescence compensation and sensitivity. The fluorescent distribution of both control and test cells is then analysed.

During intra-erythroid development of the blood phase of malarial infection, there are three distinct morphological stages of the parasite: rings, trophozoites and schizonts. Ring stages contain a single parasite nucleus which during the intra-erythroid cycle undergoes asexual schizogony to produce eight to 32 daughter merozoites in the mature schizont. Ring-stage parasites give rise to a single peak or red fluorescence of low intensity. The peak fluorescence for the schizont stage occurs at a higher fluorescence intensity thus the stage of infection may be determined.

Summary

The use of flow cytometry to measure cell function has developed over the past few years. Many assays of cell function have required the use of radio-isotopes with its obvious drawbacks. There is no doubt that non-radioactive assays, including those flow cytometric techniques described here, will prove to be the preferred procedures of the future.

References

Amann RI, Binder BJ, Olson RJ, Chisholm SW, Devereux R, Stahl DA (1990) Combined 16s rRNA-targeted oligonucleotide probes with flow cytometry for analysing mixed microbial populations. *Appl. Environ. Microbiol.* **56**: 1919–1925.

Amasino RM (1986) Acceleration of nucleic acid hybridisation rate by polyethylene glycol. *Anal. Biochem.* **152**: 304–307.

Andreef M, Bartal A, Feit C, Hirshaut Y (1985) Clonal stability and heterogeneity of hybridomas: analysis by multiparameter flow cytometry. *Hybridoma* **4**: 277–287.

Angerer LM, Cox KH, Angerer RC (1987) Demonstration of tissue-specific gene expression by *in situ* hybridisation. *Methods Enzymol.* **152**: 649–661.

Antonaci S, Polignano A, Ottolenghi A, Torterello C, Schena FP (1992) Redistribution of natural killer (NK) cell frequency and NK cytotoxic activity in primary IgA nephropathy. *Cytobios* **69**: 27–34.

Balaban EP, Simon TR, Frenkel EP (1987) Toxicity of InIII on the radiolabelled lymphocyte. *J. Nucl. Med.* **28**: 229–234.

Bauman JGJ, Bentvelzen P (1988) Flow cytometric detection of ribosomal RNA in suspended cells by fluorescent *in situ* hybridisation. *Cytometry* **9**: 517–524.

Bayer JA, Bauman GJ (1990) Flow cytometric detection of beta-globin mRNA in murine haemopoietic tissue using fluorescent *in situ* hybridisation. *Cytometry* **11**: 132–143.

Beck WT (1990) Mechanism of multidrug resistance and its circumvention. *Eur. J. Cancer* **26**: 513–515.

Berger CN (1986) *In situ* hybridization of immunoglobulin-specific RNA in cells of the B-lymphocyte lineage with radiolabelled DNA probe. *EMBO J.* **5**: 85–93.

Berman E, McBride M (1992) Comparative cellular pharmacology of daunorubicin and idarubicin in human multidrug-resistant leukaemia cells. *Blood* **79**: 3267–3273.

Bonavida B, Bradley TP, Grimm EA (1983) The single cell assay in cell mediated cytotoxicity. *Immunol. Today* **4**: 196–199.

Boye E, Lobner-Olesen A (1990) Flow cytometry: illuminating microbiology. *New Biol.* **2**: 119–125.

Brissinck J, Demanet C, Moser M, Leo O, Thielemans K (1991) Treatment of mice bearing BCL1 lymphoma with bispecific antibodies. *J. Immunol.* **147**: 4019–4026.

Butcher BA, Sklar LA, Seamer LC, Glew RH (1992) Heparin enhances the interaction of infective *Leishmania donovani* promastigotes with mouse peritoneal macrophages. A fluorescence flow cytometric analysis. *J. Immunol.* **148**: 2879–2886.

Butcher EC, Weissman IL (1980) Direct fluorescent labelling of cells with fluorescein or rhodamine isothiocyanate. I. Technical aspects. *J. Immunol. Methods* **37**: 97–108.

Callewaert DM, Radcliff G, Waite R, LeFevre J, Poulik MD (1991) Characterisation of effector–target conjugates for cloned human natural killer and human lymphokine activated killer cells by flow cytometry. *Cytometry* **12**: 666–676.

Carmicheal J, Degraff WG, Gazdar AF, Minna JD, Mitchell JB (1987) Evaluation of a tetrazolium based semiautomated colorimetric assay: Assessment of chemo-sensitivity testing. *Cancer Res.* **47**: 936–942.

Chaudhury PM, Roninson IB (1991) Expression and activation of P-glycoprotein, a multidrug efflux pump, in human haematopoietic stem cells. *Cell* **66**: 85–94.

Cohen CY, Saher E (1989) Rapid flow cytometric bacterial detection and determination of susceptibility to amikacin in body fluids and exudates. *J. Clin. Microbiol.* **27**: 1250–1256.

Deuchars KL, Ling V (1989) P-glycoprotein and multidrug resistance in chemotherapy. *Semin. Oncol.* **16**: 156–165.

Duarte AJ, Vasconcelos DM, Sato MN (1990) Common variable immunodeficiency (hypogammaglobulinemia of late onset or acquired hypogammaglobulinemia) initial follow up of 11 cases. *Rev. Hosp. Clin. Fac. Med. S. Paulo* **45**: 95–104.

Durrant LG, Robins RA, Baldwin RW (1989) Flow cytometric screening of monoclonal antibodies for drug or toxin targeting to human cancer. *J. Natl Acad. Inst.* **81**: 688–695.

Franklin RM, Brun R, Grieder A (1986) Microscopic and flow cytophotometric analysis of parasitaemia in cultures of *Plasmodium falciparum* vitally stained with Hoechst 33342: applications to studies of antimalarial agents. *Z. Parasitenkd.* **72**: 201–212.

French BT, Maul HM, Maul GG (1986) Screening cDNA expression libraries with monoclonal and polyclonal antibodies using an amplified biotin–avidin-peroxidase technique. *Anal. Biochem.* **156**: 417–423.

Gall JC, Pardue MI (1969) Formation and detection of RNA–DNA hybrid molecules in cytological preparations. *Proc. Natl Acad. Sci. USA* **63**: 378–383.

Gerlach JH, Kartner N, Bell DR (1986a) Multidrug resistance. *Cancer Surv.* **948**: 25–46.

Gerlach JH, Endicott JA, Juranka PF *et al.* (1986b) Homology between P-glycoprotein and a bacterial haemolysin transport protein suggests a model for multidrug resistance. *Nature* **324**: 485–489.

Gheuens EE, Bockstaele DR, Keur M, Tanke HJ, Oosterom AT, Bruijn EA (1991) Flow cytometric double labelling technique for screening multidrug resistance. *Cytometry* **12**: 636–644.

Green LM, Reade JL, Ware CF (1984) Rapid colorimetric assay for cell viability: Application to quantitation of cytotoxic and growth inhibitory lymphokines. *J. Immunol. Methods* **70**: 257–268.

Haber DA (1992) Multidrug resistance (MDR 1) in leukaemia: Time to test. *Blood* **79**: 295–298.

Harris N, Wilkinson DG (eds) (1990) In situ *Hybridisation: Applications to Developmental Biology and Medicine*. Cambridge University Press, Cambridge.

Hayes JD, Wolf CR (1990) Molecular mechanism of drug resistance. *Biochem. J.* **272**: 282–295.

Herweijer H, Engh G, Nooter K (1989) A rapid and sensitive flow cytometric method for the detection of multidrug-resistant cells. *Cytometry* **10**: 463–468.

Hidaka Y, Amino N, Iwatani Y *et al.* (1992) Increase in peripheral natural killer cell activity in patients with autoimmune thyroid disease. *Autoimmunity* **11**: 239–246.

Honig MG, Hume RI (1986) Fluorescent carbocyanine dyes allow living neurones of identified origin to be studied in long term culture. *J. Cell Biol.* **103**: 171–176.

Horan PK, Slezak SE (1989) Stable cell membrane labelling. *Nature* **340**: 167–168.

Hseuh CM, Lorden JF, Hiramoto RN, Ghanta VK (1992) Acquisition of enhanced natural killer cell activity under anaesthesia. *Life Sci.* **50**: 2067–2074.

Hubbard BB, Glacken MW, Rogers JR, Rich RR (1990) The role of physical forces on stability of cytotoxic T-cell–target cell conjugate stability. *J. Immunol.* **144**: 4129–4138.

Huet O, Petit JM, Ratinaud MH, Julien R (1992) NADH-dependent dehydrogenase activity estimation by flow cytometric analysis of 3-(4,5-dimethylthiazolyl-2-yl)-2-5-diphenyltetrazolium bromide (MTT) reduction. *Cytometry* **13**: 532–539.

Jacobs DB, Pipho C (1983) Use of propidium iodide staining and flow cytometry to measure antibody-mediated cytotoxicity: resolution of complement-sensitive and resistant target cells. *J. Immunol. Methods* **62**: 101–108.

Jacobs RM, Boyce JT, Jociba GJ (1986) Flow cytometric and radioisotopic determinations of platelet survival time in normal cats and feline leukaemia virus infected cats. *Cytometry* **7**: 64–70.

Jacobson KC, Fletcher RC, Kuhn RE (1992) Binding of antibody and resistance to lysis of trypanomastigotes of *Trypanosoma cruzi*. *Parasitol. Immunol.* **14**: 1–12.

Janse CJ, Vianen PH, Tanke HJ, Mons B, Ponnudurai T, Overdulve JP (1987) *Plasmodium* species: flow cytometry and microfluorometry assessment of DNA content and synthesis. *Exp. Parasitol.* **64**: 88–94.

Jiang XR, Macey MG, Newland AC (1991) Multidrug resistance in haematological malignancies. *Med. Lab. Sci.* **48**: 261–270.

Kane SE, Pastan I, Gottesman MM (1990) Genetic basis of multidrug resistance of tumour cells. *J. Bioenerg. Biomem.* **22**: 4593–4618.

Kell DB, Ryder HM, Kaprelyants AS, Westerhoff HV (1992) Quantifying heterogeneity: flow cytometry of bacterial cultures. *Antonie van Leeuwenhoek; J. Microbiol. Serol.* **60**: 145–158.

Keller GH, Manak MM (eds) (1989) *DNA Probes*. Macmillan, pp. 1–27.

Kiderlen AF, Kaye PM (1990) A modified colorimetric assay of macrophage activation for intracellular cytotoxicity against *Leishmania* parasites. *J. Immunol. Methods* **127**: 11–18.

Koch JE, Kolvraas S, Petersen KB, Gregersen N, Boland L (1989) Oligonucleotide-priming method for the chromosome labelling of alpha satellite DNA *in situ*. *Chromosoma* **98**: 259–265.

Kolvraa S, Koch J, Gregersen N *et al.* (1991) Applications of fluorescence *in situ* hybridisation techniques in clinical genetics. *Clin. Genet.* **39**: 278–286.

Koolwijk P, Rozemuller E, Stad RK, De Lau WBM, Bast B, JEG (1988) Enrichment and selection of hybrid hybridomas by percoll gradient centrifugation and fluorescent activated cell sorting. *Hybridoma* **7**: 217–225.

Krishan A, Ganapathi R (1980) Laser flow cytometric studies on the intracellular fluorescence of anthracyclines. *Cancer Res.* **40**: 3895–3900.

Krishan A, Sauertig A, Stein JH (1991) Comparison of three commercially available antibodies for flow cytometric monitoring of *p*-glycoprotein expression in tumour cells. *Cytometry* **12**: 731–742.

Landgent JE, Jansen in de Wal N, Baan RA, Hoeijmakers JHJ, Ploeg van der M (1984) 2-Acetylaminofluorene-modified probes for the indirect hybridocytochemical detection of specific nucleic acid sequences. *Exp. Cell Res.* **153**: 61–72.

Lane HC (1992) Immunoregulation, immune defects and clinical strategies in HIV infection (clinical conference). *Mt Sinai J. Med.* **59**: 244–252.

Lanier LL, Warner NL (1981) Paraformaldehyde fixation of haematopoietic cells for quantitative flow cytometry (FACS) analysis. *J. Immunol. Methods* **47**: 25–30.

Leary JF, Brigati DJ, Ward DC (1983) Rapid and sensitive colorimetric method for visualising biotin labelled DNA probes hybridised to DNA or RNA immobilised on nitrocellulose: Bio-blots. *Proc. Natl Acad. Sci. USA* **80**: 4045–4049.

Lichter P, Ward D (1990) Is non-isotopic *in situ* hybridisation coming of age? *Nature* **345**: 93–94.

Lippold HJ (1982) Quantitative succinic dehydrogenase histochemistry. *Histochemistry* **76**: 381–405.

Luce GG, Sharrow SO, Shaw S, Gallop PM (1985) Enumeration of cytotoxic cell–target cell conjugates by flow cytometry using internal fluorescent stains. *BioTech* **3**: 270–272.

Luk CK, Tannock IF (1989) Flow cytometric analysis of doxarubicin accumulation in cells from human and rodent cell lines. *J. Natl Cancer Inst.* **81**: 55–59.

Macey MG, Allen PD, Kelsey SM, Newland AC (1992) Flow cytometric bio-assay for the measurement of TNF function and cell free cytotoxicity. In: *Proceedings of the 24th Congress of the International Society of Haematology*. Blackwell Scientific Publications, Oxford, 214 (Abstr.)

Makler MT, Lee LG, Recktenwald D (1987) Thiazole orange: a new dye for *Plasmodium* species analysis. *Cytometry* **8**: 568–570.

Manafi N, Kneifel W (1991) Fluorogenic and chromogenic substrates: a promising tool in microbiology. *Acta Microbiol. Hung.* **38**: 293–304.

Mansour JD, Robson JA, Arndt CW, Schulte TH (1985) Detection of *Escherichia coli* in blood using flow cytometry. *Cytometry* **6**: 186–190.

Marder P, Maciak RS, Fouts RL, Baker RS, Starling JJ (1990) Selective cloning of hybridoma cells for enhanced immunoglobulin production using flow cytometric cell sorting and automated laser nephelometry. *Cytometry* **11**: 498–505.

Mariani E, Facchini A, Honorati MC *et al.* (1992) Immune defects in families and patients with xeroderma pigmentosum and trichothiodystrophy. *Clin. Exp. Immunol.* **88**: 376–382.

McConway MG, Chapman RS (1986) Application of solid-phase antibodies to radio-immunoassay. Evaluation of two polymeric microparticles, Dynospheres and nylon activated by carbonyl-diimidazoyle or tresyl chloride. *J. Immunol. Methods* **95**: 259–266.

McGinnes K, Chapman G, Marks R, Penny R (1986) A fluorescence NK assay using flow cytometry. *J. Immunol. Methods* **86**: 7–15.

Meinicoff MJ, Page SM, Jensen BD, Breslin EW, Horan PK (1988) *In vivo* labelling of resident peritoneal macrophages. *J. Leuk. Biol.* **43**: 387–397.

Meinicoff MJ, Horan PK, Breslin EW, Page SM (1989) Maintenance of peritoneal macrophages in the steady state. *J. Leuk. Biol.* **44**: 367–375.

Miller JS, Quarles JM (1990) Flow cytometric identification of micro-organisms by dual staining with FITC and PI. *Cytometry* **11**: 667–675.

Mitchell BS, Dhami D, Schumacher U (1992) *In situ* hybridisation: a review of methodologies and applications in the biomedical sciences. *Med. Lab. Sci.* **49**: 107–118.

Mogensen J, Kolvraa S, Hindkjaer J *et al.* (1991) Non-radioactive, sequence-specific detection of RNA *in situ* by primed labelling (PRINS). *Exp. Cell Res.* **196**: 92–98.

Molenaar D, Abee T, Korings WN (1991) Continuous measurement of the cytoplasmic pH in *Lactococcus lactis* with a fluorescent pH indicator. *Biochem. Biophys. Acta* **14**: 78–83.

Monfort P, Baleux B (1992) Comparison of flow cytometry and epifluorescence microscopy for counting bacteria in aquatic ecosystems. *Cytometry* **13**: 188–192.

Morale MC, Batticane N, Cioni M, Marchetti B (1992) Upregulation of lymphocyte beta-adrenergic receptor in Down's syndrome: a biological marker of neuroimmune deficit. *J. Neuroimmunol.* **38**: 185–198.

Nair S, Singh SV, Krishan A (1991) Flow cytometric monitoring of glutathione content and anthracycline retention in tumor cells. *Cytometry* **12**: 336–342.

Nelson D, Bathgate AJ, Poxton IR (1991) Monoclonal antibodies as probes for detecting lipopolysaccharide expression on *Escherichia coli* from different growth conditions. *J. Gen. Microbiol.* **137**: 2741–2751.

Niks M, Otto M, Busova B, Stefanovic J (1990) Quantification of proliferative and suppressive response of human T lymphocytes following Con-A stimulation. *J. Immunol. Methods* **126**: 263–271.

Nir R, Yisraeli Y, Lamed R, Sahar E (1990) Flow cytometry sorting of viable bacteria and yeasts according to beta-galactosidase activity. *Appl. Environ. Microbiol.* **56**: 3861–3866.

Noonan KE, Beck C, Holzmayer TA *et al.* (1990) Quantitative analysis of MDR1 (multidrug resistance) gene expression in human tumors by polymerase chain reaction. *Proc. Natl Acad. Sci. USA* **87**: 7160–7164.

Obernesser MS, Socransky SS, Stashenko P (1990) Limit of resolution of flow cytometry for the detection of selected bacterial species. *J. Dent. Res.* **69**: 1592–1598.

Ogden RC, Adams DA (1987) Electrophoresis in agarose and acrylamide gels. *Methods Enzymol.* **152**: 61–87.

Oiszewski WL (1987) *Lymphocyte Traffic in Neoplastic Disease in* in vivo *Migration of Immune Cells.* CRC Press, Boca Raton, FL, pp. 149–222.

Oxholm P, Pedersen BK, Horrobin DF (1992) Natural killer cell functions are related to the cell membrane composition of essential fatty acids: differences in healthy persons and patients with primary Sjögren's syndrome. *Clin. Exp. Rheumatol.* **10**: 229–234.

Pardue ML (1985) *In situ* hybridisation. In: Hames BD, Higgins SJ, eds, *Nucleic Acid Hybridisation, A Practical Approach.* IRL Press, Oxford, pp. 179–202.

Pattanapanyasat K, Webster HK, Udomsangpetch R, Wanachiwanawin W, Yong-vanitchit K (1992) Flow cytometric two colour staining technique for simultaneous determination of human erythrocyte membrane antigen and intracellular malarial DNA. *Cytometry* **13**: 182–187.

Perez P, Bluestone J, Stephany DA, Segal DM (1985) Quantitative measurements of the specificity and kinetics of conjugate formation between cloned cytotoxic T lymphocytes and splenic target cells by dual parameter flow cytometry. *J. Immunol.* **134**: 478–485.

Persidsky MD, Baillie GS (1977) Fluorometric test of cell membrane integrity. *Cryobiology* **14**: 322.

Pinder AC, Purdy PW, Poulter SA, Clark DC (1990) Validation of flow cytometry for rapid enumeration of bacterial concentrations in pure cultures. *J. Appl. Bacteriol.* **69**: 92–100.

Pinkel D, Gray JW, Trask B, Engh van den G, Fuscoe J, Dekken van H (1986) Cytogenetic analysis by *in situ* hybridisation with fluorescently labelled nucleic acid probes. *Cold Spring Habour Symp. Quant. Biol.* **51**: 151–157.

Pross H, Callewaert D, Rubin P (1986) Assays for NK cell cytotoxicity; their values and pitfalls. In: Lotzova E, Herbermann RB (eds), *Immunobiology of Natural Killer Cells*, Vol. 1. CRC Press, Boca Raton, FL, pp. 1–23.

Raphael S, Eitan F (1991) Quantitative flow cytometric analysis of ABO red cell antigens. *Cytometry* **12**: 545–549.

Roberts K, Lotze MT (1988) Interleukin-2 promotes conjugate formation by purified LAK precursors and T lymphocytes: evaluation of conjugates using flow cytometric techniques. *J. Biol. Response Mod.* **7**: 249–266.

Robertson BR, Button DK (1989) Characterising aquatic bacteria according to population, cell size and apparent DNA content by flow cytometry. *Cytometry* **10**: 70–76.

Ross DD, Ordenez JV, Joneckis CC, Testa JR, Thompson BW (1988) Isolation of highly multidrug-resistant P388 cells from drug-sensitive P388/S cells by flow cytometric cell sorting. *Cytometry* **9**: 359–367.

Ross DD, Joneckis CC, Ordonez JV et al. (1989a) Estimation of cell survival by flow cytometry quantification of fluorescein diacetate/propidium iodide viable cell number. *Cancer Res.* **49**: 3776–3782.

Ross DD, Thompson BW, Ordenez JV, Joneckis CC (1989b) Improvement of flow cytometric detection of multidrug resistant cells by cell-volume normalisation of intracellular daunorubicin content. *Cytometry* **10**: 185–191.

Rothenberg M, Ling V (1989) Multidrug resistance: Molecular biology and clinical significance. *J. Natl Cancer Inst.* **81**: 90–91.

Sambrook J, Fritsch EF, Maniatis D (1989) Preparation of single stranded probes. In: *Molecular Cloning. A Laboratory Manual*, 2nd edn, Vol. 2. pp. 18–37.

Sanders CA, Yajko DM, Hyun W et al. (1990) Determination of guanine-plus-cytosine content of bacterial DNA by dual-laser flow cytometry. *J. Gen. Microbiol.* **136**: 359–365.

Shalaby MR, Shepard HM, Presta L et al. (1992) Development of humanised bispecific antibodies reactive with cytotoxic lymphocytes and tumor cells over expressing the HER2 protooncogene. *J. Exp. Med.* **175**: 217–225.

Schattner A, Tepper R, Steinbock M, Hahn T, Schoenfeld A (1990) TNF, interferon-gamma and cell mediated cytotoxicity in anorexia nervosa; effect of refeeding. *J. Clin. Lab. Immunol.* **32**: 183–184.

Shi T, Eaton AM, Ring DB (1991) Selection of hybrid hybridomas by flow cytometry using a new combination of fluorescent vital stains. *J. Immunol. Methods* **141**: 165–175.

Slezak SE, Horan PK (1989) Cell mediated cytotoxicity: A highly sensitive and informative flow cytometric assay. *J. Immunol. Methods* **117**: 205–214.

Storkus WJ, Balber AE, Dawson JR (1986) Quantitation and sorting of vitally stained natural killer cell–target cell conjugates by dual beam flow cytometry. *Cytometry* **7**: 163–170.

Suresh MR, Cuello AC, Millstein C (1986) Advantages of bispecific hybridomas in one-step immunocytochemistry and in immunoassay. *Proc. Natl Acad. Sci. USA* **83**: 7989–7993.

Suzuki Y, Hoshi K, Matsuda T, Mizushima Y (1992) Increased peripheral blood gamma delta+ T cells and natural killer cells in Behçet's disease. *J. Rheumatol.* **19**: 588—592.

Thiebaut F, Tsuruo T, Hamada H, Gottesman MM, Pastan I, Willingham MC (1989) Immunohistochemical localisation in normal tissues of different epitopes in the multidrug transport protein P170: Evidence for localisation in brain capillaries and cross-reactivity of one antibody with a muscle protein. *J. Histochem. Cytochem.* **37**: 159—164.

Thompson J, Gillespie D (1987) Molecular hybridisation with RNA probes in concentrated solutions of guanidine thiocyanate. *Anal. Biochem.* **163**: 281—291.

Tice DG (1992) Natural killer activity is down-regulated following allogeneic small bowel transplantation. *Transplant. Proc.* **24**: 1135—1136.

Trask B, Engh van der G, Pinkel D *et al.* (1988) Fluorescence *in situ* hybridisation to interphase cell nuclei in suspension allows flow cytometric analysis of chromosome content and microscopic analysis of nuclear organisation. *Human Genet.* **78**: 251—259.

Trinchieri G (1989) Biology of natural killer cell. *Adv. Immunol.* **47**: 187—376.

Van Dilla M, Langlois RG, Pinkel D, Yajko D, Hadley WK (1983) Bacterial characterisation by flow cytometry. *Science* **220**: 620—621.

Velardi D, Grossi CE, Cooper MD (1985) A large population of lymphocytes with T-helper phenotype (Leu3/T4$^+$) exhibits the property of binding to NK cell targets and granular lymphocyte morphology. *J. Immunol.* **134**: 58—64.

Vitale M, Zamai L, Neri LM *et al.* (1991) Natural killer function in flow cytometry; identification of human lymphoid subsets able to bind to the NK sensitive target K562. *Cytometry* **12**: 717—722.

Vitale M, Zamai L, Papa S *et al.* (1992) Natural killer function in flow cytometry. III Surface marker determination of K562-conjugated lymphocytes by dual laser flow cytometry. *J. Immunol. Methods* **149**: 189—196.

Whaun JM, Rittershaus C, Ip SHC (1983) Rapid identification and detection of parasitised human red cells by automated flow cytometry. *Cytometry* **4**: 117—122.

Wong JT, Colvin RB (1987) Bi-specific monoclonal antibodies: Selective binding and complement fixation to cells that express two different surface antigens. *J. Immunol.* **139**: 1369—1374.

Yang H, Mitchel R, Lemaire I (1990) The effects of *in vitro* hypothermia on natural killer activity from lung, blood and spleen. *J. Clin. Lab. Immunol.* **32**: 117—122.

Yeaman MR, Sullam PM, Dazin PF, Norman DC, Bayer AS (1992) Characterisation of *Staphylococcus aureus*-platelet binding by quantitative flow cytometric analysis. *J. Infect. Dis.* **166**: 65—73.

Young RC, Ozols MD, Myers CE (1981) The anthracyclines antineoplastic drugs. *N. Engl. J. Med.* **305**: 139—153.

Zarcone D, Tilden AB, Cloud G, Friedman HM, Landay A, Grossi CE (1986) Flow cytometry evaluation of cell-mediated cytotoxicity. *J. Immunol. Methods* **94**: 247—255.

Zarda B, Amann R, Wallner G, Schleifer KH (1991) Identification of single bacterial cells using digoxigenin-labelled, rRNA targeted oligonucleotides. *J. Gen. Microbiol.* **137**: 2823—2830.

Zimmerman GA, Prescott SM, McIntyre TM (1992) Leukocyte—endothelial cell interactions. *Immunol. Today* **13**: 93—112.

Appendix 1
Manufacturers' Addresses

UK	USA	Europe
Amersham		
Amersham International plc Lincoln Place Green End Aylesbury Bucks HP20 2TP 0296 395222	Amersham N. America 2636 S. Clarebrook Drive Arlington Heights IL 60005 708 593 6300	Amersham Buchat Giefelweg W-3300 Braunschweg Germany 495 3072060
Amgen Ltd 321 Cambridge Science Park Milton Rd Cambridge CB4 4WD 0223 420305	Amgen Inc Amgen Centre 1840 De Havilland Drive Thousand Oaks CA 91320−1789 805 499 5725	Amgen-Roche Produits Roche SA 52 Boulevard du Parc F-92521 Neuilly sur Seine Cedex France 331 4640 5000
AMS		
AMS Biotechnology (UK) Ltd Unit 6 Tannery Yard Witney Street Burford OX8 3DN 0993 706500	AMS Biotechnology USA 23251 Los Alisos Boulevana No 8 Lake Forest CA 92630 714 472 3513	AMS (Switzerland) Centro Nord-Sud Stabile 3/Entrata A 6934 Bioggio-Lugano 091 591742
Becton Dickinson (UK) Ltd Between Towns Road Cowley Oxford OX4 3LY 0865 777722	Becton Dickinson Immunology to Chemistry Systems PO Box 7375 Mountain View CA 94039 800 223 8226	N.V. Becton Dickinson Denderstraa 24 PO Box 13 9440 Erembodegorn-Aaist Belgium 01608 37720

UK	USA	Europe
Bio-Rad Laboratories Ltd	Bio-Rad Chemicals	Laboratories
Mayland Avenue	1414 Harbour Way South	Bio-Rad SA
Hemel Hempstead	Richmond	5 Bis Rue
Herts	CA 94804	Maurice Rouvier
HP2 7TD		F-75014 Paris
	415 232 7000	France
0442 232552		
		45 45 50 10

Boehringer-Mannheim Biochemica

BCL	7941 Castleway Drive	PO Box 310120
Boehringer-Mannheim	Indianapolis	D-6800
Bell Lane	IN 46250	Mannheim 31
Lewes		Germany
East Sussex	800 428 5433	
BN7 1LG		0621 7591
0273 471611		

Bibby

Bibby Sterilin Ltd	Azlon	Bibby Dunn Labortechnik
Tilling Drive	205-I Kelsey Lane	GmbH
Stone	Tampa	Postfach 1104
Staffs	FL 33619	5464 Asbach
ST15 0SA		Germany
	813 621 2230	
0785 812121		02683 43306

British Bio-technology Ltd
410 The Quadrant
Barton Lane
Abingdon
Oxon
OX14 3YS

0865 748747

Coulter

Coulter Electronics	Coulter Corporation	Coulter Electronics
Northwell Drive	440 West 20th Street	Nederland
Luton	Hialeah	Industrieweg 42
Beds	FL 33010	3641 RM Mijdrecht
LU3 3RH		Netherlands
	800 526 6932	
0582 491414		31 2979 88578

Siba Corning	Siba Corning	Siba Corning
Colchester Road	63 North Street	Industries 11
Halstead	Medfield	DW-6301
Essex	MA 02052 1688	Fernwald 2
CO9 2DX		Giessen
	508 359 7711	Germany
0787 472461		
		641 400 30

UK	USA	Europe
CP Pharmaceuticals Ashroad North Wrexham Industrial Estate Wrexham Clwyd LL13 9UF 0978 661261		

....

UK	USA	Europe
DAKO Diagnostics Ltd Denmark House Angel Drive Ely Cambs CB7 4ET 0353 669911	DAKO Corporation 6392 Via Real Carpinteria CA 93013 805 566 6655	DAKO AS Produktionsvej 42 PO Box 1359 DK-2600 Glostrup Denmark 44 92 00 44

....

UK	USA	Europe
Dynal (UK) Ltd 24–26 Grove St New Ferry Wirral L62 5AZ 051 644 6555	Dynal Inc 45 North Station Plaza Great Neck NY 11021 516 829 0039	Dynal AS PO Box 158 Skøyen N-0212 Oslo 2 Norway 472 50 78 00

....

Ealing Beck Ltd
Greycaine Rd
Watford
WD2 4PW

....

Flow Cytometry Standards Corporation (FCSC)

From Becton Dickinson or	FCSC PO Box 12621 Research Triangle Park NC 27709 919 976 9345

....

UK	USA	Europe
Gelman Sciences Brackmills Business Park Caswell Road Northampton NN4 0EZ 0604 765141	Gelman Sciences 6005 Wagner Rd Ann Arbor MI 48106 313 665 0651	Gelman Sciences Medical Device Division 1M Gewerbepark A 158400 Regensburg Germany 49 941 44692

....

Gibco

UK	USA	Europe
Life Technologies Ltd Trident House PO Box 35	Life Technologies Inc 8400 Helgerman Court Gathersburg	Life Technologies GmbH Postfach 1212 Diselstrasse

UK — *USA* — *Europe*

UK	USA	Europe
Renfrew Road	MD 20877	5,7514
Paisley		Eggenstein
PA3 4EF	301 840 8000	Germany
0800 269210		0721 780444

....

Hoechst

Hoechst Pharmaceuticals	Calbiochem-Behring	Calbiochem GmbH
PO Box 18	PO Box 12087	Postfach 110360
Hounslow	San Diego	D-6300
Middx	CA 92112	Giessen
TW4 6JH		Germany
	800 854 9256	
081 570 7712		0641 71059

....

HV Scan Ltd
425–433 Stratford Rd
Solihull
West Midlands
B90 4AE

....

ICN Biomedicals Ltd	ICN Biomedicals	ICN Biomedicals
Eagle House	3300 Hyland Ave	Muehlgrabenstrasse 10
Peregrine Business Park	Costa Mesa	D-5309 Meckanheim-bie-
Gomm Rd	CA 92626	Bonn
High Wycombe		Germany
Bucks	714 545 0100	
HP13 7DL		492 225 88050
0494 443826		

....

Imagenetics
150 West Warrenville
   Road
PO Box 3011
Napierville
IL 60566–7011

708 420 3841

....

Integrated Genetics
One Mountain Road
Framingham
MA 01701

508 872 8400

....

ISCO

	Instrument Specialities	ISCO Europe AG
	Company (ISCO)	Bruschstrasse 17
	4700 Superior	CH-8708
	Lincoln	Mannedorf
	NB 68504	Switzerland
	402 464 0231	411 920 2425
	800 288 4250	

298

APPENDIX 1
Manufacturers'
Addresses

UK	USA	*Europe*

Kodak Ltd
Kodak House
Station Road
Hemel Hempstead
Herts
HP1 1JU

081 748 7979

Eastman Kodak Co
343 State St
Rochester
NY 14650

716 214 4000

Kodak
Postfach 600345
7000 Stuttgardt
Germany

49711 4060

Medarex Inc
12 Commerce Avenue
West Lebanon
NH 03784

603 298 8456

Mercia

Mercia Diagnostics
Mercia House
Boadford Park
Shalford
Guildford
Surrey
GU4 8EW

0483 505255

Centocor Inc
200 Great Valley Parkway
Malvern
PA 19355–1307

Centocor Diagnostics
Europe
Desguinlel 50
B-2018
Antwerp
Belgium

Merck Sharp & Dohme
Hertford Rd
Westhill
Hoddesdon
Herts
EN11 9BU

0992 467272

Merck & Co Ltd
1 Merck Drive
Whitehouse Station
NJ 088 8920100

908 423 1000

Merck Sharp & Dohme BV
Chaussée de Waterloo 1135
B-1180
Brussels
Belgium

32 2373 4211

Molecular Probes
4849 Pitchford Avenue
Eugene
OR 97402

503 344 3007

National Collections of
Type Cultures (NCTC)
Central Public Health
Laboratory (CPHL)
61 Colindale Avenue
London
NW9 5HT

081 200 4400

Nyegaard

Nycomed (UK) Ltd	Accurate	Nyegaard & Co AS
Nycomed House	Chem & Scientific Corp	Diagnostic
2111 Coventry Rd	300 Shames Drive	Postbox 4220
Sheldon	Westbury	Torshou
Birmingham	NY 11590	N-0401 Oslo 4
B26 3EA		Norway
	516 433 4900	
021 742 2444		472 644000

....

Ortho

Ortho Diagnostic Systems	Ortho DS Inc	Ortho Diagnostic Systems
Enterprise House	Route 202	Casella Postale 17171
Station Road	Rantan	20170 Milan
Loudwater	NJ 08869	Italy
Bucks		
HP10 9UF	800 631 5807	392268131
0494 442211		

....

Oxoid

Unipath Ltd	Unipath Inc	Unipath GmbH
Wade Road	217 Colonade Rd	AM Lippegglacis 628
Basingstoke	Nepean	Postfach 1127 4230
Hants	Ontario K2E 7K3	Wesel
RG24 0PW	Canada	Germany
0256 841144	613 226 1318	49281 1520

....

Pharmacia

Pharmacia Ltd	Pharmacia LKB	Pharmacia LKB
Pharmacia LKB	Biotech Inc	Biotech AB
Pharmacia House	800 Centennial Ave	Bjorkgatan 30
351 Midsummer	PO Box 1327	75182 Uppsala
Boulevard	Piscataway	Sweden
Central Milton Keynes	NJ 08855−1327	
MK9 3YY		081 16 30 00
	201 457 8000	
0908 661101		

....

	Phoenix Flow Systems Inc	
	11575 Sornento Valley	
	Road	
	Suite 208	
	San Diego	
	CA 92121	
	602 453 5095	

....

UK	USA/Canada	Europe
Polysciences		
Polysciences Ltd 24 Low Farm Place Moulton Park Northampton NN3 1HY 0604 646496	Polysciences Inc 400 Valley Road Warrington PA 18976 215 663 6484	Polysciences Ltd Niederlassang St Goar Postfach 64, Ulmenhof 28 D5401 St. Goar Germany 0 6741 2081
Sigma Chemical Company Ltd Fancy Road Poole Dorset BH17 7NH 0800 447788	Sigma St Louis 3050 Spruce Street St Louis MO 63103 800 325 3010	Sigma Chemie Grünwalder Weg 30 W-8024 Deisenhofen Germany 089 613 01 0
Sysmex UK Ltd Sunrise Parkway Linford Wood Milton Keynes		
Vector Laboratories Ltd 16 Wulfric Square Bretton Peterborough PE3 8RF 0733 265530	Vector Laboratories, Inc 30 Ingold Road Burlingame CA 94010−9976 800 227 6666	Biosys SA 21 Quai du Clos des Roses 60200 Compiègne France 44 86 22 75
Whatman Scientific Whatman House Leonards Road Maidstone Kent ME16 0LS 0622 674823	Whatman Sci., Inc PO Box 1359 Hillsboro OR 97123 9981 503 648 1434	Prolabo BP 369 77526 Paris Cedex 11 France 1 49 23 15 00
	Zynaxis Cell Science Inc 371 Phoenixville Pille Malvern PA 19355 800 232 5212 *Also available from Sigma*	

Appendix 2
Additional CD Classification of Leucocyte Antigens Defined at the Vth International Workshop on Leucocyte Differentiation Antigens

Table A2.1 New CD antigens

Antigen	Other names	Mol wt (kD)	Main cellular distribution	Comments
CD79a	MB1, BPC#1alpha	33, 40	B lymphocytes	Alpha subunit of molecule
CD79b	B29, BPC#1beta	33, 40	B lymphocytes	Beta subunit of molecule
CD80	BB1, BPC#2	45–65	B lymphocytes	B7 molecule, co-stimulatory molecule
CD81	BCP#3	22	B lymphocytes	TAPA-1 molecule
CD82			B lymphocytes	Molecule involved in signal transduction
CD83	HB15, BCP#5	43	B lymphocytes	Antigen on dendritic cells
CDw84	BCP#6	74	B lymphocytes	Function unknown, also on monocytes and platelets
CD85	BCP37	72	B lymphocytes	Also on plasma cells and monocytes
CD86		80	B lymphocytes	Function unknown
CD87	UPA-R	50–65	Myeloid cells	Urokinase plasminogen activator receptor
CD88	C2aR, GR10	40	Monocytes, macrophages	Receptor for complement component C5a
CD89	Fc alpha-R	5–70	Monocytes	Fc receptor for IgA
CDw90	Thy-1		Early myeloid cells	Human equivalent to mouse Thy-1
CD91	ALPHA2M-R	500	Myeloid cells	Receptor for alpha$_2$ macroglobulin
CDw92	GR9	70	Myeloid cells	Function unknown
CDw93	GR11	190, 180, 140	Myeloid cells	Function unknown
CD94	Kp43	70	Natural killer cells	Function unknown
CD95a	TACTILE	240, 180, 160	Natural killer cells, T lymphocytes	T-cell late activation expression
CD95b	TACTILE	240, 180, 160	Natural killer cells, T lymphocytes	T-cell late activation expression
CD98			T cells	Function unknown, associated with kinases
CD99	E2	32	T cells	Associated with the E2 molecule which is the product of the MIC2 gene. Antibodies block E-rosette formation

Antigen	Other names	Mol wt (kD)	Main cellular distribution	Comments
CD100	BD-16		T cells	Two isotypes, increased by activation, function unknown
CDw101			Restricted expression on CD4 and CD8	Co-expressed with CD28. Function unknown, also expressed on platelets and granulocytes
CD102	ICAM2	60	T cells	Associated with adhesion
CD103	HML-1	175	T cells	Human mucosal lymphocyte antigen
CD104	Beta4	160	T cells	Beta4 integrin associated with adhesion
CD107a	LAMP-1	110	Platelets	Lysosomal associated membrane protein 1. Associated with activation
CD107b	LAMP-2	110	Platelets	Lysosomal associated membrane protein 2. Associated with activation
CD105	VCAM-1 INCAM-110	99, 93	Endothelium	Associated with activation
CDw108		80	Endothelium	GP1-activated. Associated with adhesion
CDw109	GR56	165	Endothelium	Associated with activation
CD115	G-CSF-1r		Wide distribution particularly myeloid cells	Receptor for granulocyte colony stimulating factor
CD117	SCFR, CKIT	145	Stem cells, mast cells	Receptor for stem cell factor. Important for haemoipoiesis
CD118	INFalpha R		Wide distribution	Receptor for interferon (g/b). Modulates IR
CD119	INFgamma R	90	Wide distribution	Receptor for interferon (b). Modulates IR
CD120a	TNFR-55KD	55	Wide distribution	Receptor for tumour necrosis factor alpha. Important in inflammatory response
CD120b	TNFR-75KD	75	Wide distribution	Receptor for tumour necrosis factor beta
CDw121a	IL-1R type 1		Wide distribution	Receptor for interleukin-1 alpha
CDw121b	IL-1R type 2		Wide distribution	Receptor for IL-1 beta
CD122	IL2r	75	L-2 activated lymphocytes	Receptor for IL-2
CD123	IL3r		Stem cells, early progenitor cells	Receptor for IL-3, important for cell differentiation
CD124	IL4r		T and B lymphocytes	Receptor for IL-4, important for Ig synthesis
CD125	IL5r		T lymphocytes, mast cells	Receptor for IL-5, important for eosinophil differentiation and function

Table A2.1 Continued

Antigen	Other names	Mol wt (kD)	Main cellular distribution	Comments
CD126	IL6r	80	Wide distribution	Receptor for IL-6, promotes differentiation of numerous cell types
CD127	IL7r		T and B lymphocytes	Receptor for IL-7, important for the differentiation and activation of T and B cells
CD128	IL8r		Wide distribution	Receptor for IL-8, important for chemotaxis
CDw130	gp130	130	Wide distribution	

Table A2.2 Alterations to some existing CD numbers

Antigen	Comments
CD15	Acquires a subgroup CD15s due to selective binding to granulocytes, monocytes and myeloid cell lines. Negative on eosinophils, lymphocytes, and epithelia
CD20	Acquires subgroup CD20cy for cytoplasmic binding antibodies
CD29	Now known to be ß1 integrin chain
CD42	GP1b/IX complex subdivided into: CD42a GP-IX CD42b & c GP-1bß CD42d GP-V
CD44	Acquires a subgroup CD44R
CD49a	VLAα1
CD49b	VLAα2
New CD49c	VLAα3
CD49wd	Becomes CD49d VLAα4
CD49e	VLAα5
CDw49f	Becomes CD49f VLAα5
CDw50	Is ICAM3
CD62	Subdivided into: CD62P P-selectin CD62E E-selectin CD62L L-selectin

Index

304